Teaching Nursing: The Art and Science
(It's All About Student Success!)

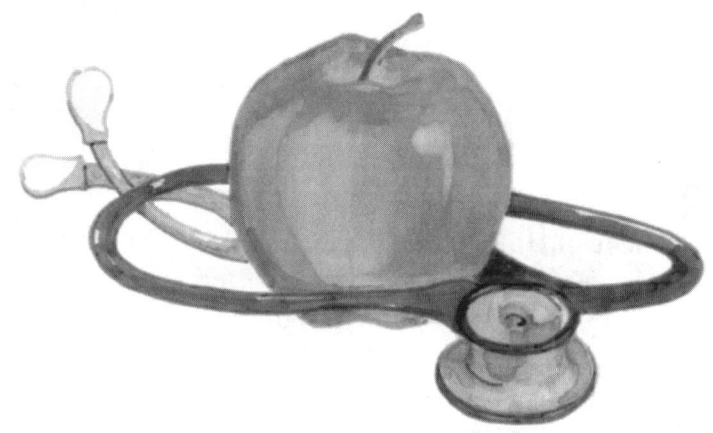

Linda Caputi, MSN, EdD, RN, CNE
Professor of Nursing
College of DuPage
Glen Ellyn, Illinois

Lynn Engelmann, MSN, EdD, RN
Professor of Nursing
College of DuPage
Glen Ellyn, Illinois

Volume 4

College of DuPage Press

College of DuPage Press
425 Fawell Blvd.
Glen Ellyn, Illinois 60137

Project Administrator: Joseph Barillari
Project Manager: Linda Caputi
Designer: Janice Walker
Typesetter: Janice Walker
CD Designer: Janice Walker
Production Coordinator: Janice Walker
Editor: Jim Vondran
Editor: Eleanor Donlon

About College of DuPage: For more than 15 years College of DuPage has been a leader in publishing learning materials for nursing education including multimedia computer programs, an on-line student self-assessment tool, videos, books, board games, and other print materials. We are committed to providing the highest quality products in the most appropriate format for our colleagues. Visit the College of DuPage website at www.dupagepress.com for information on all our products.

© 2008, College of DuPage Press

ISBN: 978-1-932514-12-4

Printed in the United States of America

All rights reserved. No part of this publication may be reproduced, stored in a retrieval system, or transmitted in any form or by any means, electronic or mechanical, including photocopying, recording, or otherwise without permission in writing from College of DuPage.
Request permission at 1-800-290-4474.

Acknowledgements

Since writing our first book, *Coaching Your Students to NLCEX® Success*, we have been dedicated to the notion of student success. Truly, teaching nursing is ALL about student success. As we explored this topic in some detail, we quickly realized the myriad of variables that impact student success. How to effect student success became our overriding quest. We greatly appreciate Joseph Barillari's unending support and encouragement of this new quest. True to form, he enabled us to engage in discovering the art and science of nursing education that fosters student success.

We would like to acknowledge our four reviewers who provided their insights and helpful commentary: Donna Henry, Anita Kinser, Elizabeth Stokes, and Diane Whitehead. We also appreciate the efforts of the support staff in information technology at College of DuPage who helped maintain a smooth, efficient production process: Gail McPike, Cathy Russo, and Sue Puccinelli. We are also grateful for the dedication and creative talent of our book designer and CD developer, Janice Walker.

Finally, we would like to thank our families for their unending support. Our husbands, Victor Caputi and Gary Engelmann, and our children, Linnea Caputi-Favela and Vince Caputi, and Christina, Brett, and Elliot Engelmann, have sustained us in this undertaking.

Yours in Nursing,
Linda Caputi and Lynn Engelmann

Preface

The goal of nursing education is to graduate competent, safe practitioners. Positioning student nurses for success from the beginning to the end of a nursing program poses a remarkable challenge for nurse educators, a challenge we think is possible to meet with the right plan in mind.

To that end, we have designed a book totally devoted to student success. Background information for this book was based on an extensive review of the literature and a number of research studies we conducted specifically for this book. Our four reviewers represent a wealth of experience and diverse backgrounds; and, therefore, provided four unique perspectives as they reviewed each chapter. From this we wrote a Student Success Program that details a plan nurse educators may modify to meet the needs of their student population. Due to the diverse nature of each nursing program, no one plan fits all. However, the Student Success Program presented in this book provides an organizing framework and essential elements to consider when designing a Student Success Program.

The overall character of ***Teaching Nursing: The Art and Science, Volume 4, It's All About Student Success*** is friendly, but professional, so sit back and enjoy!

Forward

This book represents a comprehensive undertaking to research, construct, and explain a Student Success Program that faculty can adapt for their undergraduate nursing students. As you read this book, it is our hope that you will be thinking about how the content might apply to you, your students, and your nursing program.

Special features of this book include integrative reviews and research conducted to further explore the many facets of student success and *The Hypothetical School of Nursing,* a hypothetical school depicting application of the content for Chapters 2 through 10 to illustrate how to develop a Student Success Program.

Teaching Nursing: The Art and Science, Volume 4, It's All About Student Success, is a book whose value lies in both its practical and theoretical applications. To that end, we have created a CD-ROM that holds valuable supplemental material that we and other educators have designed.

Where you see this symbol:

you may refer to the CD-ROM to explore these additional materials. Please feel free to use these tools in your role as a nurse educator. These items are copyrighted as noted.

Authors

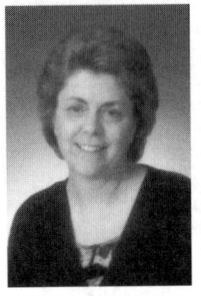

Linda Caputi, MSN, EdD, RN, CNE
Dr. Caputi was awarded a BSN from Northern Illinois University and an MSN from Loyola University. She holds a Doctor of Education in Instructional Technology. She is certified as a Certified Nurse Educator (CNE) from the National League for Nursing. Dr. Caputi has authored over 25 educational multimedia programs, nursing education books, produced and developed videotapes, and published book chapters, journal articles, and board games for nursing education. She is co-editor of *Teaching Nursing: The Art and Science (Volumes 1 & 2)* and editor of *Teaching Nursing: The Art and Science (Volume 3)*. She has presented her work nationally for over 15 years on many nursing education topics. Her work has won six awards from Sigma Theta Tau, two from American Journal of Nursing Company, and one from The Association for Educational Communication and Technology. Dr. Caputi was acknowledged for teaching excellence in the 1998, 2002, and 2005 editions of *Who's Who Among America's Teachers*. Dr. Caputi was named Educator of the Year for 2004 by the National Organization of Associate Degree Nursing. She is on the editorial staff of *Advance for Nurses* and serves on the Board of Governors for the National League for Nursing. She is a member of Sigma Theta Tau International Honor Society of Nursing. She is a Professor of Nursing at College of DuPage in Glen Ellyn, Illinois with 25 years of teaching experience. Dr. Caputi is a consultant to undergraduate nursing programs in the areas of curriculum, student success, and effective teaching strategies in the classroom, the nursing laboratory, and clinical and to graduate programs with a specialty in nursing education.

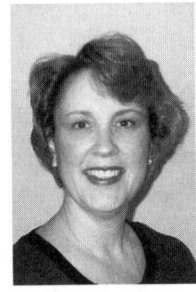

Lynn Engelmann, MSN, EdD, RN
Dr. Engelmann was awarded a B.S.N. from Marycrest College and an M.S.N. from Case Western Reserve, Francis Payne Bolton School of Nursing. She holds a Doctor of Education in Adult and Continuing Education from Northern Illinois University. She is co-editor of *Teaching Nursing: The Art and Science (Volumes 1 & 2)*. Dr. Engelmann serves on the Editorial Board of *Teaching and Learning in Nursing*. She is an NLN task force member exploring Excellence in Nursing Education and an NLN Ambassador. Dr. Engelmann is a member of Sigma Theta Tau International Honor Society of Nursing, Kappa Delta Pi, International Honor Society in Education, and was acknowledged for teaching excellence in Who's Who Among America's Teachers, 2005. She was also acknowledged in Who's Who of American Women, 2007. Dr. Engelmann is a Professor of Nursing at College of DuPage in Glen Ellyn, Illinois.

Contributing Author

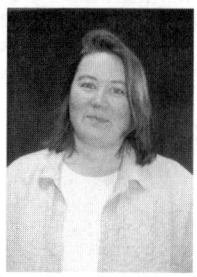

Jennifer L. Bissett was awarded a B.A. in biology and psychology from the University of St. Thomas (Houston), and an M.Ed. in Counseling and a Ph.D. in Counseling Psychology from the University of Houston. Dr. Bissett has worked in college/university student retention for over 10 years, and has worked specifically in the area of nursing student retention since 2003. Her efforts in nursing programs have been very successful, with evidence of as much as 20 percent increases in student retention in programs where she has consulted and worked.

Reviewers

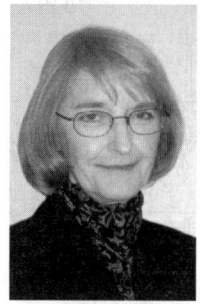

Donna Henry, MS, RN, CHTP, AHN-BC, is Associate Dean of Nursing and Allied Health at Illinois Eastern Community Colleges. She has been the Associate Dean for 8 years. Prior to that time, she was an instructor in the Associate Degree Nursing program. Her clinical experience includes cardiac critical care, women's health, AIDS counseling and testing, and crisis intervention for teens. She has been a certified Healing Touch Practitioner for 10 years and is also board-certified Advanced Holistic Nurse.

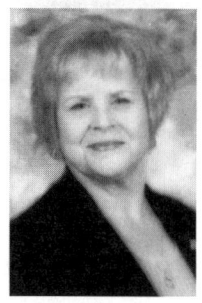

Anita Kinser, EdD, RN, BC, has over 26 years experience in nursing with over 10 years as an educator in ADN, BSN, and MSN programs. She is board certified by the American Nurses Credentialing Center (ANCC) in Nursing Informatics and is a member of the ANCC's Content Expert Panel for Nursing Informatics. She is an Associate Professor and ADN Department Chair for Riverside City College, School of Nursing, Riverside, CA, and adjunct professor for Western University of Health Sciences, Pomona, CA. As a Nursing Education Resource Specialist, her focus has been on assessment and remediation of at-risk nursing students, and integration of technology into nursing education curriculum. Dr. Kinser was acknowledged for teaching excellence in the 2003 and 2005 editions of *Who's Who Among America's Teachers*. She has presented nationally at a number of conferences; her publications include articles in the *Journal of Nursing Education* and *Nurse Educator*. She recently co-authored *Start Right in Nursing School*, a nursing student assessment software program with Dr. Linda Caputi.

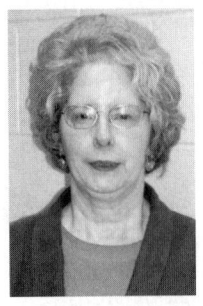

Elizabeth N. Stokes, EdD, RN, CNE, has an educational and experiential background in adult health and gerontological nursing. Her primary teaching areas are research, role development, and the care of the chronically ill. She is also a consultant on curriculum, instruction, and evaluation to both undergraduate and graduate nursing programs. A Professor Emeritus, Dr. Stokes is currently teaching as adjunct faculty at Arkansas State University and continuing professional service and scholarship activities.

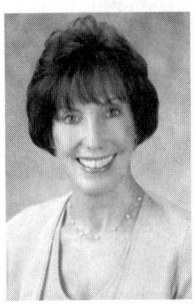

Diane Whitehead, MSN, EdD, RN earned an MSN from the University of Miami and an EdD from Florida International University. She has experience in ICU and home health care. She has been both faculty and administrator in associate degree, baccalaureate, and masters nursing programs. In 2002, Dr. Whitehead developed the nursing program at Nova Southeastern University (NSU). She currently serves as Associate Dean for Nursing at NSU. Dr. Whitehead has numerous publications and presentations. Her textbook, *Essentials of Nursing Leadership and Management*, was selected as an American Journal of Nursing textbook in 2002. Now in its 4th edition, this textbook is widely used in community college nursing programs throughout the country and in Europe. Dr. Whitehead chairs a national task force on nursing faculty leadership for the National League for Nursing. She was funded for a National League for Nursing Research Grant on this topic in 2005.

Table of Contents

Chapter 1: Introduction to the Process of Developing a Plan for Student Success 1

Chapter 2: Identifying Your At-Risk Students 17

Chapter 3: Formulating an Admissions Policy 50

Chapter 4: Planning a Student Success Program 78

Chapter 5: Elements of a Student Success Program Prior to Entering a Nursing Program 115

Chapter 6: A Student Success Program for Currently Enrolled Students 145

Chapter 7: A Case Study: Creating a Success Program for Nursing Students 226

Chapter 8: Passing, Failing, and Readmitting 264

Chapter 9: A Model for NCLEX® Success 295

Chapter 10: An NCLEX® Success Course 338

Tables and Figures 363

Index 367

Chapter 1: Introduction to the Process of Developing a Plan for Student Success

As an academic nurse educator, a priority goal is to promote nursing student success. To that end, you continuously expand and update your knowledge of nursing practice and nursing education. To that end, you continuously update your knowledge of healthcare and nursing research. To that end, you continuously update your knowledge of the students entering nursing education. To that end, you go to work each day and you learn.

Student success is a broad term. In this book, the general term student success is used to address success in completing a nursing program and passing the NCLEX. These two aspects of success exist in tandem; both are required for students to be successful in meeting their goal of becoming a licensed nurse.

The overall goal for this book is to:

Provide a model that all faculty can adapt to develop a Program Plan for Student Success in an undergraduate nursing program.

The word **all** means this prescriptive model must be flexible so all faculty will find the plan adaptable for their specific program, philosophy, and student demographics.

This approach is akin to a nursing student writing a patient care plan. The student uses nursing care plan books to provide the basic approach to planning care. The care plan books provide interventions that must be adapted to the individual client. We take great care to ensure that our students individualize their plans of care. Faculty must do likewise if they are to foster student success.

With this analogy in mind, the models proposed in this book are ones that provide direction and guidance, yet are flexible so all faculty – regardless of program philosophy and student demographics – can individualize their overall plan for success to meet their needs.

This chapter lays out some important foundational information on which the rest of the book builds. It provides a succinct look at the bigger picture, pointing out the classification of variables that influence student retention. The chapter ends with an explanation of the methods used to collect, analyze, and report the myriad of data that impacts nursing student retention and presents a beginning model of the elements of a program plan for student success.

Broadening the Scope of Student Success

In the year 2000, *Coaching Students to NCLEX Success* was published. At the time that book was written, NCLEX scores in schools across the country had dropped. Many schools were concerned about their decreasing pass rates and were looking for ways to help their students succeed on that examination. The intent of the book, *Coaching Students to NCLEX Success*, was to provide a plan – an approach – which could be used to help students do just that – successfully pass the NCLEX on the first attempt.

Faculty from many schools incorporated the ideas, processes, and suggestions outlined in that earlier book. They reported the strategies were helpful in developing their overall approach to raising their NCLEX scores. We were delighted.

Now, a number of years later, we realize there was a fundamental flaw in the thinking that went into *Coaching Students to NCLEX Success*. That flaw is this: the only students who benefited from a faculty devised plan for successfully passing NCLEX were those students who **first** successfully completed their course of study in a nursing program. That is, they first had to earn the degree! Therefore, this book, *Teaching Nursing: The Art and Science, Volume 4, It's all about Student Success*, considers the usefulness of a plan for success for students while they are **enrolled** in a nursing program, not just as they are nearing the end of their studies. This book provides a more thorough presentation by looking at **all** aspects of success for nursing students. To that end, the chapters include:

- Chapter 1: Introduction to the Process of Developing a Plan for Student Success
- Chapter 2: Identifying Your At-Risk Students
- Chapter 3: Formulating an Admissions Policy

Chapter 1: Introduction to the Process of Developing a Plan for Student Success

- Chapter 4: Planning a Student Success Program
- Chapter 5: Elements of a Student Success Program Prior to Entering a Nursing Program
- Chapter 6: A Student Success Program For Currently Enrolled Students
- Chapter 7: A Case Study: Creating a Success Program for Nursing Students
- Chapter 8: Passing, Failing, and Readmitting
- Chapter 9: A Model for NCLEX® Success
- Chapter 10: An NCLEX® Success Course

Sorting through the Data

The literature is replete with articles, books, dissertations, and documents addressing the topic of student success from a variety of perspectives. Those perspectives represent an extensive and impressive assortment of nursing programs, student demographics, faculty credentials, and nursing education philosophies. This wide array of literature presented a challenge. We realized we needed an approach for writing this book; an approach that would analyze all this literature in a systematic manner, sort through the literature with an unbiased eye, then add to that body of knowledge with original research. But first, we must present a framework for clearly presenting the bigger picture of success in a nursing program and success on NCLEX along with related factors.

The Bigger Picture

Many variables and topics are discussed under the umbrella concept of **student success**. Some factors refer to the individual student such as personal, environmental, and psychosocial factors. Other factors relate to the nursing program, its policies and procedures, and faculty expertise. It is fairly easy to get caught in a web of variables and experience difficulty when attempting to sort out which variables influence student success in the nursing program and which influence student success on NCLEX. Some factors relate solely to success in a nursing program, some to success on

NCLEX, and many to both. There are occasions when it may be helpful for faculty to determine which aspect of student success a variable influences. Determining the effect of a specific factor may be desirable when developing program policies or guidelines for faculty teaching. Let's look at an example. Table 1.1 contains a sampling of the many topics that influence student success which are discussed throughout this book. The first column in Table 1.1 lists some nursing program policies or faculty guidelines that may impact student

Table 1.1 – Example Variables Influencing Student Success

Variable	Program Success	NCLEX Success
Admission testing. Purposes: • Admission criteria • Advisement	Determines if student is ready for nursing studies. Directs student support services	Not predictive of NCLEX success
Student self-assessment (on entry to a nursing program) Purpose: Identify factors affecting success	Identifies helpful and interfering variables to success in a nursing program	Not predictive of NCLEX success
Setting a minimum pass rate for **each** nursing exam.	Ensures prerequisite knowledge and skills are learned for success in subsequent nursing courses	Provides information for ongoing remediation for success on NCLEX
Comprehensive final exams for all nursing courses	Ensures prerequisite knowledge and skills are learned for success in subsequent nursing courses	Provides information for ongoing remediation for success on NCLEX
Midcurricular exam administered by external entity	Ensures prerequisite knowledge and skills are learned for success in subsequent nursing courses	Provides information for ongoing remediation for success on NCLEX
Nursing specialty exams administered by external entity	Ensures prerequisite knowledge and skills are learned for success in subsequent nursing courses	Provides information for ongoing remediation for success on NCLEX
Summer bridge course	Ensures prerequisite knowledge and skills are learned for success in subsequent nursing courses	Provides information for ongoing remediation for success on NCLEX
Standardized testing at the end of a nursing program	Not related to students' success in a nursing program but may be used to determine progression to graduation.	Predicts student readiness to take NCLEX. Identifies gaps in curriculum that can be addressed prior to student graduation.

Chapter 1: Introduction to the Process of Developing a Plan for Student Success

success. Columns 2 and 3 suggest what impact each of the items in Column 1 has on a student's success in a nursing program and/or on NCLEX. Sorting out these factors and how each factor might affect student success decreases confusion, thereby enhancing the goal of promoting student success among faculty. This sorting out process also assists with determining cause and effect. Faculty can now ask, "If a policy is enacted, what is the cause and effect related to student success?" Although the cause and effect relationship may be speculative when a policy is first implemented, it can be extremely useful when analyzing data that impacts future decisions.

Throughout each chapter, these and many other factors affecting student success are discussed. As you read through each chapter and determine which factors are important to your nursing program, differentiate to which aspect of success the factor relates.

Each chapter presents these factors in the form of a model. A step-by-step example of how to use these models is presented at the end of each chapter to assist faculty in using the information discussed. Feel free to use these models as you develop your Program Plan for Student Success.

Quality Assurance Interventions

To meet the desired outcome of student success, faculty may institute some general quality assurance interventions. Faculty interventions are an important aspect of a Program Plan for Student Success, demonstrating that student success is two-sided. One side is the student and the other side is the faculty. Student characteristics and behaviors influence student success. Faculty behaviors and expertise also influence student success. It is common opinion that faculty don't pass or fail students, rather students pass or fail themselves; however, faculty **can** pass or fail students, many times unintentionally. For example, faculty who lack skills in test item writing may write a test at a level that is much higher than the students' abilities. This same faculty may then fail to consider this position and take action to correct the situation. All faculty have a responsibility to be the best teacher possible, yet none of us is perfect. As with all professionals, we must each consider our abilities and shortcomings and correct any shortcomings so we do not become the factor that interferes with student success.

Examples of quality assurance interventions are faculty guidelines for instruction that will assure quality learning. All faculty should meet and discuss

Table 1.2 – Variables Influencing Quality Assurance

Quality Assurance Variable	Program Success	NCLEX Success
Ensure that test questions are valid and reliable	Tests accurately reflect students' understanding of content	Students experience quality testing resembling NCLEX
All faculty grade subjective assignments in the same way	Grading accurately reflects program outcomes	Provides information for ongoing remediation for success on NCLEX
Clinical instruction: Skills blitz at the beginning of each term	Ensures prerequisite knowledge and skills are learned	Provides information for ongoing remediation for success on NCLEX
Incorporate critical thinking activities in all learning activities	Meet program outcomes related to high-level thinking	Prepared to take application/analysis level questions on NCLEX
Incorporate different ways of thinking – i.e. concept maps	Meet program outcomes related to high-level thinking	Prepared to take application/analysis level questions on NCLEX

these interventions and arrive at a consensus regarding which interventions should be instituted across the curriculum. A sampling of quality assurance variables is shown in Table 1.2. These interventions are discussed throughout the book to use when developing your Program Plan for Student Success.

Collecting Data

After much reflection and discussion with colleagues around the country, we realized that no one methodology for collecting data for writing this book would do justice to the broad topic of nursing student success. A variety of intellectual activities were needed to produce the information. Three specific methodologies emerged:
1. Review the literature over the prior ten years
2. Conduct new research studies applicable to selected areas of interest
3. Conduct disciplined integrative reviews of salient topics

Review the Literature Over the Prior Ten Years

A general literature review was conducted that included peer-reviewed journal articles, books, and dissertations from the last ten years. The literature

Chapter 1: Introduction to the Process of Developing a Plan for Student Success

review also covered gray or fugitive literature such as conference proceedings and web sites. The literature was read and reviewed from our perspective as the authors of this book. Simply stated, we read the literature, organized the information, and repackaged it for readers to digest. This methodology yields a discussion of topics based on the authors' interpretation of the literature.

It is important to note that personal perspectives may influence a general literature review. Consider the following example of a personal perspective:

> Sherlock Holmes and Dr. Watson went on a camping trip. As they lay down for the night, Holmes asked: "Watson, look up into the sky and tell me what you see."
> Watson: "I see millions and millions of stars."
> Holmes: "And what does that tell you?"
> Watson: "Astronomically, it tells me that there are millions of galaxies and potentially billions of planets. Theologically, it tells me that God is great and that we are small and insignificant. Meteorologically, it tells me that we have a beautiful day tomorrow. What does it tell you?"
> Holmes: "Somebody stole our tent."
> — Author Unknown

All authors writing from the perspective of a literature review have an obligation to avoid bias in the interpretation and rendering of their reporting. We believe we have an ethical responsibility to put forth much effort to hold true to this obligation, yet personal perspectives may unknowingly influence our interpretation of the literature.

As stated earlier, the literature reviewed for this book included articles, books, dissertations, and gray literature that discussed ideas that were implemented and led to improvements in learning. This is the humanistic approach to educational research (Burkhardt & Shoenfled, 2003). A critical appraisal of the literature is required to assess its plausibility, internal consistency, and fit with the educational strategies in current use. Our goal is to implement that critical appraisal in such a way that yields additional insights not previously considered.

Conduct New Research Studies

As Tanner (2004) notes, there is a great need for nursing education research to justify the cost of a nursing education and to accommodate a greater number of students. In addition, Tanner (1999) also asks who will develop the science of nursing education. As a discipline, nursing education must encourage its members to become scholars and researchers. Diekelmann and Ironside (2002) applaud nursing faculty for their creative, innovative approaches to solving educational problems. But they propose that what is lacking is the research that supports the effectiveness and usefulness of these innovative practices that might lead to a practice base for nursing education. The National League for Nursing (2005), in their *Scope of Practice for Academic Nurse Educators*, addresses educational research. They note that "Faculty and students contribute to the development of the science of nursing education through the critique, utilization, dissemination, or conduct of research" (p. 10). Throughout this book we attempt to critique, utilize, and disseminate research, as well as conduct research to add to the science of nursing education.

Research Studies

To help widen the scope of literature that is empirically based, we conducted some simple research studies on various topics covered in this book. During the review of the literature, we identified topic areas that piqued our interest. We then conducted various types of research on those topics: surveys, phenomenological research, a case study, descriptive research, and integrative reviews.

It is our hope that in conducting new research for this book, we encourage other nurse educators to think like researchers. For the body of knowledge to grow, we must **all** think like researchers. Small studies are a great start! Research studies can be generated in one's own school. These studies focus attention and yield additional questions for future research. After feeling comfortable with this type of research, faculty can proceed to larger multi-site, multi-method, and multi-paradigmatic studies. This is a priority identified by the National League for Nursing in its priorities for research in nursing education (National League for Nursing, 2003). If evidence-based nursing education is to grow, all faculty must contribute to the body of knowledge through research.

Chapter 1: Introduction to the Process of Developing a Plan for Student Success

The research studies conducted for this book were designed to build on the existing body of knowledge. The studies include:
1. Six surveys sent to individual nursing faculty that addressed the following topics:
   o Implementation of a student success program and the components of the program
   o Assessment and teaching of critical thinking
   o Characteristics of the student at-risk for failing a nursing course
   o Assessment of and information about students' learning styles
   o Interventions to help students prepare for NCLEX
   o Use of a test to predict NCLEX Success
2. A descriptive research study that reviewed the admission criteria of 80 nursing programs
3. A case study of one nursing program that implemented an inclusive student success program
4. A phenomenological research study using conversation circles to discover the needs of the non-English language background nursing student

Each of these research studies is addressed in this book in the chapter in which that topic is discussed. Complete information on how these studies were conducted and analyzed is located on the CD-ROM accompanying this book. We encourage readers to use this information as they develop their own nursing education research studies. We also encourage readers to contact us with any questions and comments related to these studies.

Conduct Disciplined Integrative Reviews

The third methodology used to collect data to write this book involved conducting integrative reviews on salient topics. Tanner (2004) cites the U. S. Department of Education's *Strategic Plan for 2002-2007*:

> Unlike medicine, agriculture, and industrial production, the field of education operates largely on the basis of ideology and professional consensus. As such, it is subject to fads and is incapable of the cumulative progress that follows from the application of the scientific method and from the systematic collection and use of objective information in policy

making. We will change education to make it an evidence-based field (p. 50).

To achieve the cumulative progress that Tanner mentions, we must do more than conduct and report individual research studies. All research on one topic must be considered in the aggregate and analyzed for application to practice. Integrative reviews provide such an avenue for this type of work.

The overall purpose of an integrative review can be conceptualized as an analysis of related research studies that on their own are not necessarily useful but when evaluated in the aggregate can be processed to yield effective, useful pedagogy. This process is the foundation for an evidence-based practice which is the basis of a science of nursing education.

A Closer Look at Integrative Reviews

Evidence-based nursing education requires a systematic review of research. Isolated research studies can be enlightening, but do not provide a basis for an evidence-based profession. An important step in developing evidence-based nursing education is to sort through the research, systematically analyze and interpret the studies, synthesize the findings into a comprehensive whole, then develop best practice guidelines that faculty can use. This links evidence to action – action faculty take when planning and implementing learning activities. Faculty who use these best practice guidelines further advance the notion of evidence-based teaching practice by serving as role models.

Students benefit when faculty use new teaching methods that encourage students to use new ways of thinking, observing, learning, and practicing. These activities carry over into the clinical setting which improves patient care (National League for Nursing, 2004). This role modeling promotes the importance of an evidence-based practice for graduates to consider when molding their own evidence-based practice as nurses.

Perhaps integrative reviews can be challenged as not being empirical – merely another review of the literature. However, true integrative reviews are indeed different because they systematically compare and contrast reported research. Integrative reviews are crafted to provoke thinking (Diekelmann & Ironside, 2002). They consider multi-method studies to explore various types of evidence available and make meaningful the aggregate. They challenge accepted pedagogy by exploring and constructing new approaches.

An integrative review typically looks at research studies rather than anecdotal reports, and is based on a strict scientific design aimed at minimizing bias and ensuring reliability. An integrative review provides a systematic analysis of the research about a particular topic then conceptualizes relationships among the findings of these studies. Finally, an integrative review offers best practice guidelines for evidence-based instructional strategies. This can be perceived as a repackaging of the collection of research studies for the purpose of clearly communicating knowledge and its implications.

The end product of an integrative review is a best practice guideline that directs faculty in their practice. This is an evidence-based guideline because it is based on a systematic review and processing of the literature. Faculty can then use this best practice guideline to direct their teaching/learning practice. This leads to best practice recommendations and evidence-based practice guidelines.

Thus the science of nursing education is built. The saying, "In God we Trust, Everyone else must bring the data!" (Melnyk, 2005) best illustrates this methodology. The end product is a synthesized review that is translated into a model that can be used to guide practice decisions and actions.

Looking at the Art and Science

The use of evidence-based guidelines in nursing practice is taking on an added dimension incorporating the expertise of the practitioner and preferences and values of the patient. Melnyk (2005) states:

> "Evidence-based practice (EBP) is a problem solving approach to clinical practice that integrates the conscientious use of best evidence in combination with a clinician's expertise as well as patient preferences and values to make decisions about the type of care that is provided."

Melnyk shrouds this combination of best practice guidelines, clinician's expertise, and patient preferences and values in a context of caring to achieve quality patient outcomes. This approach draws on a range of evidence to facilitate the application of evidence-based guidelines derived from research. This is a melding of the art and science of nursing practice.

Figure 1.1. – The Merging of the Art and Science of Nursing Education

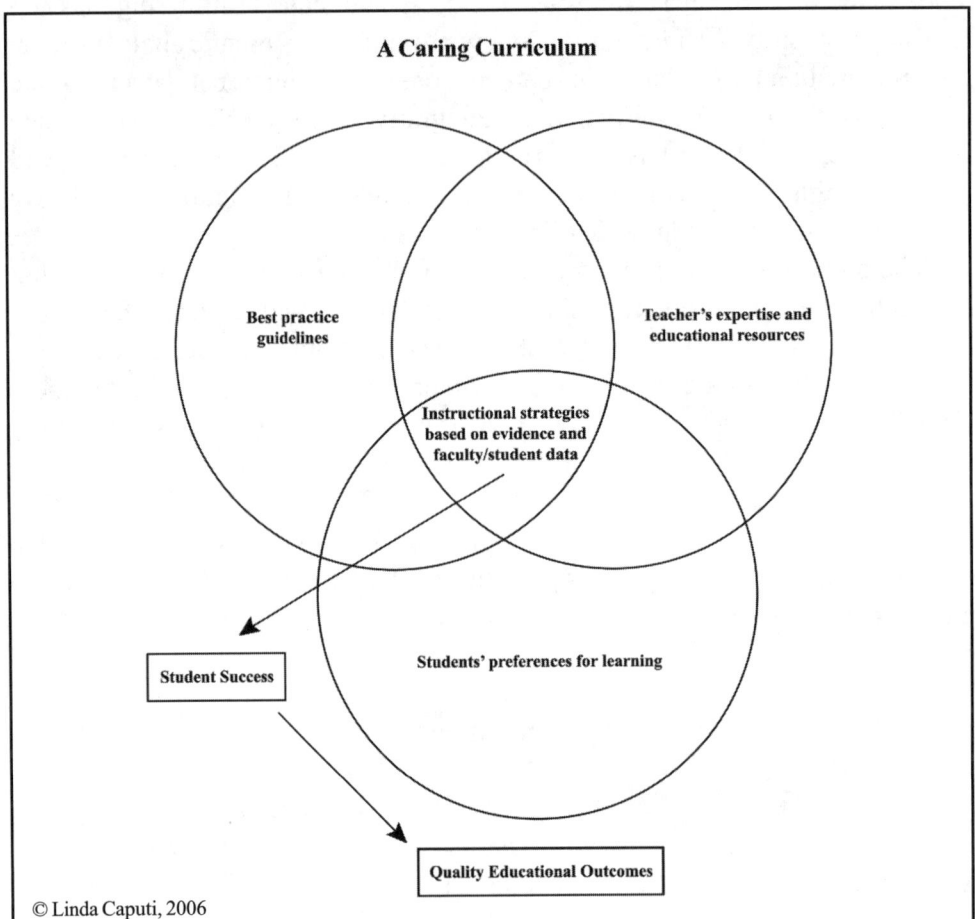

This same approach can be applied to nursing education. Figure 1.1 demonstrates the relationship of similar components within a caring curriculum, resulting in the merging of the art and science of nursing education.

This model demonstrates how the three factors overlap to produce student success all within the context of a caring curriculum.

The integrative reviews conducted for this book explored the following topics:
- concept maps to foster critical thinking
- collaborative testing
- peer tutoring

Chapter 1: Introduction to the Process of Developing a Plan for Student Success

The integrative reviews are addressed in the chapters of this book where the topic of the review is discussed, to enrich the discussion and provide a careful systematic look at the topic. For information on the process of how these integrative reviews were conducted, refer to the CD-ROM accompanying this book.

Developing an Individualized Program Plan for Student Success

These three approaches for data collection to write this book yielded a phenomenal amount of varying types of data. The primary challenge was to sort through, process, and analyze all the information then use it to develop models of the various aspects of nursing student success. Figure 1.2 is a graphic illustration of the methodologies used to write this book and their relationship to the development of a model for student success.

Figure 1.2 – Graphic Representation of Methodologies

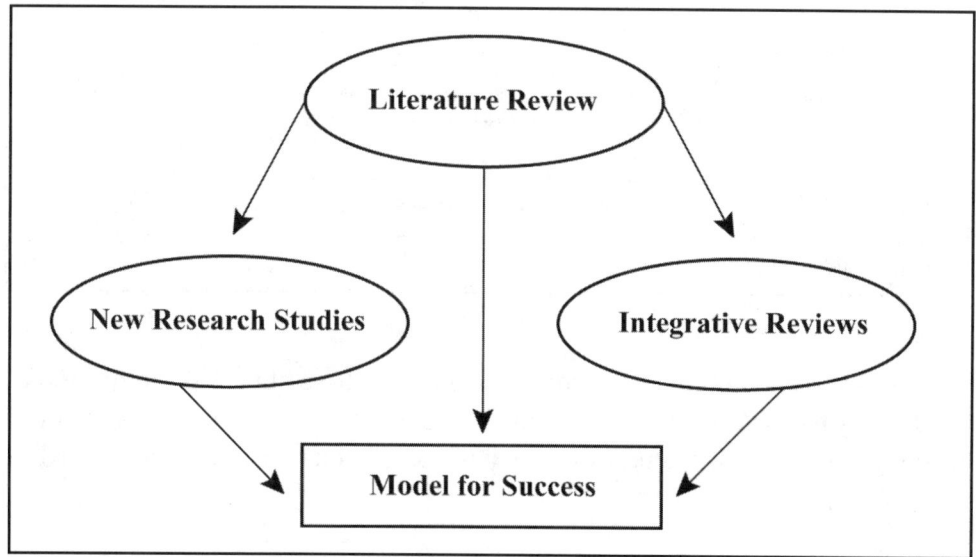

Each chapter in this book provides pieces of the unfolding Model for Student Success. These models are presented for faculty to use as they build their own individualized Program Plan for Student Success. In each chapter, the model is presented and then applied to a hypothetical nursing program to illustrate how the model can be used by nursing faculty. This illustration gives faculty an opportunity to examine how the model can be used in a simulated real-world context.

As you develop your own Program Plan for Student Success, remember that such a plan must be individually developed within your own school's context of practice, taking into account all the demographic variables about your students, curriculum, characteristics of individual faculty, and knowledge of teaching/learning strategies. Figure 1.3 illustrates the relationship of these elements leading to a Program Plan for Student Success.

Figure 1.3 – Elements of a Program Plan for Student Success

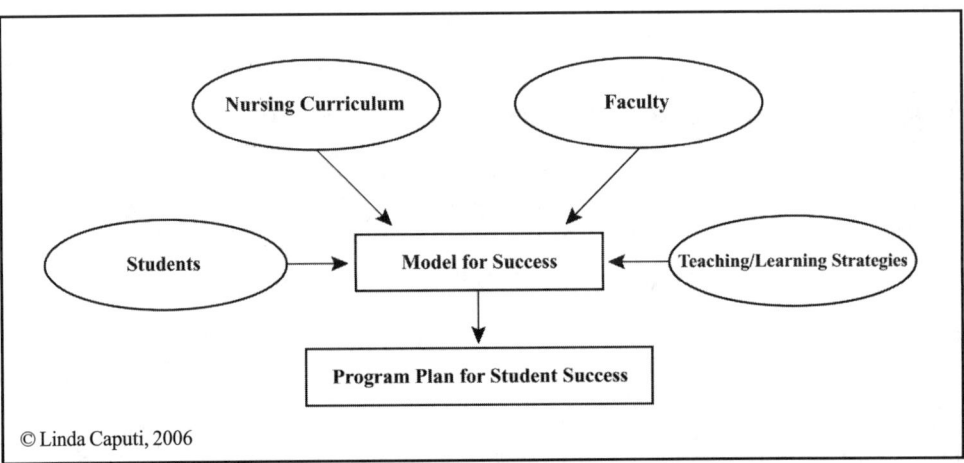

Each of the elements in Figure 1.3 will be discussed throughout this book. Faculty then use their Program Plan for Student Success to plan and implement learning experiences, evaluate those experiences, then revise the plan as needed.

Closing Thoughts

Our hope is you will use the information discussed throughout this book to design your Program Plan for Student Success. Once you have developed your

Chapter 1: Introduction to the Process of Developing a Plan for Student Success

plan, you will put it to the test. You will develop approaches for implementing your plan, develop teaching/learning strategies specific for your student population, and apply new pedagogies all within the context of a caring curriculum. You will also conduct research studies addressing questions that arise from your work then revise, revise, revise. As you work through this process, we encourage you to dialogue with other nurse educators. In doing so, you will learn from them and they will learn from you as we all work together to develop an evidence-based program for student success.

Learning Activities

1. Identify two variables from your nursing program policies that directly relate to student success in your nursing program. Identify two variables from your nursing program policies that directly relate to student success on NCLEX.
2. Locate the information about integrative reviews on the CD-ROM accompanying this book. Applying the process used to conduct integrative reviews for this book, conduct an integrative review on a topic of interest to you. Ask a colleague to join you in your research efforts.
3. Write an article discussing the results of your integrative review from activity #2. Submit the article to a nursing education journal for publication.

References

Burkhardt, H., & Shoenfled, A. H. (2003). Improving educational research: Toward a more useful, more influential and better-funded enterprise. *Educational Researcher, 32*(9), 3-14.

Diekelmann, N., & Ironside, P. (2002). Developing a science of nursing education: Innovation with research. *Journal of Nursing Education, 41,* 379-380.

Melnyk, B. M. (2005). *Igniting evidence-based practice in clinical and educational settings.* Plenary address at Sigma Theta Tau International's 16th International Nursing Research Congress, Kona, Hawaii.

National League for Nursing (2003). Priorities for Research in Nursing Education. www.nln.org.

National League for Nursing (2004). Evidence-based teaching practice: An interview with Dr. Lin Jacobson. *Shaping the Future, 5,* 2-3.

National League for Nursing (2005). *The scope of practice for academic nurse educators*. New York: Author.

Tanner, C. (1999). Developing the new professorate. *Journal of Nursing Education, 38,* 51.

Tanner, C. (2004). Nursing education: Investing in our future. *Journal of Nursing Education, 43,* 99-100.

Chapter 2: Identifying Your At Risk Students

Predicting whether a student will successfully complete a nursing program can be a challenge for faculty. Faculty should approach this problem armed with reliable data that can be equally applied to all applicants. The overall goal of identifying which students are at-risk for failing a nursing program is to provide assistance to those students possessing the identified "at-risk" characteristics. The outcome is to improve retention of these students in the nursing program. Retention is important because of its impact on students, the institution, and the nursing shortage. Early identification facilitates efficient academic support and enhances the students' chances for academic success. Students are assessed, their individual characteristics identified, and plans for retention are established. These steps help meet the overall goal of retention.

This chapter examines the characteristics of today's nursing students, then focuses on the specific characteristics that can be used to predict which students are at risk for not completing a nursing program. Faculty use this information to formulate predictions for success, counsel students on how to be successful in their nursing program, and establish a Student Success Program specific to their students.

The Traditional Student

The traditional undergraduate nursing student is described as an eighteen-year-old entering college directly from high school with no financial or family responsibilities (AACN, 2003). These are students of the past. Consider for a moment nursing schools from the 1960s, a time when many current faculty were students. Obvious characteristics of nursing students from that era included:
- single; never married
- young
- female

- no financial or family responsibilities
- lived in school housing
- had established curfews each night

Do these characteristics describe the students currently in the nursing classes you teach?

The Nontraditional Student

Nearly 73% of undergraduate students are now considered nontraditional (AACN, 2003). The nursing education literature is full of references classifying current nursing students as nontraditional. An early definition of the nontraditional student was offered by Bean and Metzner (1985) who defined the nontraditional student as older than 24 years, a commuter, or a part-time student. More recently, Jeffreys (2004) expanded that definition of the nontraditional undergraduate nursing student as one "who meets one or more of the following criteria: (1) age 25 years or older, (2) commuter, (3) enrolled part-time, (4) male, (5) member of an ethnic and/or racial minority group, (6) speaks English as a second (other) language, (7) has dependent children, (8) has a general equivalency diploma (GED), and (9) required remedial classes" (pg. 7). Overall, nontraditional students have complex lives that include family responsibilities, jobs, long commutes, and part-time student status. These students are typically older and financially independent. Because of the competing responsibilities of these nontraditional students, the number of part-time students has tripled since 1970. For the nontraditional student, certain socioeconomic factors weigh heavily on success. These students rank family responsibilities and family crises as having the greatest impact (Jeffreys, 1998).

In the past, many nontraditional students lacked basic skills necessary for college-level work (Levine and Cureton, 1998). However, this may be changing. In a recent study presented at the 2005 Sigma Theta Tau International Research Conference, Prevost reported that incoming baccalaureate nursing students' educational preparation and academic performance had increased from the year 2002 to 2004. This nontraditional group may also be a dynamic group that changes with the passage of time.

Chapter 2: Identifying Your At Risk Students

Characteristics of Current Nursing Students

In general, the current nursing student population has been described as diverse. Larger numbers of students who represent minority groups or whose first language is different than the predominant language in the educational institution are enrolling in nursing programs (Guhde, 2003). This diversity is also evident on other dimensions such as educational background and socioeconomic status (Tracey, 2003). The following characteristics illustrate this diversity:

1. Less prepared academically. It is estimated that between 33 and 75% of all students need remediation and developmental support (Tracey, 2003; Candela, et al, 2004).
2. Employed full time
3. Attending school part time
4. Earning a second degree
5. Lacking adequate study time. Although students may be advised that every hour of college credit requires three hours per week of preparation and study time, most students carrying 12 to 15 credit hours spend less than a total of 15 hours per week studying (AACN, 2003).
6. Older age. The average age of nursing students in all programs is 30.9 years, an increase of seven years from ten years earlier (AACN, 2003).
    a. *Negative influences.* Older students may have many responsibilities that can interfere with time spent studying. Adult students returning to school must deal with various transitions and adjustments in their lives that can be stressful. Not all adult learners are the same; they enter school with an inordinate amount of variety in their backgrounds. Even their ages vary tremendously – the adult learner can range from age 20 to over 60 years of age. This variation in age and developmental stages affects their ability to perform well in a nursing program (Patton & Goldenberg, 1999). These variations represent serious challenges for nursing faculty.
    b. *Positive influences.* However, the whole picture may not be bleak. Students older than 22 years of age have been found to perform better than students aged 17 to 21 years (Houltram, 1996). Patton and Goldenberg (1999) talked about older students being hardier and more experienced in implementing

effective coping strategies. Hardiness refers to their commitment to handling stressful life events, maintaining control in the face of stressful events, and handling the challenge of returning to the college environment. This hardiness is a result of experience implementing effective coping strategies in other areas of their lives that they can now use when faced with the stresses of nursing school. Younger students may not have developed these coping strategies.

Older students who have made a decision to alter their lives and return to school are often highly motivated, self-directed, and committed. Past experiences that have contributed to their return-to-school decision are strong motivators to do well.

Traditional vs. Nontraditional or Good vs. Bad

From this discussion, the question beckons: "Is 'traditional' all good and 'nontraditional' all bad?" There are no absolutes. Perhaps the most important reason for making the point about the term nontraditional is to help **faculty** better understand students and know that students of today are very different than students of the recent past and, quite likely, different than when faculty themselves attended nursing school. To label students nontraditional is not to stereotype but to alert faculty that students have changed and so must our image of what a nursing student should be.

It is important to understand the differences that have been reported between traditional and nontraditional students. For example, Tinto's (1987) model suggests that the integration of academic and social factors of the campus environment is extremely important. When students do not feel socially integrated into the campus environment the likelihood of withdrawal increases, even for students with satisfactory academic performance. However, Wells (2003) suggests that this may not be the case with current nontraditional students because they are likely to live off campus and have many other commitments. Therefore, the campus environment is of less concern to these students.

Chapter 2: Identifying Your At Risk Students

Proposing a New Term to Describe All Nursing Students

At this point we would like to suggest that the tendency to label nursing students as traditional or nontraditional contributes to vagueness and possibly false assumptions about students. The discussion up to this point illustrates that because of the many characteristics that are used to categorize a student as nontraditional, these nontraditional students have only one thing in common: they are all labeled nontraditional. Each student may have needs very different from all the other students in the nontraditional group and still be considered nontraditional. Likewise, we would suggest the same for traditional students. Although they may have some of the same characteristics as their peers, they may each have very different needs. This is not to say that both groups do not have much in common; it is to say that we cannot make assumptions about a student because that student is labeled traditional or nontraditional. We must take what is known about traditional and nontraditional students and ascertain what actually applies to any one student. And, we must keep our minds open to learning about factors in any one student's life that may make that student at-risk for failing; some of the factors may not fall neatly into the category of traditional or nontraditional. Therefore, we would like to propose the abandonment of the terms traditional and nontraditional and replace those terms simply with the term diverse. It may be more productive to realize that today's nursing students are diverse, then work from that point to determine what characteristics are unique to the student and to the group the faculty are currently teaching. This approach prevents making assumptions that are inherent in the traditional and nontraditional labels, and frees faculty to look at each student as an individual and each group of students as unique.

The Impact of Attrition

As many as 33 to 46% of students entering college are considered at-risk for academic failure (Candela, et. al, 2004; Sandiford & Jackson, 2003). These and other characteristics of nursing students place these students in need of additional academic help and other support services to be successful. It is vital to address the potential for failure because academic failure has widespread impact.

Impact on Students

At heart, faculty are very student supportive. It is our goal to help students succeed. When students fail they experience some very negative consequences, including:
- loss of self-esteem
- embarrassment
- hopelessness
- loss of potential occupational, monetary, and societal rewards

Students who attrite also experience financial consequences such as early repayment of student loans (Wells, 2003) and nonpayment of employee tuition benefits because of not completing the course.

Impact on Educational Institutions

Money is and has been tight in higher education for many years. The current economic status does not indicate this situation will improve any time soon. Institutions must be fiscally responsible ensuring their dollars are spent in the best possible way. High attrition rates drain financial and other resources from the educational institution. The high cost of academic preparation for nursing students mandates efforts to help students succeed so education dollars are not wasted. Students who do not complete a program of study put strain on the financial resources of an institution because the student must repeat a course, or does not graduate thus decreasing by one the potential supply of licensed nurses. The National League for Nursing Accrediting Commission (NLNAC, 1996a, 1996b) suggests schools maintain a retention rate of 80%. An institutional goal of recruiting qualified students and graduating 80% of those students can be a challenge. Identifying predictors of success that are dependable in describing students most likely to succeed would support a selection process that maintains student retention at an acceptable level.

Failure also conflicts with the mission statement of most institutions. Colleges and universities exist to provide an education for students, not to fail students. A high rate of attrition may also impact accreditation status, or at the very least, reflect poorly on the school.

Impact on the Nursing Shortage

Over the past few decades the supply of licensed nurses has experienced many peaks and valleys. Currently there is a severe nursing shortage that is expected to persist for many years. Students who start a program but do not graduate drain resources without contributing to the supply of nurses.

Characteristics That Contribute to At-Risk Status

We have established that current nursing students are nontraditional. Also, we have established that it is undesirable to have a high attrition rate. So the question still remains, "How do you define an at-risk nursing student?"

A review of the literature (Abdur-Rahman & Gaines; 1999; Candela, Kowalski, Cyrkiel, & Warner, 2004; Guhde, 2003; Hegge, et al, 1999; Hunt, 1995; Jeffreys, 2004) revealed factors that interfere with learning. We have grouped these factors as academic, personal, and environmental factors. They are presented in Table 2.1.

Stress – An Important Factor

Stress, and the student's ability to deal with stress, can be a major factor contributing to poor performance in nursing school. A high degree of stress from the academic environment can interfere with learning. Sources of academic stress for nursing students include fear of poor evaluations, test anxiety, lack of self-confidence, clinical concerns about safe practice, study skills, and excessive academic load (Bolan & Grainger, 2003). Students often underestimate the workload and discover that it is much heavier or more difficult than they expected. Life stresses such as financial concerns and family situations impact on the student in addition to the stress of nursing school.

Students must identify ways to cope with stress (Gaze, 2000). One way to cope is to have a close friend or family member with whom to talk about the stress. Faculty can assist students by teaching ways to protect and maintain mental health and deal with stress and then help students identify what works for them. For some it may be a good cry, for others it may mean taking a few hours to engage in a pleasurable activity, a few moments of quiet, or a yoga class. These lessons can carry over into their practice as a nurse.

Table 2.1 – Factors Interfering with Learning

Academic Factors	Test anxiety and test-taking
	Critical thinking
	Reading comprehension
	Note-taking
	Personal Feelings about Teachers
	Integration
	Loneliness; isolation
	Difficulty coping with amount of coursework
	Dissatisfaction with program requirements
	Inadequate preparation
	Transportation; traveling distance
Personal Factors	Personal feelings about college
	Attitude toward attendance
	Attitude toward study skills
	Lack of pre-entrance counseling
	Non-English language background
	Time management
	Stress management
	Motivation
	Perseverance
	Self-confidence; low self-esteem
	Health problems
Environmental Factors	Hours of employment
	Finances
	Job obligations
	Family, home responsibilities
	Family problems
	Church, community activities/commitments

Positive Factors

Positive factors affecting student retention have been identified (Jeffreys, 2001; Maxwell, 2000; Tracey, 2003).

Academic variables have a strong influence on academic success. The personal study habits of students and faculty advisement are ranked by students as the two top academic factors affecting success in a nursing program (Jeffreys, 1998). Faculty who provide assistance and support exert a positive influence on student retention (Shelton, 2003). Academic factors also include school facilities and services, as well as social interaction with other students.

Positive personal factors can help balance negative ones. For example, motivation has a strong influence on success and can balance negative academic factors. Many students who may have been academically ill-prepared for nursing school can overcome this barrier if motivated to do so.

Table 2.2 lists these and other factors that positively influence student success.

Table 2.2 – Positive Factors

Academic Factors	Collaborative learning environment
	Good student to faculty rapport
	Faculty guidance and support
	Frequent student-faculty interaction
Personal Factors	Recognition of personal worth
	Motivation
Environmental Factors	Formal campus learning activities
	Social support system
	Study groups
	Good student-to-student rapport
	Involvement with campus activities

Table 2.3 shows a summary of select studies that indicate additional positive predictors for success. The table itself illustrates the diversity and complexity of the topic of predicting success.

Table 2.3 – Summary of Select Studies Indicating Predictors of Success

Study	Factors that positively influence success	Factors that negatively influence success
Aber & Arathuzik (1996) (baccalaureate students)	High self-efficacy (ability to help oneself).	
Byrd, Garza, & Nieswiadomy (1999) (baccalaureate students)	Prenursing: Higher cumulative science GPA; younger age. After admission: grade in introduction to nursing course and first med/surg course.	
Ehrenfeld, Rotenberg, Sharon, & Bergman (1997) (baccalaureate students)	Older students more persistent; younger students performed better academically during the first year.	
Jeffreys (1998) (associate degree students/nontraditional)	Realistic self-assessment of academic supports and need for preparation.	Self-assessment as "supremely" efficacious: overestimated their academic supports and underestimated need for preparation.
Lewis & Lewis (2000) (transfer nursing students)	Completion of the total requirement of anatomy and physiology courses.	
Manifold & Rambur (2001) (American Indian students)	Increasing age positively correlated with completion of a program for American Indian students. High school GPA was not a significant predictor. High Test of Adult Basic English (TABE) language scores.	
Potolsky, Cohen, & Saylor (2003) (baccalaureate students)	Prerequisite science course grades B or higher.	
Sandiford & Jackson (2003) associate degree students	Pre-semester GPA 2.5 and above; college level language skills.	Pre-semester GPA 2.0 – 2.49
Shelton (2003) associate degree students	Function and psychological support from faculty.	

Uniqueness of Nursing Education

Most faculty agree that nursing school is a unique educational experience with its multifaceted academic requirements that impose additional stress to the typical demands of college courses. The workload may be overwhelming, especially for beginning nursing students who are shocked at how different nursing courses are from their previous coursework. Attrition rates in the beginning fundamentals in nursing course can range from 0 to 50%.

Many students are reluctant to openly talk about their stress and how to handle their situation. Because of this reluctance, students do not know that other students are feeling the same way. And, there is no taking a "mental health" day; absences are discouraged. In some nursing programs, more than two days of clinical absence per term means dismissal from the nursing program.

Conflicting Data

Interestingly, research continues to yield conflicting data. Sandiford and Jackson (2003) studied first year associate degree nursing students in a community college with an open door policy. These researchers found that some nonacademic factors typically associated with failing a nursing program were not supported by their study. They found that the number of hours worked in a week, financial difficulty while attending college, and motivation to achieve were not significant predictor variables. What they did find to be significant predictor variables were college level language abilities and pre-semester grade point average. Students with college level language skills had lower attrition rates than students with language skills below the college level. Students with a pre-nursing grade point average of 2.5 and above had lower attrition than students with a grade point average between 2.00 and 2.49. It may appear that the students who are most prepared academically are most likely to be successful.

Perhaps there are so many variables and occasionally conflicting data because each sample of nursing students is somewhat unique. For example, influences such as geographical location, predominate socioeconomic group, minority status, and use of the English language, to name a few, are factors unique to any given sample studied which can influence the results of the study.

Once again this makes the case for identifying nursing students as diverse then closely studying the characteristics of your own students. Next, determine if those characteristics have a positive or negative influence on the students' success in your nursing program. Awareness of identified at-risk factors is a start, a knowledge base from which to work.

Surveying Nurse Educators

As this chapter reports, the literature is replete with an abundance of characteristics that describe a student at-risk for failing a nursing program. These are, of course, the findings of faculty researchers who study student retention and publish their work. What would be the opinions of a randomly selected sample of nursing faculty? Would their ideas be similar to what is in the literature?

To address this question, we developed a survey and administered it via a blind mailing to 204 randomly selected nursing faculty from all levels of undergraduate, pre-licensure, registered nurse programs. A total of 45 faculty completed the survey for a response rate of 22%. The details of how the survey was constructed and administered, the survey instrument, and the complete results can be found on the CD-ROM accompanying this book. Table 2.4 lists the comments of 38 faculty answering the question: What is your definition of the "at-risk" student – the student who is at risk for not successfully completing your nursing program?

Table 2.4 – Definition of the "At-Risk" Student

What is your definition of the "at-risk" student – the student who is at risk for not successfully completing your nursing program?

Associate Degree Nursing Programs

Have not written a "definition". Factors that we consider are 1) students who have difficulty passing A&P on the first try or who manage to barely pass with a C-, 2) ESL student population, 3) students who attempt to work too many hours while in the program.

Academic under-preparedness; social issues.

Student with time requirements outside of nursing school which limit the

Chapter 2: Identifying Your At Risk Students

amount of outside time the student has to study to less than 15 hours per week. We are currently looking at diversity issues that may put the student at risk for unsuccessful performance in nursing school.

Working in addition to school and family situations (single parent, marital/relationship discord, aging parents). Reading comprehension difficulties. Test-taking difficulties. ESL students. Having to take core classes with nursing classes. Previous failures in nursing program or history of taking core classes multiple times in order to pass.

One who does not think critically; does not have the capability or does not put forth the effort required.

Students considered at risk are those who scored just over the minimal number of points for (reading, math, sciences including A&P, Nelson-Denny reading test). Also considered at risk are those who have many responsibilities outside of nursing school—single parent, family member seriously ill, working full or part time. Unfortunately we also have some students who do not read assigned readings and depend entirely on instructor lessons to pass tests. I am not talking about the aforementioned students, I am speaking about those who are young, primarily, and have an active social life.

A student who has an educational history, personal or emotional fragile characteristics or impaired physical health that high stress, demanding schedule and mental challenges will overwhelm.

Usually one with no background in biologic sciences and poor math skills; these usually serve as good predictors.

A student whose average is below 74% on didactic testing, or a student who has more than 18 hours of missed clinical hours logged. We also pay close attention to those students experiencing personal crisis.

Students who are unable to meet the minimum curriculum standards.

Students who must take remedial courses before entering; we have many single parents with low incomes also and little outside support (financial or social).

Student who: (a) has had difficulty with science and math courses, (b) is ESL, or is (c) working full time.

An at-risk student is one who is demonstrating less than satisfactory performance in either the clinical component or academic component of the course.

One who cannot focus for long periods of time, made good grades in high school but does not know how to study.

A "C" or below in a course grade.

The "at-risk" student has difficulty translating theory into practice. They may struggle to maintain a passing average. They [are] not consistent in their delivery of nursing care - have unsafe practices. Some tend not to seek help.
The student who has the pre-reqs but barely, along with borderline SAT scores, and high school grades, but great motivation.

Baccalaureate Degree Nursing Programs

Students who lack the ability to use critical thinking; don't have good study or test-taking skills.

Student may be unable to academically succeed in meeting the course requirements or is unable to accommodate to their perception of the role of RN.

Students who have less than a 3.0 GPA and receives multiple C's in courses or fails a course.

English as a second language. Working full-time. Less than 75% didactic scores.

The student who is overwhelmed with family responsibilities. The student with poor boundaries between self and patient, a pattern of behavior. A student who believes they know exactly what they need to learn and so is closed to the variety of experiences offered in their education. The entitled student, who believes they do not need to participate to gain knowledge. The angry, hostile, tightly defended student who is challenged.

A student who is a "loner," who works at a full-time job in addition to going to school, or who speaks English as a second language.

Someone who has a GPA of below a 2.75; who is unable to receive a passing score on level comprehensive exams and the NLN Diagnostic, or the HESI exams in the Senior Level.

Chapter 2: Identifying Your At Risk Students

Scoring below 78% on test or assignments in theory or not meeting clinical competencies.

Excessive work hours or personal/family commitments, lower GPA on prerequisite classes - particularly the sciences, lower SAT score, history of educational experiences in a setting that did not teach/demand critical thinking, history of a course or clinical failure while in the nursing program.

At-risk students are those who are not prepared academically or psychosocially to meet the demands of the program.

Students with low reading skills.

One that is struggling with A&P/chemistry who need to repeat those classes especially more than once. Students who routinely "just squeak in" with a passing grade in nursing courses. Transfer students who have not passed sciences or nursing courses at another facility.

A student who has had a nursing course failure or needs remediation in reading and/or math. We do not accept students who have less than a grade of C in science courses.

Early signs of failure; i.e. difficulty with first basic nursing courses.

At risk students are those who with additional concentrated effort from the instructors remain didactically challenged and/or who have not developed the clinical skills to provide a safe environment and/or safe care or environment for their clients.

Students who are having personal problems or struggling with health issues or feel overwhelmed by the assignments and work load.

We do not have a definition. But any student in a didactic course who is receiving less than a 75% in any exam or an average of 75% based on grading in the course would be considered "at risk." For clinical performance it would be a student who is not receiving satisfactory levels weekly on their clinical evaluation tool.

Students who have had to repeat their science courses to enter the program, students who have multiple outside factors (economic, family responsibility, work full-time); immaturity; poor work ethic; those who 'just pass' most of their exams or courses.

Diploma Nursing Program

Student with SAT scores below 850; science course grades at "C" or below; repeat of science courses; below 50th national percentile on TEAS entrance test; also students with multiple personal/ family responsibilities.

Accelerated Bachelors/Masters (Second Degree)

Disorganized and not able to articulate concepts, synthesis, critical thinking in both oral and written form.

(All text in the above table is drawn from a survey and is presented verbatim.)

As the responses indicate, the faculty who completed this survey reported a myriad of variables they believe contribute to at-risk status. Nursing students are diverse, which is why there is no universal definition of the at-risk student.

A second question asked on that same survey yielded very interesting responses. The question was: Based on your assessments, what do you believe is the NUMBER ONE reason students are at-risk for not completing your nursing program? The responses are reported in Table 2.5.

Table 2.5 – Number One Reason Students are At-Risk

Question: Based on your assessments, what do you believe is the NUMBER ONE reason students are at risk for not completing your nursing program?

Associate Degree Nursing Programs

Inability to develop critical thinking skills, remaining on a concrete level.

Time allotment to the curriculum.

Lack of time to study outside of class time.

Extenuating life circumstances (relationship/family/financial issues).

Chapter 2: Identifying Your At Risk Students

For most of our students, the major issue is time - time to devote to nursing studies along with work and family obligations.

Trying to do too many other activities while in school.

Now that we have the pre-RN test I think mental fragileness and lack of earnestness.

Poor high school preparation.

Poor reader.

Working too much; poor reading comprehension skills; poor study skills.

The inability to make the switch from knowledge based testing in other courses to the application level testing in nursing theory.

Lower GPA standards (the nursing college has just increased the standard for admission from a 2.0 to 2.5). Stats will be followed for 3 years to see if this increases completers.

Financial/social support (go hand in hand).Poor background in math and science.

Not investing enough effort. Most high-risk students do not read the text, study consistently, or dedicate the necessary time out of the classroom.

Personally I think it is the cell phone. Too little time to concentrate on studies without phone ringing. Not enough three-hour study sessions without interruptions.

Study habits are poor.

They lack the ability to process all the information that is required, cognitive, affective and psychomotor. I am referring to those who are not successful on the second try.

Not understanding the commitment and study it takes, not only to learn but change behavior.

Baccalaureate Degree Nursing Program

Poor basic skills.

Their expectations of the role or the requirements to meet that role are unrealistic. (Nursing as it is portrayed in the media is not often realistic).

Lack of a sound prenursing knowledge base.

Grasp of English language.

Unable to retain content.

Disabling. Weak interpersonal skills.

Large number of hours worked at a job.

Students are not reading or studying enough either because they are not focused, or they are working full or part-time that may interfere with their studies. Many students also have family issues that affect their studies and place them at risk, such as illness of a family member, children, or illness of their own.

Priority decisions.

Inexperience with critical thinking in previous educational experiences (not knowing how to take NCLEX style tests).

Poor academic background. Low scores in English and sciences.

Difficulty meeting course objectives for any of the above mentioned reasons. My clinical students, displaying difficulties, are provided learning opportunities and support prior to any decision to terminate.

Underprepared in High School and work and personal responsibilities that interfere with adequate study.

Unable to adequately pass the sciences - if they struggle there, they will struggle with pathophysiology/pharmacology/assessment, which are a big base for all the clinical courses.

Generally weak academically when entering college.

Academic failure.

Science GPA.

Chapter 2: Identifying Your At Risk Students

> Academically weak performances.
>
> Unrealistic expectations of nursing!
>
> Personal problems.
>
> Need for accommodations due to learning disabilities. Our students are nontraditional students (not right out of high school). Many of our students have multiple roles: married, children, working which can impact their educational process. But we as a faculty on our campus work extremely hard to retain our students. Tutorial Services is another service offered where they can access NCLEX practice questions in their weak areas.
>
> ### Accelerated Bachelors/Masters (Second Degree)
>
> Trying to work too many hours and too many outside commitments to devote the time needed for an accelerated program.
>
> ### Faculty Teaching in both a BSN and MSN Program
>
> Students who cannot think logically and critically.

(All text in the above table is drawn from a survey and is presented verbatim.)

Again, there was no consensus on the number one reason students are not successful. Nursing students are a diverse group of people.

Most of the responses are ones that have been noted previously in the literature with the exception of one response:

> Personally I think it is the cell phone. Too little time to concentrate on studies without phone ringing. Not enough three-hour study sessions without interruptions.

This was a very insightful response that illustrates the concept that our student population has changed over time, and we must be acutely aware of those changes. As we witness every day, people are constantly talking on their cells phone and our students are no exception. Students in the past were not so accessible and could plan study times when they were not interrupted by phone calls. This is no longer the case. Perhaps we should advise students to turn off their cell phones when they are studying.

It was interesting that the respondents to the questions posed in Tables 2.4 and 2.5 did not have a specific definition of the at-risk student. Although we did not ask if their nursing school had a specific definition of the student at-risk to fail, it is not evident from the responses that such a definition existed in any of the 45 schools represented. Faculty may want to consider taking a close look at their student population and crafting a definition of their at-risk student. This definition can then be used to develop advising for prospective students, admission requirements, and support for students before and after entering a nursing program. Figure 2.1 shows this relationship.

Figure 2.1 – Relationship of Definition for At-Risk Student and Admission Components

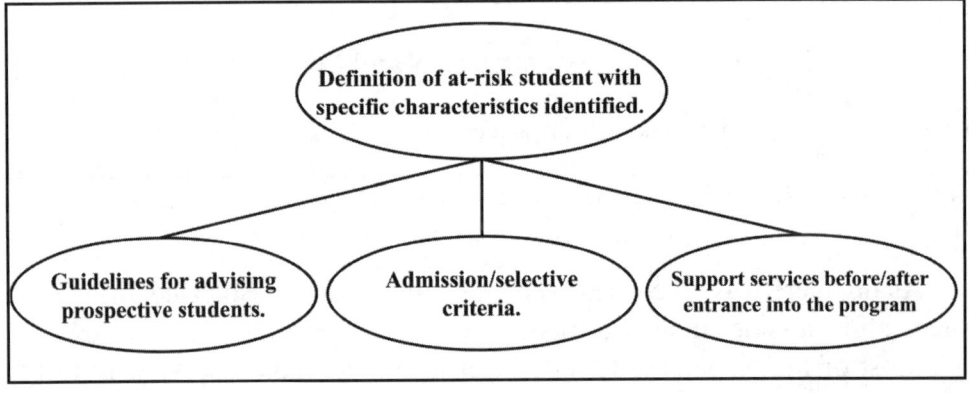

Figure 2.1 is important to consider for two reasons. The first reason is that some schools look to predictors of success as a means for determining admission criteria. This is considered in depth in Chapter 3 of this book. The second reason to identify predictors of success is to establish support services ready to assist students throughout their nursing education. These predictors can identify which students will have the most difficulty succeeding and what measures can be instituted to help them succeed.

Admission and selective criteria can be used for two reasons. The first reason is used to restrict enrollment to those most likely to succeed; the second reason is to expand enrollment to those who may have difficulty succeeding in a

Chapter 2: Identifying Your At Risk Students

nursing program and then plan strategies to help them succeed. These represent two very different perspectives. The first represents a philosophy of selective enrollment. The second represents a philosophy of what we propose to be called supportive enrollment. For example, Holyoke Community College uses the philosophy of supportive enrollment. Holyoke Community College actively recruits students who are traditionally underrepresented in nursing and traditionally at-risk for failure. Awareness of the factors that put these students at risk for failure helps focus support to provide services to help these students succeed (Anonymous – Nursing Education Perspectives, 2002). Many of these students would not succeed without these support services. Over a 12 year period, the number of underrepresented students in Holyoke's nursing program increased from 3.2% to 27% of the nursing class, largely in part to measures instituted to help this group of students succeed.

Identifying YOUR At-Risk Students

The faculty of a nursing program must examine the characteristics of their nursing student population and determine what factors predict success for their very unique student body. Although research on attrition and retention of nursing students has been conducted for decades, little research focuses on specific at-risk variables for a specific student population. Therefore, faculty must determine what factors influence success for their students. Also, faculty must be aware that these predictors change with time. Predictors of student success 10 years ago may not be accurate predictors in the current student and nursing environment. Examining and choosing predictors is an ongoing process subject to revisions as new characteristics arise.

With extensive diversity among nursing students, faculty must consider the unique aspects of their students' culture to provide effective instruction. Any analysis of student characteristics must always include cultural factors such as social roles, family values, religion, and the world view of all the cultural groups represented in your student population. Ethnicity and its many facets impact retention (Manifold & Rambur, 2001).

Another factor to consider when looking at your own local students is at what point the student entered your program. Whether the student entered at the beginning of the program or transferred from another school may be a factor that impacts success. Oftentimes transfer students struggle because they come from a variety of institutions with various levels of preparation. Faculty may find it difficult to assimilate these students into their general population of students. Faculty may want to assess individually these students to find the best fit in their program for entry.

Developing a Definition of "At-Risk" for Your School

The first step in identifying the "at-risk" student in your nursing program is to determine the outcomes you consider indicators of success. You may want to set an acceptable graduation rate within a certain number of years or establish a retention rate. With your goals set, you then consider all the predictors that have been discussed in this chapter and determine which ones apply to your student population. You will develop a profile of what you believe makes your students at-risk for not meeting your indicators of success. Quantifying criteria that serve as the best predictors of success are identified and applied to your applicants. The purpose is again twofold:

1. Develop admission and selective criteria so those most likely to be successful are admitted into the nursing program. (Of course, this must be in agreement with your program's philosophy. You may have a philosophy that does not restrict enrollment and takes all students without applying any selective criteria other than first come, first admitted.)
2. Provide early intervention that will improve performance and facilitate retention.

If factors that interfere with success are identified, then the school has an obligation to provide support, or at the very least make students aware that if they enter the program they may have difficulty passing if they possess the identified characteristics.

When you consider positive and negative influences and determine predictors, if these predictors are used for admission criteria, they may not be predictive of the students' success in all nursing courses. Gallagher, Bomba, and Crange (2001) found that admission scores were not good predictors of success in the final nursing course. Therefore, students who minimally meet the admission criteria may pass the initial nursing courses but need support and assistance throughout the nursing program to be successful in the higher-level nursing courses.

Chapter 2: Identifying Your At Risk Students

From all this information, develop a definition that works for your students. Use the checklist in Table 2.6. Add to the table any additional factors you identify as important for your students. Look at each item on the checklist and determine to what degree that item influences success for each student. This is a subjective decision on your part, based on your assessment of the individual student's profile. Will you place more emphasis on academic factors, personal factors, or environmental factors? Do the negatives outweigh the positives? If yes, the student is "at-risk." If no, the student is not "at-risk." Use this checklist as a guide to talk with students one-on-one. This table is on the CD-ROM that accompanies this book. You may use this table or revise it to fit your needs.

Some of the factors on the chart may be difficult to include as admission or selective criteria. For example, motivation and/or desire may tip the scales to either the positive or negative side. You may have had experience with students who have beaten the odds by passing their courses while working 30 hours a week and caring for several dependent children, all while lacking a personal support system. Even though motivation was the key to this student's success, it would have been difficult to measure accurately motivation at the time of admission.

Another intervening factor is self-efficacy. Self-efficacy refers to a sense of confidence that a task can be completed. Students who rate high on self-efficacy feel confident in their ability to succeed. Aber & Arathuzik (1996) reported that students who ranked high in self-efficacy were able to succeed in spite of personal burdens such as family and child care responsibilities requiring up to 44 hours per week of the students' time.

Nursing Faculty Behaviors as a Factor Contributing to At-Risk Status

An interesting area to explore that may factor into the students' at-risk to fail equation is faculty behavior. Are we contributing to our students' failure rate? Condon (1996) studied 770 culturally diverse nursing students. When asked what factors received high priority by nursing students as important for academic success and progress, they all agreed that caring nursing faculty who are willing to give academic or clinical help to students was very important. Interestingly, Tracey (2003) found that students reported they would go to a friend or family member before they would go to a teacher for help with their studies. If students

Table 2.6 – Checklist of Positive and Negative Factors

Classification of Factors	Place a Checkmark if Positive Factor Applies	Positive Factors	Place a Checkmark if Negative Factor Applies	Negative Factors
Academic/School-Related		Academically well prepared – acceptable pre-nursing GPA		Less academically prepared overall – low prenursing GPA
		Acceptable science scores		Low science scores: biological science; social science; chemistry
		Acceptable math scores		Low math scores
		Reading at college level		Reading below college level
		Studies at least 3 hours per credit hour per week		Studies less than 3 hours per credit hour per week
		Positive attitude toward educators		Negative attitude toward educators
		Previous degree		No prior college experience
		Pre-entrance counseling		Lack of pre-entrance counseling
		Good test-taking skills		Test anxiety
		Critical thinker		Difficulty with critical thinking
		Good time management skills		Difficulty with time management
		< 20 minute travel to school		> 20 minute travel to school
Personal Factors		Very motivated		Lacks motivation
		Strong social support		Lack of social support
		Manages stress well		Difficulty dealing with stress
		Age on entry		Age on entry
		High self-efficacy		Low self-efficacy
		Self-confident		Low self-esteem
		No health problems		Health problems
Environmental Factors		Minimal church, community commitments		Many church, community commitments
		No family responsibilities		Has family responsibilities
		No issues with child care		Problems with child care
		No family problems		Family problems

identify a helpful teacher as important to their success, they must feel comfortable approaching that teacher for help.

Condon (1996) recommends that students can benefit from support, encouragement, and help provided by involved, caring nursing faculty. Shelton (2003) reported that students were more likely to persist to graduation in a nursing program when they perceived both functional and psychological support from faculty. Functional support refers to supportive behaviors directed at the achievement of educational tasks to reach the students' goals. Types of behaviors classified as functional support include monitoring academic progress, providing help with course content, referring to appropriate academic resources within the school, and facilitating goal setting and problem solving. Psychological support refers to behaviors that encourage a sense of competency and self-worth and includes being available, approachable, and demonstrating respect by correcting students without belittling them (Shelton, 2003).

Faculty can directly facilitate student success and program completion through frequent and supportive interactions with students. Faculty should reach out to a student who is having difficulty and not wait for the student to contact them. When faculty provide such support, students perceive that the faculty care. Caring is an essential part of the student-faculty relationship and models behaviors that can transfer to the student-client relationship.

When students have an opportunity to exchange suggestions with faculty, useful ideas may be gleaned for course and curricular improvement. Thus, development of a positive interaction among students and faculty may not only benefit the students' educational experience, but the entire program.

Students also report that positive factors influencing retention include congruence between classroom and clinical learning experiences as well as the pace and content of a course (Bolan & Grainger, 2003). Faculty can look at these factors and consider them when planning courses.

Putting the Parts Together

Figure 2.2 presents a model illustrating how the components discussed in this chapter relate. The model illustrates how that information feeds into an admission policy. Formulating an admission policy is discussed in Chapter 3.

Figure 2.2 – Identifying Your At-Risk Student: The At-Risk Model

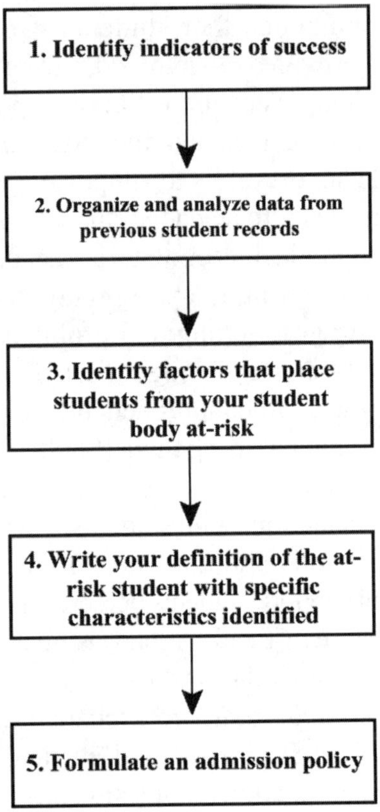

```
1. Identify indicators of success
          ↓
2. Organize and analyze data from previous student records
          ↓
3. Identify factors that place students from your student body at-risk
          ↓
4. Write your definition of the at-risk student with specific characteristics identified
          ↓
5. Formulate an admission policy
```

A Hypothetical Example Using the At-Risk Model

This section presents a hypothetical school named Hypothetical Nursing School demonstrating application of the At-Risk Model in Figure 2.2.

1. Identify Indicators of Success

The faculty established that students must earn a C in all nursing courses to progress to the next nursing course and to graduate. Therefore, the first indicator of success is that the student will earn a grade of C or higher. The second indicator of success is a retention rate of 85% on-time graduation and 15% graduation with one step-out.

Chapter 2: Identifying Your At Risk Students

2. Organize and Analyze Data from Previous Student Records

The second step in the model is to organize and analyze data from previous student records. The example reports information from records of 40 students from the past five years who earned a grade of D, F, or W (withdrew). Table 2.6 was slightly modified for this example and the numbers of students for each positive and negative factor were entered. The results are presented in Table 2.7.

Entering the numbers in the table provides an organized presentation of data that can be easily studied. The data in the completed table indicate the following:
1. Factors that present problems for this group of students in this specific nursing program
2. Information on some factors is unavailable by reviewing student files. In the future, this information should be collected before the student enters the nursing program or while enrolled in nursing courses.

3. Identify Factors that Place Students from Your Student Body At-Risk

Once the data collection was complete, the faculty studied the information and identified factors that place their students at-risk for earning a grade of D, F, or W. The faculty first determined what would be an acceptable number in any one of the cells in Table 2.7. Once that number is exceeded, it then becomes a risk factor. The faculty at Hypothetical Nursing School determined that any negative factor representing 20 or more students is a factor indicating the student is at-risk for not completing a nursing course.

4. Write Your Definition of the At-Risk Student with Specific Characteristics Identified

Using the information from steps 2 and 3, the faculty developed their definition of the at-risk student with specific characteristics identified.

Using the guideline "20 or more students with a negative factor," the definition for a student at-risk was written as follows:

A student entering the Hypothetical Nursing School is considered at-risk for failing a nursing course if one or more of the following factors apply to that student:
1. Low GPA

Table 2.7 – Numbers of Students with Positive and Negative Factors from Hypothetical Nursing School

Classification of Factor	Number of students with D, F, or W	Positive Factors	Number of students with D, F, or W	Negative Factors
Academic/School-Related	10	Academically well prepared – acceptable pre-nursing GPA	30	Less academically prepared overall – low pre-nursing GPA
	18	Acceptable science scores	22	Low science scores: biological science; social science; chemistry
	30	Acceptable math scores	10	Low math scores
	8	Reading at college level	32	Reading below college level
	UD	Studies at least 3 hours per credit hour per week	UD	Studies less than 3 hours per credit hour per week
	UD	Positive attitude toward educators	UD	Negative attitude toward educators
	15	Previous degree	25	No prior college experience
	UD	Pre-entrance counseling	UD	Lack of pre-entrance counseling
	UD	Good test-taking skills	UD	Test anxiety
	12	Critical thinker as per clinical evaluation	28	Difficulty with critical thinking as per clinical evaluation
	20	Good time management skills	20	Difficulty with time management
	UD	< 20 minute travel to school	UD	> 20 minute travel to school
Personal Factors	UD	Very motivated	UD	Lacks motivation
	UD	Manages stress well	UD	Difficulty dealing with stress
	27	Age on entry > 25	13	Age on entry =< 25
	UD	High self-efficacy	UD	Low self-efficacy
	UD	Self-confident	UD	Low self-esteem
	37	No health problems	3	Health problems
Environmental Factors	8	No family responsibilities	32	Has family responsibilities
	UD	Strong social support	UD	Lack of social support
	30	No issues with child care	10	Problems with child care
	UD	No family problems	UD	Family problems
	UD	Minimal church, community commitments	UD	Many church, community commitments

(UD = Unable to Determine)

Chapter 2: Identifying Your At Risk Students

2. Low science grades
3. Reading score below college level
4. No prior college experience
5. Difficulty with critical thinking
6. Difficulty with time management
7. Multiple family responsibilities
8. Works 20 or more hours per week

These preceding steps guide the faculty to a clear vision of what puts their students at-risk for failure. This information is critical for developing the school's admission policy. Formulating the admission policy is covered in Chapter 3.

Closing Thoughts

As Campbell & Dickson (1996) reported nearly a decade ago, nursing education research continues to be unable to identify consistent predictors of success in a nursing program. This is still true today. There are two absolutes that can be drawn from this chapter:
1. Today's students are very diverse.
2. Tomorrow's students will be different from today's students.

Therefore, faculty must continuously analyze what factors are applicable to their own student population. Helpful to the effort of identifying factors that place your students "at-risk" would be multi-site studies conducted collaboratively among comparable institutions with similar student populations. This approach may yield more consistent and reliable findings. Until then, faculty must identify for themselves what predictors can be used with their students.

Once the at-risk predictors are identified, faculty must decide what to do with that information. One use as indicated in the model in Figure 2.2 is to relate these factors to admission and selective criteria so these criteria are based on data gleaned from the school's specific student body. They are also used to plan interventions that are focused on specific student needs. These topics are covered in the following chapters.

Finally, the identified predictors and your definition of the at-risk student should be evaluated on an ongoing basis. Student characteristics change over time. These evaluations relate to your program outcomes set for the purpose of program evaluation. For example, you may set an 85% retention rate as a program outcome. You have your definition of at-risk, your predictive factors based on your individual student population, set standard for rate of retention, and the data that shows if your established criteria are reliable, valid, and trustworthy. This data can be collected, analyzed, aggregated, and trended as the basis for decision-making for your program.

Learning Activities

1. Using Table 2.7 conduct a retrospective study of students who graduated from your nursing program during the last year. (An electronic version of this table is located on the CD-ROM accompanying this book). Complete another table for students who earned a grade of D, F, or W in the last year. Compare the numbers you entered in each table. What conclusions can you make?
2. Using the information you collected in activity #1, develop a definition of the student at-risk for failing your nursing program.

References

AACN, (2003). White Papers, Faculty Shortages. Retrieved January 28, 2005, from aacn.nche.edu/Publications/WhitePapers/FacultyShortages.htm.

Aber, C., & Arathuzik, D. (1996). Factors associated with student success in a baccalaureate nursing program within an urban public university. *Journal of Nursing Education, 35*(6), 285-288.

Abdur-Rahman, V., & Gaines, C. (1999). Retaining ethnic minority nursing students (REMNS): A multidimensional approach. *The ABNF Journal, 10*(2), 33-36.

Bean, J. P., & Metzner, B. (1985). A conceptual model of nontraditional undergraduate student attrition. *Review of Educational Research, 55,* 485-540.

Bolan, C. M., & Grainger, P. (2003). High school to nursing. *Canadian Nurse, 99*(3), 18-22.

Byrd, G., Garza, C., & Nieswiadomy, R. (1999). Predictors of successful completion of a baccalaureate nursing program. *Nurse Educator, 24,*(6), 33-37.

Campbell, A. R., & Dickson, C. J. (1996). Predicting student success: A 10-year review using integrative review and meta-analysis. *Journal of Professional Nursing, 12*(1), 47-59.

Candela, L. L., Kowalski, S., Cyrkiel, D., & Warner, D. (2004). Meeting the at-risk challenge: Empowering nursing students through mentoring. *International Journal of Nursing Education Scholarship, 1*(1), 1-13.

Condon, V. M. M. (1996). Student identified factors related to the academic success or progress of culturally diverse baccalaureate nursing students. (Doctoral dissertation, Claremont Graduate School, 1996).

Ehrenfeld, M., Rotenberg, A., Sharon, R., & Bergman, R. (1997). Reasons for student attrition on nursing courses: A study. *Nursing Standard, 11*(23), 34-38.

Gallagher, P., Bomba, C., & Crane, L. (2001). Using an admissions exam to predict student success in an ADN Program. *Nurse Educator, 26*(3), 132-135.

Gaze, H. (2000). All business and no pleasure? *Nursing Times*, 96(19), 30-31.

Guhde, J. A. (2003). English-as-a-second language nursing students: Strategies for building verbal and written language skills. *Journal of Cultural Diversity*, 10(4), 113-117.

Houltram, B. (1996). Entry age, entry mode and academic performance on a Project 2000 Common foundation programme. *Journal of Advanced Nursing, 23,* 1089-1097.

Jeffreys, M. R. (1995). Joining together family, faculty, and friends. New ideas for enhancing nontraditional student success. *Nurse Educator, 20*(3), 11.

Jeffreys, M. R. (2001). Evaluating enrichment program study groups: Academic outcomes, psychological outcomes, and variables influencing retention. *Nurse Educator, 26*(3), 142-149.

Jeffreys, M. R. (2004). Nursing student retention: Understanding the process and making a difference. New York: Springer.

Levine, A., and Cureton, J. S.(1998).*When hope and fear collide: A portrait of today's college student*. San Francisco: Jossey-Bass.

Lewis, C., & Lewis, J. (2000). Research brief. Predicting academic success of transfer nursing students. *Journal of Nursing Education*, 39(5), 234-236.

Manifold, C., & Rambur, B. (2001). Predictors of attrition in American Indian nursing students. *Journal of Nursing Education*, 40(6), 279-281.

National League for Nursing Accrediting Commission. (1996a). *Criteria and guidelines for the evaluation of associate degree programs in nursing 1996* (NLN Publication No. 23-6983). New York: Author.

National League for Nursing Accrediting Commission. (1996b). *Program evaluator's report: Baccalaureate and higher degree programs, 1996 criteria.* New York: Author.

Patton, T., & Goldenberg, D. (1999). Hardiness and anxiety as predictors of academic success in first-year, full-time and part-time RN students. *Journal of Continuing Education in Nursing*, 30(4), 158-167.

Potolsky, A., Cohen, J., & Saylor, C. (2003). Academic performance of nursing students: Do prerequisite grades and tutoring make a difference? *Nursing Education Perspectives*, 24(5), 246-50.

Prevost, S. (2005, July). *Nursing students: A constantly changing audience.* Paper presented at the meeting of the Sigma Theta Tau International Honor Society of Nursing, 16th International Nursing Research Congress, Waikoloa, HI.

Sandiford, J., & Jackson, K. (2003). *Predictors of first semester attrition and their relation to retention of generic associate degree nursing students.* East Lansing, MI: National Center for Research on Teacher Learning. (ERIC Document Reproduction Service No. ED481947)

Shelton, E. N. (2003). Faculty support and student retention. *Journal of Nursing Education, 42*(2), 68-76.

Spahr, A. (1995). Predicting graduation status of nursing students using entering GPA and grades in algebra, biology, and chemistry. *U.S. Illinois*, 6 pages.

Tinto, V. (1993). *Leaving college: Rethinking the causes and cures of student attrition.* Chicago: University of Chicago Press.

Tracey, G. (2003). A national study of support programs (efforts) in baccalaureate and associate degree nursing programs to enhance retention and success of students. (Doctoral dissertation, University of Central Florida, 2003). *Dissertation Abstracts International, 64*(2598).

Wells, M. (2003). An epidemiologic approach to addressing student attrition in nursing program. *Journal of Professional Nursing, 19*(3), 230-236.

Chapter 3:
Formulating an Admissions Policy

A review of the literature quickly reveals that almost every conceivable variable has been considered as a factor influencing admission and selective criteria for entrance into an undergraduate nursing program. These factors have been used singly or in a variety of creative ways to determine which students should be admitted and to predict who would be most successful in achieving an on-time graduation.

In this chapter, the many variables used as admission and selective criteria are reviewed. After a brief discussion of these variables, elements of an admission policy are examined using these variables.

Differentiating Terms

There are several terms used when discussing student admission to a nursing program. All members of a nursing faculty should agree on the definition of these terms to facilitate clear communication.

Admission Criteria

The term "admission criteria" refers to the criteria the student must meet to be admitted into the nursing program. Admission criteria include the requirements for general admission into the institution as well as additional requirements specifically for admission into the nursing program.

General institutional admission requirements, such as a specific grade point average (GPA) or score on the ACT, apply to all students entering the school. The requirements for general admission may be different than those of the nursing school. For example, a general college admission requirement may be a GPA of 2.0. The school of nursing may require a GPA of 2.5. When a specific program such as a nursing program within a larger institutional setting establishes higher admission criteria for applicants than other students must meet, that program is often said to have "selective admission." These criteria are termed selective or even highly selective depending on the number of factors used and the standards represented by these factors.

There are two categories of admission criteria for a nursing program:
1. Required prerequisite courses to ensure students are prepared for the nursing coursework. Examples include courses such as biology, chemistry, and medical terminology.
2. Factors used as predictors of success to select students most likely to pass nursing courses

Admission Criteria Used as Predictors of Success

Some admission criteria are used as predictors of success in a nursing program. When used as predictors of success, the criteria may serve as information for advising students. For example, an admission criterion may be that the students complete a microbiology course with a grade of C or better. The specific grade the student earned in that microbiology course may also be used as a predictor of successful completion of the nursing program. That is, if the student earned a grade of A in microbiology, the student is more likely to be successful in nursing courses than the student who earned a C in microbiology. Both students meet the admission criteria; however, the student who earned an A in microbiology is predicted to be more likely to pass the nursing courses than the student who earned a C in the same microbiology course.

For required prerequisite courses, an important consideration is to determine how many times the student has taken a required course. For example, many students may retake a required course to earn an acceptable grade for admission. However, some students may have earned an acceptable grade but may retake a course to raise a grade, such as a B to an A to increase their chances of admission. A higher grade may earn the student more points toward admission. However, some schools actually subtract points in their point system when a student repeats a course, even if the reason for repeating the course was to raise a B grade to an A grade.

Selective Criteria

Selective criteria are different from admission criteria. Because many more qualified candidates are seeking admission to a nursing program than available positions in that program, all applicants meeting the admission criteria may be further considered using selective criteria. Selective criteria used by nursing schools are many and varied. In an attempt to quantify and objectify the selection process, a point system may be used. This yields what is sometimes referred to as a Selective Criteria Score. Table 3.1 shows an example point system.

Table 3.1 – Example Point System for Selective Criteria Score

Selective Criteria	Points Earned
ACT Composite 30 + 4 points 26 – 29 3 points 22 – 25 2 points 18 – 21 1 point	
GPA 3.7 – 4.0 4 points 3.3 – 3.6 3 points 2.9 – 3.2 2 points 2.5 – 2.8 1 point	
Previous College Degree Previous degree 1 point No previous degree 0 points	
Reading Exam Score High score 2 points Middle range 1 point Low score 0 points	
Biology Grade A 2 points B 1 point C 0 points	
Chemistry Grade A 2 points B 1 point C 0 points	
Total Points (Selective Criteria Score)	

Each student who meets the admission criteria is assigned a Selective Criteria Score. Students are rank-ordered for admission using these scores and admitted from the highest score down until all slots are filled.

Additional Admission Requirements

Once students have met all the admission requirements and selective criteria, they are accepted into the nursing program. However, their admission may be contingent on completing additional requirements. Some schools call this status Conditional Acceptance or Tentative Admission. If the student completes these additional requirements, the student is admitted; if not, the student is not admitted. Schools that operate in this manner often have a "waiting list" of students who meet the admission requirements but who earned a lower Selective Criteria Score than that earned by the students who were admitted. The students on the waiting list are admitted when other students fail to complete these additional requirements. Some of these requirements might include:
- certification as a nursing assistant
- certification in basic life support
- clearance with a criminal background check
- clearance with drug screening
- completion of a prerequisite nursing course or other related course such as medical terminology or anatomy and physiology

Students must complete all the additional requirements before admission into the nursing program. If they fail to complete these additional requirements, they are taken out of the pool of applicants.

A school may opt to include these additional requirements as admission requirements. This is a decision each school must make based on the effect these additional admission requirements will have on their applicants and the educational community. For example, if a school has 300 applicants but can only admit 50, it may not be fair or feasible to require all applicants to complete a Certified Nursing Assistant (CNA) course knowing that only one in six will be admitted. Also, does the school or the community have the resources to educate 300 students at the CNA level or offer certification in basic life support? These are important considerations when deciding what criteria to use for admission, selection, and additional requirements after acceptance.

A Review of the Literature

From the preceding definition of terms and discussion, it is apparent that determining admission and selective criteria are not easy tasks. A review of the literature can actually complicate the process because of the many suggested criteria and combinations of these criteria. Table 3.2 lists some of the common criteria used for admission cited in the literature.

Table 3.2 – Criteria Commonly Used as Admission Criteria

Admission Criteria
GPA

Standardized Tests
 • ACT
 • Nursing School Entrance Exams
     o HESI
     o NET
     o NLN
 • Test of English as a Foreign Language (TOEFL)

Previous Coursework Grades   • Algebra   • Anatomy & Physiology   • Biology   • Chemistry   • Social Sciences
Mathematic Computation Ability
Reading Score
Essay
Personal Interest Inventory
Personal Interview
Professional References
Work Experience in a Healthcare or Related Field

A Brief Discussion of Admission Criteria

Once characteristics that place a student at-risk for failing a nursing program are identified, faculty should use those characteristics to determine criteria for admission for their student body. Because enrollment in nursing programs is typically limited by many forces, those admitted must be carefully selected. Admission criteria should identify those students most likely to complete successfully the nursing program, yet not inadvertently restrict admission to any particular group of students.

Grade Point Average (GPA)

Grade point average (GPA) is probably the most universally used criteria. GPA is used extensively in schools of nursing because research and anecdotal evidence indicate a positive correlation between previous academic performance and success in a nursing program (Bolan & Grainger, 2003; Jeffreys, 2004). Tracey (2003) reported that required minimal GPA ranges from 2.00 to 3.00 with 2.50 being the most frequently used. Sandiford & Jackson (2003) found that students entering a nursing program with a grade point average of 2.5 and above had lower attrition than students with a grade point average between 2.00 and 2.49. Students who earn below average grades in the first nursing courses typically have low high school and prerequisite course grades (Potolsky, Cohen, & Saylor, 2003). Nursing schools should consider a minimum of 2.5 for an entry GPA.

Science Courses

Grades in science courses such as biology, chemistry, and anatomy and physiology have long been used to predict success in nursing courses. Generally speaking, the higher the grade in these courses, the better the chance for success in nursing courses (Byrd, Garza, & Nieswiadomy, 1999). Therefore, faculty may want to require a prerequisite science course grade of B or higher. Or, faculty may choose to use grades in science courses as an indicator for remediation. Students with lower science scores may benefit from remediation in those sciences so a firm knowledge base is formed prior to entering nursing courses.

Nursing Entrance Examinations

To help faculty sort through all the variables that can be considered for admission criteria, a number of companies and organizations have developed entrance examinations based on many of the factors listed in Table 3.2. Some of these tests are so inclusive they provide "one stop shopping." Schools can simplify the admission process by requiring a minimal GPA combined with a specific score on one of these entrance examinations. Furthermore, a standardized test may be preferable over requiring a certain grade in a prerequisite science course. Compare the student who earned an A after seeking out an "easy" teacher with the student who earned a C in the same subject but with a more challenging teacher. The C student may be more prepared to take nursing courses than the A student. A standardized test may be a better indicator of the actual knowledge level of these two students.

One example of an entrance examination is the Admission Assessment (A^2) by Health Education Systems, Inc. (HESI). This test covers the areas of:
- Anatomy and physiology
- Biology
- Chemistry
- Grammar
- Math
- Reading
- Vocabulary and general knowledge

A school using the A^2 examination can specify some or all of the above categories to be used for the test administered to their students. A study guide is available to help students review for this examination.

The scores on the A^2 examination may be used in a variety of ways. Some schools find the overall grade helpful as a predictor; however, for many, the reading comprehension score may be the most useful indicator. This reading comprehension score is used to establish a minimum score below which students will not be admitted.

Depending on one indicator as the only criterion for admission is practical and time-efficient, but may eliminate many capable students from admission. Use of a single criterion, such as an entrance exam, may eliminate students who do not test well. Many nursing schools rely solely on objective tests as the measure of a student's success in each nursing course; therefore, ability to test well may be an important factor.

To yield reliable predictor data without undertaking a formidable task, you may consider using two indicators such as a standardized entrance exam and GPA or reading level and GPA. GPA may be further refined by requiring a certain GPA in prerequisite courses rather than a cumulative GPA. Using several factors and providing preadmission remediation for low scorers may be a more viable option.

Research Study – A Closer Look at What Schools are Doing

The websites of 86 pre-licensure registered nursing schools from all regions of the United States were randomly chosen to determine the kind of admission criteria currently in use. The findings are listed in Table 3.3.

Most schools in the study with selective criteria used a combination of factors. Some used strictly hard criteria. Some combined hard and soft criteria.

Hard Criteria

Hard criteria are those criteria that are quantifiable. These criteria include objective data such as GPA, course grades, ACT scores, SAT scores, and nursing entrance exam scores.

Soft Criteria

Soft criteria are those that are difficult to quantify. These are subjective in nature and include criteria such as an essay, professional references, work experience, and personal interview.

Personal Interview

Some faculty believe a personal interview is an extremely helpful mechanism for determining who may be a good fit for the nursing profession. Other faculty believe this type of subjective evaluation tool is vague and litigious. All faculty who conduct student interviews should follow an established protocol and ensure interrater reliability. A personal interview is

Table 3.3 – Summary of Admission Criteria from 86 Schools of Nursing

Admission Criteria	Comments
Type of Admission Selective Admission = 70 schools Open Admission = 16 schools	Selective = ranges from selective to highly selective (very high requirements). Ranges from only requiring a GPA higher than that required for general college entrance to a complex ranking system. Open = uses only college-wide admission requirements.
GPA (minimum required for admission) GPA Number of Schools 2.0 6 2.3 1 2.5 25 2.6 2 2.65 1 2.7 7 2.75 5 2.8 1 3.0 2 3.3 1	

ACT   10 schools
SAT   9 schools
High School Ranking > 50th
Critical Thinking Score 2 schools
Nursing School Entrance Exams
   o HESI 4 schools
   o NET 8 schools
   o NLN 8 schools
   o TEAS by ATI 3 schools
   o Some mentioned a prenursing entrance exam but didn't specify which one
Test of English as a Foreign Language (TOEFL) = 4 schools mentioned specifically but many mentioned that if English is not the first language the student must take TOEFL.
	Some school set minimum requirements; some merely require the scores to be submitted; some give points if higher than a certain number such as > 19 on ACT.

Previous Coursework Grades • Anatomy and Physiology • Biology • Chemistry	Most schools required some or all of these as prerequisites. The majority stated C minimum; some C- minimum; a few B minimum.
Mathematic Computation Ability	Some schools set a minimum on their math entrance exam. Sometimes the math test is part of a required nursing entrance exam.
Reading Score	Some schools set a minimum on their reading entrance exam. Sometimes the reading test is part of a required nursing entrance exam.
Essay 2 schools	
Personal Interview 5 schools	
Professional References 10 schools	
Work Experience in a Healthcare Field	3 schools required work experience; many gave points for experience which added to the applicant's chances for admission.
CNA required = 6 schools	

very helpful if questions are carefully asked. Asking why the person chose nursing can be informative but may elicit a pat answer such as, "I want to help people." Although that may be true, that answer does not hold much predictive value. Perhaps a more valuable line of questioning would involve an efficacy appraisal to ascertain the individual's perception of their ability to perform (Jeffreys, 1998). Questions that can address the applicant's perceptions relate to:

- ability to perform academically
- difficulty of the course of study in a nursing program
- amount of energy available to devote to the study of nursing
- any external assistance such as financial assistance, tutoring, personal support system
- prior experiences with successes and failures in school
- the degree to which the student will seek support

One key to student success is the student's ability to assess accurately when to seek support. Ofori and Charlton (2002) found that if a student seeks support for learning difficulties, this support-seeking had a direct effect on performance in a nursing program. In fact, learning behaviors such as support-seeking can compensate for deficiencies in other areas. To seek support, the student must have a realistic perception of when help is needed.

Another approach to use during a student interview is to provide interviewees with a typical week in the life of a nursing student and elicit the applicants' perception of how that week would fit into their lives. Students with answers that indicate an overly supreme opinion of their abilities may indicate unrealistic perceptions which may result in failure and discouragement (Bandura, 1986). Learning, as with most things in life, is greatly influenced by perception (Knowles, 1980). According to Jeffreys (1998) students who are supremely efficacious and overestimate their academic abilities and underestimate their need for preparation can be considered at-risk for failing in a nursing program. If students with supremely efficacious opinions of themselves are admitted into the nursing program, faculty should work with these students to help them develop a realistic self-appraisal so they can maximize their strengths and identify areas of weakness that need to be addressed. Examples of problems typical for the school's nursing students can be presented with applicants challenged to explain how they would deal with these situations.

Other Soft Criteria

While perusing the websites of the 86 schools of nursing, other soft criteria were noted. These criteria included statements such as:
- mentally capable to provide patient care
- physically capable with a physical activity (strength) classified as medium by the Department of Labor
- emotional ability to carry out nursing activities
- satisfactory physical and mental condition
- possess certain abilities and skills in the areas of intellect, sensory function, communication, physical abilities, and behaviors

Although these types of requirements were listed on some websites, there was no information about how they would be measured. If faculty choose to use these types of soft criteria, it would be extremely prudent to delineate specific ways in which the criteria are measured and then ensure consistent measurement with each and every applicant.

Required Advising Sessions

Almost all 86 schools noted applicants must attend a required advising session as part of the admission process. These sessions appeared to be group advising sessions. Group advising sessions are preferable at this point because they are time efficient in that a number of students can be served at one time. Another advantage is that students will learn from other students' questions. One school required the student to complete an online test after attending the advising session.

Selective Criteria Score

Approximately 30% of the websites reviewed mentioned using a point system for determining a selective criteria score to rank students for admission. Some schools outlined in detail the components of the system and how many points would be given for each component. However, a few schools mentioned they would be assigning points to each applicant and the applicants would be admitted based on their points, but there was no explanation of the point system. With a point system, it is possible that some students may earn the same number

of points. The faculty need to have an established tiebreaker policy. Example tiebreakers include:
- highest GPA
- date when application was completed (first applied; first qualified)
- number of degree applicable courses completed. Some mentioned no points would be given if a prerequisite course was repeated.

Determining Predictors of Success

As previously mentioned, many academic indicators have been considered as predictors for success including GPA, ACT, science grades, social science grades, and assessment tests. Factors which can be used to predict success in a nursing program have been the subject of research studies and publications for decades with the ongoing suggestion: Future research is needed to determine more specifically the variables to use to predict success for nursing students.

We propose that the issue is not to predict success but to predict success **specifically** for **your** nursing students. Scrutinize and study all the research reported in the literature for the purpose of planning an approach for determining the best predictors for **your** students. It would be very difficult if not impossible to read a research study and declare, "Yes, these are the criteria we will use." It is better to read a research study and then ask which criteria reported in the study is best for your particular student population. This would be an excellent topic for faculty to conduct an integrative review of the literature (as discussed in Chapter 1). Then, based on the strength of the findings, determine which criteria are appropriate to your pool of applicants.

Determining the Best Predictors for Your Students

Many individual factors have been examined for admission criteria. Combinations of those factors weaved into a matrix have been used for selective criteria. What works and what doesn't work? What is best for **your** student population? Studies have looked at attrition and retention rates of nursing students for over four decades, yet there is minimal literature reporting on specific student populations (Manifold & Rambur, 2001). The characteristics of each school's students are extremely important when formulating predictors for success. For example, in a study conducted by Manifold & Rambur (2001) a low high school GPA was not a significant predictor of completion of a nursing program for American Indian students, while studies with other student populations did find a positive correlation between high school GPA and program completion. More significant for American Indians in this study was their use of standard English. Although these students could speak English, the words and phrases are interpreted differently in their home settings than they are in academia. The standard English format used on nursing exams may present a challenge for these students' ability to comprehend the meaning of the questions. Therefore, for this group of students, an admission criterion might be a score on a test of standard English. After administering a test of standard English, interventions should be planned to provide support services to teach the student the difference between colloquial speech and that used on examinations. These students would not be asked to abandon their rich cultural language, but to adapt to the language and thinking required to read and answer exam questions accurately. This type of study of your particular student population is considered when formulating your school's admission criteria.

So what is a nursing faculty to do? How does the faculty in any one school use all this information to determine admission criteria or a selective criteria point system for their specific student body? And, does every school want a point system? What happened to the "open door" policy of community colleges and many private four-year institutions? In such institutions the philosophy may be, "No nursing student left behind!" If that's the case, and all students are allowed to enter, what is the responsibility of the faculty and the school to help students succeed? By identifying predictors of both academic success and academic failure, faculty and administration can intelligently put in place an educational support system needed to ensure success (Lewis & Lewis, 2000). Identification of predictive factors is important for schools of nursing even if they are not considering selective admission.

There is a nursing shortage – how do schools of nursing fill that need if their attrition rate is high because the "everyone should have the opportunity to be a nurse" method admits people who aren't prepared? However, restricting admission to only those with certain criteria that indicate (in your best judgment) that these people are prepared to succeed may limit opportunity for many groups of people.

The California community college system has an interesting approach to this issue. California's community colleges function under an open admission policy. Because of the nursing shortage and the need to educate more nurses, nursing programs in the California system can use a selective admission system to admit applicants they believe will successfully complete the nursing program; however, they must demonstrate they are not excluding any particular group of people (California Community Colleges Chancellor's Office, 2002).

Defining Your Purpose and Indicators of Success

One of your first tasks when considering predictors of success is to define your purpose and indicators of success. Determine your purpose for establishing admission criteria and the variables to be used to indicate student success. Then consider what admission criteria will serve that purpose. Are you looking at admission criteria to determine who will finish the program? Should criteria for entry into a nursing program be used to predict NCLEX success? Perhaps entry criteria should look at success in the program resulting in graduation. Student grades in nursing courses including performance in clinical might be a better predictor of NCLEX success.

Is success defined as:
- completion of the nursing program with "on-time" graduation?
- eventual completion of the program with no more than one "stop out"?
- eventual completion with any number of "stop outs"?

Set a graduation rate. What would be acceptable: 52%, 78%, 80% graduating with no stop-outs? Setting an acceptable graduation rate is important because once students are admitted faculty, administrators, and support personnel should all be available to ensure the graduation rate is realized. An infrastructure of support is one of the surest ways to ensure your predetermined graduation rate will become a reality.

Selecting the Criteria to Meet Your Purpose

A retrospective study of your graduates may be the best way to determine what criteria meet your purpose. Consider any and all data that may impact your students' success rate. Following are two examples.

Example #1

Currently a school has selective criteria with a 30% attrition rate. It would be important to compare the performance on the selective criteria items of those who passed with those who did not pass. That is, if the students who failed had lower numbers on their selective criteria than those who passed, these criteria may need to be reset at a higher level. If those who did not pass had similar scores on their selective criteria as those who passed, other data need to be studied to determine what other factors influenced the grade they earned. Did they have outside commitments such as family obligations or many hours of work on a job? Was test anxiety an issue? Did they fail to seek assistance early in the course?

Example #2

Another school of nursing may have selective criteria with a 100% on-time graduation rate. However, this school's NCLEX pass rate is only 80%. It may be helpful to compare the selective criteria of those who passed NCLEX with those who did not pass to determine if there is a difference; that is, if the candidates who did not pass NCLEX had lower numbers on their selective criteria, these criteria may need to be reset at a higher level. If those who did not pass had similar scores on the selective criteria, perhaps the admission criteria cannot be used as a predictor of success on NCLEX. The students' performance in their nursing courses and their clinical performance may be a better predictor of NCLEX success.

Possible Scenarios When Establishing Admission Criteria

As the preceding discussion suggests, there are many different scenarios that can lead to the need to develop admission and selective criteria within an admission policy. Let's consider a few of these scenarios.

Scenario #1

You know what your problem areas are; they are well established and identified. Therefore, your task is to select admission criteria that address these areas. For example, students who do not pass nursing courses have difficulty understanding the textbook. An entrance exam that measures reading level is appropriate.

Scenario #2

You have not been able to identify your problem areas. You do know that some students do well and some students do not do well. Also, you have more qualified applicants than you can admit. Therefore, you need a system to identify those students most likely to succeed. You look to the literature as a basis for selecting admission criteria.

Scenario #3

You have an open door policy so students are admitted without any selective admission criteria. You have a high attrition rate. You need to collect data about the students you are admitting so you can plan resources to help students succeed. This data will direct your plan for allocating resources.

Scenario #4

You have an acceptable retention rate and you have an acceptable NCLEX pass rate. You have no reason to establish selective admission criteria. Your system thus far has been to accept applicants on a first come/first serve basis after the applicant completes all prerequisite courses.

Scenario #5

Your mission is to attract students from underrepresented groups and recruit them into your nursing program. The goal is to graduate nurses who more closely reflect the general population served by your school. You collect data so you can plan resources to help these students succeed.

Developing an Admission Policy

Developing an admission policy is a very challenging task. The overall message is this: there is no magic bullet. Faculty must consider the uniqueness of their student population, school philosophy relative to student admission, and indicators of success. Each school is unique in the characteristics of its student body, geographic location, philosophy regarding selective admission, and available resources for student assistance. The most important question is, "What is your objective?" Is your objective to admit only those students most likely to succeed or is your objective to open opportunities to all segments of society so the nursing profession will more closely represent the people the profession is serving? The latter objective means attracting students from all ethnic, socioeconomic, racial, and religious groups and educational background.

A Few Suggestions

If you are establishing selective admission criteria, once you have identified the criteria, be certain these criteria have merit. At the very least have a rationale why the criteria were chosen as ones that will meet your purpose. Know why these criteria are necessary for the population of students you serve.

If you have a program that is nonselective or has an open door policy, your students may enter your nursing program without the necessary skills to be successful. Know the characteristics of your students and what kinds of problems they will encounter. You must plan interventions and identify available resources to help these students be successful.

Steps for Establishing an Admission Policy

Your written admission policy directs the specific steps of your admission procedure. When writing your admission policy consider the following.

1. Identify the Purpose of Your Admission Policy and Your Measures of Success

Be sure your admission policy reflects your nursing school's philosophy and mission. Issues to consider when formulating your purpose and measures of success may include some or all of the following:

1. If your purpose is to maintain a high retention rate, select only those students who are most apt to complete successfully the nursing program. A measure of success might be that 90% of students will graduate on time.
2. Ask if underrepresented and minority students are denied admission based on your policy. Consider providing educational opportunities for that population of students. A measure of success is that your student body reflects the diversity of the community.
3. Early identification of at-risk students is important. Early identification and early intervention are key to helping students succeed. Plan strategies during the beginning courses of the program.
4. Identify the academically strong students and plan enrichment activities to challenge these students.
5. If a predetermined first-time pass rate on NCLEX is your goal, admission criteria may not be a reliable indicator. Plan strategies throughout the nursing program to meet this goal. Chapter 9 addresses a model for NCLEX success.

2. Consider the Characteristics of Your Students

What are the major characteristics of your students as identified in Chapter 2, Table 2.6? Pull out the characteristics that would be applicable to your admission policy.

3. Identify Resources

It is unfair knowingly to admit students who are not academically prepared, and not have resources available to help those students. Consider:
1. resources to provide academic help
2. resources for financial aid
3. faculty to student ratio

4. resources to assist with personal issues
5. resources to help faculty implement success strategies

4. Develop an Admission Policy

Write your overall admission policy considering your student population, predictors of success, at-risk characteristics, and resources available to help support student success. When writing your admission policy also consider the following:

1. Consider which of the characteristics identified in Table 2.7 represent at-risk characteristics. Determine the characteristics of the students who completed the program and students who did not complete the program.
2. Plot trends in pass rate on NCLEX; determine characteristics of students who were unsuccessful on NCLEX.
3. Determine admission criteria based on the type of admission; that is, open-door or selective. If selective, develop selective admission criteria. The selective admission criteria may reflect the predictors of success, such as a GPA of 2.5. Other criteria may not align completely with predictor criteria. For example, you require a B in all prerequisite science courses but realize students who earn A's in those courses are more likely to be successful in nursing courses.

5. Develop or Locate, then Administer, a Tool for Collecting Data from Applicants

The type and specific data collection tools must be identified. You may decide to use a reading and math test already in use at your school. Or, you may decide to use one of the comprehensive nursing entrance exams discussed in Chapter 2, gleaning the reading and math scores from that comprehensive tool.

6. Consider for Admission

In this step you decide which students meet the admission criteria and which do not. Then you apply the selective criteria to the group to rank the students for admission. Any students who are not admitted should be notified. It is most helpful to those students to indicate why they were not accepted for admission and how they can prepare for reapplication to the nursing program.

7. Establish Tentative Admission Requirements

Determine what requirements, if any, students must meet before final acceptance into the nursing program. Discussed earlier in this chapter, these requirements can include completing a CNA program or consenting to a criminal background check.

8. Determine if Measures for Success are being Met

Once the admission policy is established, identify factors that may interfere with your students' successful completion of the nursing program. Determine if you are meeting the measures of success as identified in Step 1. These factors form the basis for developing your Student Success Program. Chapters 4, 5, and 6 discuss how to establish such a program.

Apply this process to **all** entering students. Understanding the characteristics of the students who are NOT at risk for failure is as important as understanding those who are at risk for failure. All students deserve attention and the stimulation of a rich learning environment to enhance their educational experience.

Your admission policy should undergo continuous scrutiny and evaluation on a regular schedule. After two to three years, use trended data to make changes. It is critical that you research the predictive value of your admission and selective criteria and determine if you are accomplishing your measures of success. How accurate were the criteria in predicting student success? Should the criteria be changed? Do the criteria continue to be appropriate for your current applicants or have your applicants changed? The answers to these questions guide the revision of your admission policy. Figure 3.1 illustrates these steps in a model or flowchart format.

Hypothetical Nursing School Example

The faculty at the Hypothetical Nursing School (HNS) developed a new admission policy based on student data. The data included information about

Figure 3.1 – A Model for Developing an Admission Policy

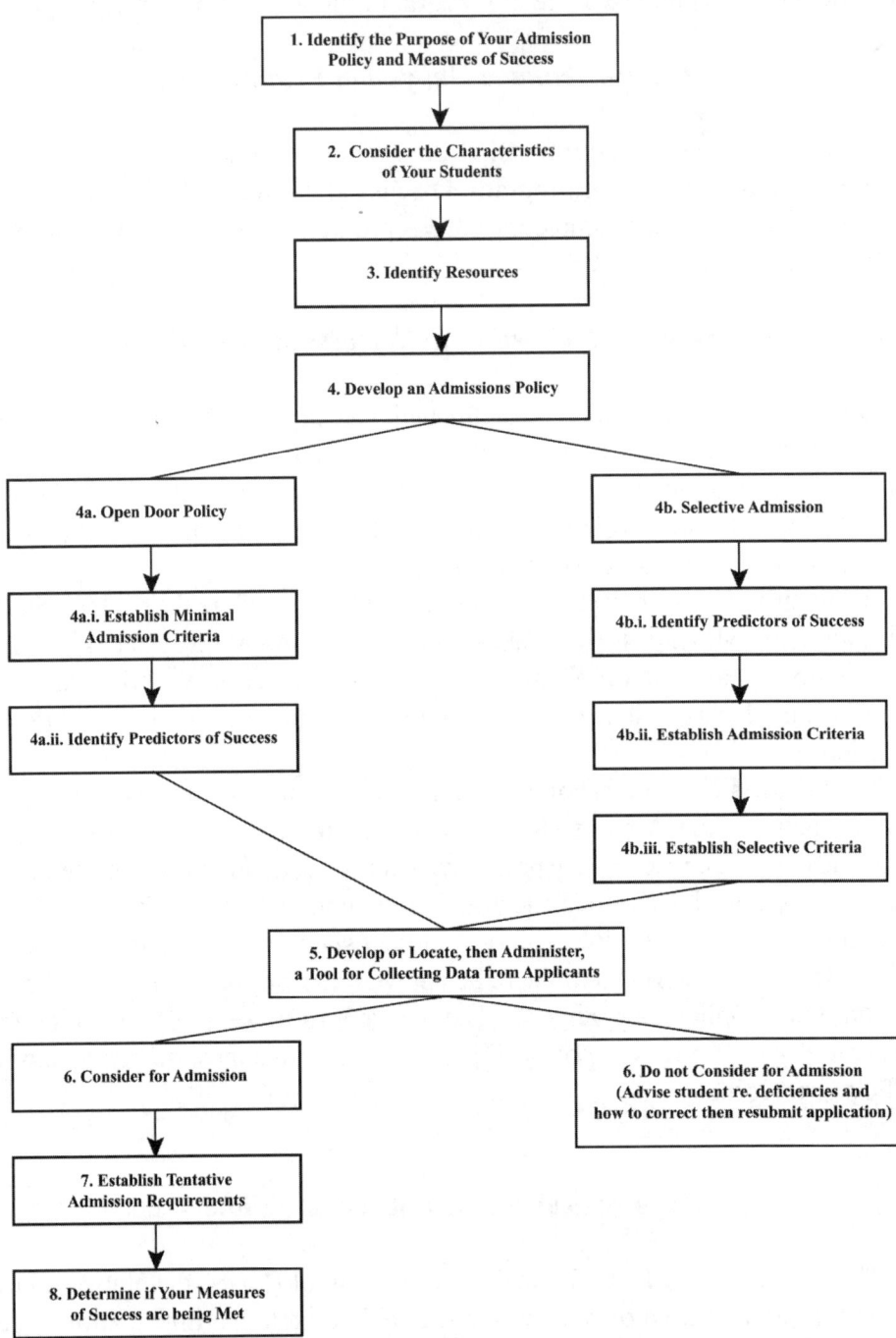

Chapter 3: Formulating an Admissions Policy

the student population and how admission and selective criteria correlated with student success. The faculty then followed the steps listed in the model in Figure 3.1 to work through the development of their admission policy.

1. Identify the Purpose of Your Admission Policy and Your Measures of Success

The faculty of HNS developed the purpose statement for their admission policy. The statement reads, "The purpose of the admission policy at the Hypothetical Nursing School is to admit students who are deemed most likely to complete successfully the nursing program and who represent the diversity of our patient population." Most students who attend HNS work in the local community upon graduation. The diversity of the local community was used as the guide for the desired diversity within the student body. Fourteen percent of the community population constitutes minority groups. The minority population is divided among African-American, Hispanic-American, and Asian-American. Therefore, the school would work to attract students from these minority groups. The faculty identified three measures of success:

1. The student will earn a grade of C or higher in each nursing course.
2. The program will have an 85% on-time completion rate. The remaining 15% of students will graduate with one stop-out.
3. The diversity of the graduating class will resemble the ethnic diversity of the community.

2. Consider the Characteristics of Your Students

The faculty at HNS used their definition of the at-risk student to develop admission and selective criteria. The characteristics of the students admitted to the HNS were studied to determine which characteristics might impact student success. The information from Table 2.7 was used. The characteristics that were identified and considered for the admission policy included:

1. High GPA (= or > 2.5)
2. Reading at college level
3. Middle to high math score
4. Previous college degree
5. Demonstrated ability to be a critical thinker

Many of the other factors identified in Table 2.7 were marked as UD – Unable to Determine. Because some of these factors may be factors interfering with successful completion of a nursing course, the faculty decided it was important to gather this information from current and subsequent students. A self-assessment tool that the student completes is one method for gathering this data. This tool will be administered either in a pre-nursing course or in the first nursing course. The Hypothetical Nursing School faculty formed a success committee to locate available data collection tools including a student self-assessment. This information will be collected and evaluated for possible at-risk factors. The HNS will use the tool *Start Right in Nursing School: A Self-Assessment Tool ™*, developed by College of DuPage. This tool collects personal and environmental data that can be used for this step in data collection.

3. Identify Resources

The HNS has access to the general college student support system. The types of support provided include reading, math, and writing assistance. The college has a department to help students whose first language is a language other than English. The advising department offers general test-taking and time management workshops. These services are not discipline-specific and are offered to all students at the college. The HNS does not have a dedicated person offering assistance specifically to nursing students. The ratio of teacher to students in lecture classes is 1 to 50 and in clinical sessions is 1 to 9. The school has a counseling department that can help students with personal problems.

4. Develop an Admission Policy

The HNS decided to have a selective admission policy. The student must meet all the general requirements of a student entering the college at large. In addition to the general requirements the student must meet the following:
1. GPA of 2.5 or higher
2. Score at the college level on a reading test
3. Score in the middle range or higher on a mathematical computation test
4. Attend a mandatory advising session prior to submitting an application

5. Complete prerequisite courses to include one semester each of biology, chemistry, and anatomy and physiology. Students must earn a C or higher in each of these courses.

In addition to the above, a point system was developed to rank selectively all applicants. When considering student characteristics, it was found that students with higher GPAs, higher scores on prerequisite courses, and previous college experience earned higher grades in nursing courses and were more

Table 3.4 – Point System for HNS

Selective Criteria	Points Earned
GPA 3.7 – 4.0 4 points 3.3 – 3.6 3 points 2.9 – 3.2 2 points 2.5 – 2.8 1 point	
Math Test Score High score 1 point Middle range score 0 points	
Previous College Experience College degree earned 2 points Some college courses 1 point No previous college experience 0 points	
Anatomy and Physiology Grade A 2 points B 1 point C 0 points Repeat course 0 points	
Biology Grade A 2 points B 1 point C 0 points Repeat course 0 points	
Chemistry Grade A 2 points B 1 point C 0 points Repeat course 0 points	
Total Points (Selective Criteria Score)	

successful. Also, while examining past student records, the students who earned higher grades in nursing courses were more apt to be successful on the NCLEX. Therefore, these criteria were included in the point system. Because skill in mathematical computation is important for medication administration, the faculty decided that students with strong math skills should earn a higher selective score than those with weaker, yet acceptable, math scores. The point system was established as shown in Table 3.4.

5. Develop or Locate, then Administer, a Tool for Collecting Data from Applicants

The type and specific data collection tools must be identified. The HNS faculty decided to use student transcripts to determine GPA and previous course grades. To determine math and reading scores, the A^2 examination from Health Education Systems, Incorporated (HESI) would be administered. This test also yields additional information that can be tracked to determine if that data would be helpful in the future. That is, the biology and chemistry scores may be used rather than previous course grades. The faculty will track this data.

6. Consider for Admission

The HNS faculty will develop a list of all applicants meeting the admission requirements then rank order them according to the selective criteria point system. If there is a tie with the number of points earned, the GPA will be used as a tiebreaker. If there is still a tie after applying GPA, the date the application was submitted will be used. Once the class is filled, the remaining students will be placed on a waiting list. Students who applied to the HNS but did not meet the criteria will receive a letter outlining their deficiencies and ways to correct those deficiencies before resubmitting an application.

7. Establish Tentative Admission Requirements

The students admitted at this point receive Tentative Admission status. Each student must meet the following requirements prior to receiving Final Admission status:
1. Complete a certified nursing assistant course and pass the certification examination

2. Complete a CPR course
3. Show evidence of immunizations required by the clinical agencies
4. Pass a drug test
5. Complete a criminal background check
6. Complete a self-assessment tool that provides students insight regarding various factors that influence their ability to perform well in school. This can be completed during a pre-nursing success course or prior to entering the first nursing course.

If the student does not complete these additional requirements, that student will be taken off the Tentative Admission list and a student from the waiting list will be admitted with Tentative Admission status. That student must meet the additional requirements before Final Admission status is granted.

8. Determine if Measures for Success are being Met

The faculty of the HNS will track the success of the students admitted under the new admissions policy. They will also compare the students' scores on the A^2 examination to the grades the students earned in the nursing courses to determine if the A^2 test should be used in the future as a better predictor of success than the criteria currently used.

Closing Thoughts

After establishing an admission policy, faculty must engage in ongoing critical evaluation of the entire process. The admission and selective criteria are evaluated for their continued predictive ability. Retrospective studies should be conducted to determine if the criteria actually predict success without restricting admission to any particular group of applicants. Nursing education research has yet to determine what characteristics best predict success in nursing school. This may be due to the diversity of the current population of nursing students as well as the lack of nursing education research. One size does not fit all. Faculty of each school must study their own student body to determine which characteristics have the most predictive value in determining success. The growing nursing shortage and limited enrollment mandate that faculty critically evaluate their admission criteria and their process for ensuring student success after admission into their nursing program.

Learning Activities

1. Read the admission policy at the school where you teach or at a local college. Does the policy include a purpose statement? What is included in that statement? What are their measures of success?
2. Interview nursing faculty from three different schools. Ask them to discuss the admission policy at their employing institutions. Compare and contrast the three admission policies.
3. Using Figure 3.1 as a guide, develop an admission policy. Provide rationale for each step of your admission policy.

References

Bandura, A. (1986). *Social foundations of thought and action.* Englewood Cliffs, NJ: Precentice-Hall.

Bolan, C. M., & Grainger, P. (2003). High school to nursing. *Canadian Nurse, 99*(3), 18-22.

Byrd, G., Garza, C., & Nieswiadomy, R. (1999). Predictors of successful completion of a baccalaureate nursing program. *Nurse Educator, 24*(6), 33-37.

California Community Colleges Chancellor's Office. (2002). *ADN Model Prerequisites Validation Study.* Accessed October 16, 2005, http://www.cccco.edu/divisions/esed/voced/grants/nursing.htm

Jeffreys, M. R. (1998). Predicting non-traditional student retention and academic achievement. *Nurse Educator, 23*(1), 42-48.

Jeffreys, M. (2004). *Nursing student retention: Understanding the process and making a difference.* New York: Springer.

Knowles, M. (1984). *Andragogy in action.* San Francisco: Jossey-Bass.

Lewis, C., & Lewis, J. H (2000). Predicting academic success of transfer nursing students. *Journal of Nursing Education, 39*(5), 234-236.

Ofori, R., & Charlton, J. P. (2002). A path model of factors influencing the academic performance of nursing students. *Journal of Advanced*

Nursing, 38(5), 507-515.

Potolsky, A., Cohen, J., & Saylor, C. (2003). Academic performance of nursing students: Do prerequisite grades and tutoring made a difference? *Nursing Education Perspectives, 24*(5), 246-250.

Sandiford, J., & Jackson, K. (2003). *Predictors of first semester attrition and their relation to retention of generic associate degree nursing students.* East Lansing, MI: National Center for Research on Teacher Learning. (ERIC Document Reproduction Service No. ED481947)

Tracey, G. (2003). A national study of support programs (efforts) in baccalaureate and associate degree nursing programs to enhance retention and success of students. (Doctoral dissertation, University of Central Florida, 2003). *Dissertation Abstracts International, 64*(2598).

Chapter 4: Planning a Student Success Program

Perhaps the greatest task faculty face in their teaching career is to assist students toward success by assessing their students' at-risk profile, framing the challenges they face, and formulating a viable plan for their success. This is not a one-size-fits-all process. Nor is it a one-time only assessment of factors related to success. This planning process must be program-long and continuous.

This chapter looks at the process of determining what information can be used to develop a Student Success Program. The approach requires a retrospective study of your student population to develop an initial plan for success. Revisions should be made as needed integrating information about the current student population. The information used includes data obtained from:
- admission criteria
- selective criteria
- student self-assessment
- learning style inventory
- curriculum choke points

After determining what information will be used to plan a Student Success Program, the next step is to identify indicators of success, as discussed in Chapter 3. These are outcome criteria that are measurable indicators that demonstrate the Student Success Program is working. Finally, the Student Success Program is developed. This chapter focuses on determining which data to use and how to use it, and identifying outcome criteria.

Collecting Data

Data collection is designed to gather information faculty need to plan their Student Success Program. Comprehensive data collection begins when students apply to a program and encompasses variables that place students at-risk for success, as discussed in detail in Chapter 2. Admission policies establish some of the characteristics students have in common when entering a program of nursing and form a basis for student assessment. For example, the selective admission requirement of a middle to high range score on the math test can be trended and evaluated. If faculty find students who score in the middle range on the math test have poor performance on dosage calculation tests, they may consider resetting the range of middle scores on the math test to a higher range or providing additional math instruction. Student assessment continues throughout the students' course of study. Evaluation of students' progress and determination of particular needs is essential for planning supportive mechanisms to foster student success. In some cases, based on past experience teaching the curriculum, faculty can identify the points at which students can be predicted to experience difficulty.

Once students are admitted, all data about the characteristics of the student population are collected and analyzed. This includes data about problems for currently enrolled students and data about curricular choke points for previously enrolled students. Using this information faculty can develop interventions to improve performance and retention. In gathering this data, faculty address the following questions:

- what are the areas of the curriculum that caused difficulty for students over the past five years?
- what problems are identified with the current student population?
- what specifically are the issues to address in a Student Success Program?

The collected data are used to identify patterns and problems that indicate students who are at-risk for failure. An analysis of the data provides concrete information that replaces hunches and intuition with fact. Problems may occur at any point during the course of study, so data collection and analysis are ongoing. A careful study of the data provides root causes that underlie manifestations of student difficulties. Sometimes these causes are student-centered and sometimes they are teacher or curriculum centered. Identifying the source of the problem is essential before formulation of interventions. Data is used to help establish valid goals and meet educational outcomes.

Figure 4.1 - Data Flow for Planning Your Student Success Program

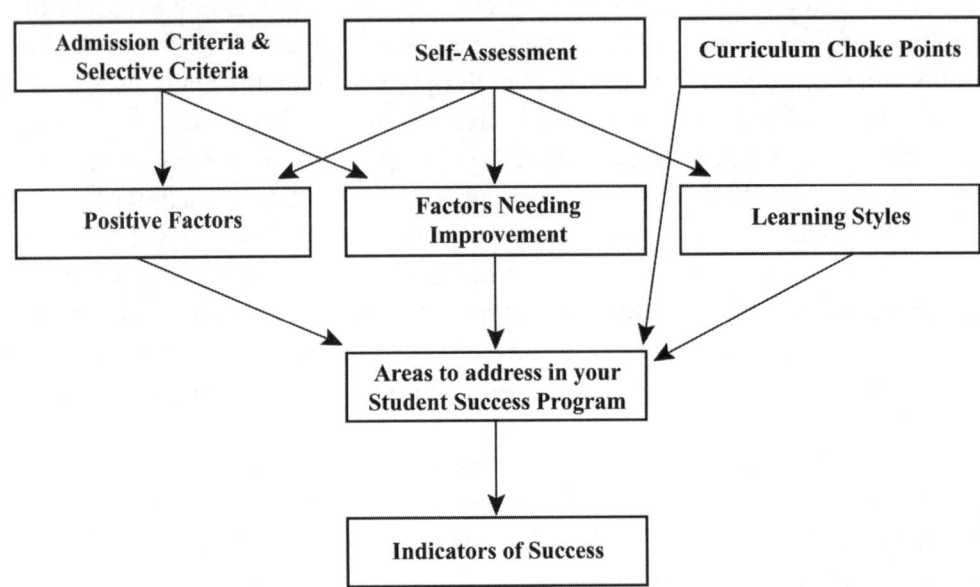

Model for Data Collection Used to Plan a Student Success Program

Figure 4.1 illustrates the flow of data that is used to identify issues to address when planning the elements of your Student Success Program.

Admission and Selective Criteria

In Chapter 3, a plan was presented for developing an admission policy using specific admission and selective criteria. Assessment data were collected during the admission and selection processes to identify needs of an academic nature. Consider the admission policy you have in place and the types of data you collect. Although a school has admission and selective criteria established, these data represent a range of possibilities. Consider the make-up of the population and determine if the students' characteristics will have a positive or negative impact on success. For example, a nursing program may have a policy to admit students with a minimum GPA of 2.5. All students meet that criterion. Consider the aggregate GPA of the incoming class. If the range of GPAs is 2.5 to

2.9, this class may have very different needs than a class with a range of GPAs from 3.4 to 4.0. Determine how this information can be used to develop a Student Success Program. Include both positive factors and those factors needing improvement.

Admission and Selective Criteria: Positive Factors

Factors with a positive impact on an academic outcome might include a cumulative GPA of 3.0 or higher, or a high score on a nursing admission test. These factors are considered in light of the other data collected about students.

Admission and Selective Criteria: Factors Needing Improvement

Consider data that may point to areas in need of improvement, such as a poor math score on an entrance exam. This low math score may indicate a need for remediation so the student will be able to perform calculations relative to medication administration.

Following is an example of one way in which data collected via an admission policy may impact student success.

Example

A school of nursing with an open admission policy requests all students to take a reading test for advisement purposes. Many of the incoming students are reading below the 12th grade level. Assistance with reading will be a major focus of the Student Success Program. On the other hand, if a school's admission policy requires a score indicating the applicant reads at the 12th grade level or above, students may not experience difficulty reading the nursing textbooks. In the latter case, assistance with reading will not be addressed in the Student Success Program.

Self-Assessment

Once the student has been selected and admission has been accepted by the student, it is an appropriate time for the student to perform a self-assessment relative to study skills and test-taking abilities. This type of self-assessment is most helpful if conducted prior to entering a nursing program. Ideally, the student reviews the self-assessment results with faculty. Together, the student and faculty outline a remediation program. This topic is covered more extensively in Chapter 5.

The act of completing a self-assessment for early identification of lack of essential skills and behaviors that may interfere with success is an important first step for students to be successful in a nursing program (Fox & Broome, 2001; Lockie & Burke, 1999). Early intervention is key. Students who identify a lack of skills and remediate prior to taking nursing courses have a greater chance for success than students who do not remediate early.

Components of a self-assessment addressed in a Student Success Program include:
- demographics
- study skills
- learning styles
- time management
- concentration
- reading
- note-taking
- test-taking strategies
- family issues
- health habits

Students may be aware these are important factors for success, but may not have given each item enough consideration to identify them as barriers to their success. Sometimes students are not realistic in their self-appraisal. A self-assessment that guides students through questions can be extremely helpful because students may be unaware of what kinds of questions to ask of themselves or unaware of the need for change. Faculty must keep in mind that a self-assessment tool depends heavily on a realistic assessment by the student.

Faculty may opt to use student assessment tools that are offered by outside sources. An example of such a tool is *Start Right in Nursing School: A Self-Assessment Tool TM* from College of DuPage. Features of this tool include:
- web-delivered, secure assessment to help nursing students gain insights to improve their study habits, manage their time, and prepare for their nursing education

- avenue for nursing faculty and nursing education administrators to understand better their students' characteristics and needs as a basis for a plan for their success
- system for teachers and advisors to analyze individual or aggregate data. Reports may be used to enhance individual student performance and provide important aggregate data for program evaluation and long-term planning.

Specifically, the *Start Right in Nursing School: A Self-Assessment Tool* collects student demographics, evaluates individual learning styles, and collects data on concentration and reading skills, time management, note-taking, test preparation, and test-taking. Also included is useful information on the impact of specific factors of the student's non-academic life on learning. Students gain practice answering the type of test items they will encounter in their nursing courses and on NCLEX. Immediately upon completion of the assessment instrument, the student receives a report containing their responses and individualized recommendations for success. Teachers, advisors, and administrators receive individual and aggregate reports containing both the assessment results and recommended activities and strategies they can use to improve student success.

Many of the factors included in a self-assessment, such as time management, test-taking strategies, and study skills including concentration, reading, and note-taking, typically comprise the foundation of a general student success program. These items directly relate to individual student abilities to manage studying and testing to produce positive results. In addition, factors such as family issues and health habits that impact a student's ability to succeed in a course of study are addressed in a Student Success Program. All these factors are discussed in greater detail in Chapters 5 and 6.

Self-Assessment: Positive Factors

Positive factors present an opportunity to capitalize on those attributes or findings that lend toward student success. Just as it is essential to understand the rationale for correct responses on a test item, it is important to know those personal characteristics that help students succeed. Positive factors were described in detail in Chapter 2. Such factors include, but are not limited to those listed in the tool presented in Table 4.1.

Table 4.1 – Organizing Data to Plan Student Success – Checklist of Positive and Negative Factors

Classification of Factors	Place a Checkmark if Positive Factor Applies	Positive Factors	Place a Checkmark if Negative Factor Applies	Negative Factors
Academic/School-Related		Academically well prepared – acceptable pre-nursing GPA		Less academically prepared overall – low pre-nursing GPA
		Acceptable science scores		Low science scores: biological science; social science; chemistry
		Acceptable math scores		Low math scores
		Reading at college level		Reading below college level
		Studies at least 3 hours per credit hour per week		Studies less than 3 hours per credit hour per week
		Positive attitude toward educators		Negative attitude toward educators
		Previous degree		No prior college experience
		Pre-entrance counseling		Lack of pre-entrance counseling
		Good test-taking skills		Test anxiety
		Critical thinker		Difficulty with critical thinking
		Good time management skills		Difficulty with time management
		< 20 minute travel to school		> 20 minute travel to school
Personal Factors		Very motivated		Lacks motivation
		Strong social support		Lack of social support
		Manages stress well		Difficulty dealing with stress
		Age on entry *		Age on entry *
		High self-efficacy		Low self-efficacy
		Self-confident		Low self-esteem
		No health problems		Health problems
Environmental Factors		Minimal church, community commitments		Many church, community commitments
		No family responsibilities		Has family responsibilities
		No issues with child care		Problems with child care
		No family problems		Family problems

* In keeping with our proposed term of diverse student populations, consideration of the student's prior educational experience, success in past educational endeavors, length of time since last exposed to coursework (high school or post- secondary), and age upon current enrollment is important (Jeffreys, 2004). Faculty may want to track these variables to determine if they impact success in their student population.

Students' sense of self-worth and accomplishments may be enhanced by concentrating on those attributes that position them well for success, such as a positive attitude and a willingness to learn. Following is an example of self-assessment data that may positively impact student success.

Example

During a self-assessment a student cites no outside work commitments and a strong base of family support. The student can call upon family to care for the student's two children after school three days a week, thus has two full days to devote to studying, and one day to complete household errands. This schedule leaves adequate family time on weekends. These two facts, no work commitment and a strong family base, help alleviate personal stress from the demands of school because the student is able to balance school and family responsibilities.

Self-Assessment: Factors Needing Improvement

In the same way that positive factors present an opportunity to promote student success, identification of factors that need improvement present an opportunity to establish interventions for student success. Faculty cannot know what to do for students until they know what problems their students face. Equally important, a plan must be in place to address the factors which need improvement. Refer to Table 4.1 for negative factors noted on a self-assessment that may impact student success.

Example

During the self-assessment, a student identifies difficulties in managing work and school commitments. The student commutes a long distance to a current job, which wastes time that could be spent on other activities. The student appears harried and has missed several assigned deadlines. Faculty suggest the student explore work-study opportunities on campus to provide an income and reduce travel time for work. The student investigates work-study positions available on campus and discovers the minimal salary reduction with work-study would be offset by reduced travel distance and expenditures for gas and car maintenance. Most importantly, three hours per day are saved by eliminating the long commute. The student decides to accept a work-study position on campus.

Two weeks later, the student appears more relaxed and reports spending more time with his family and friends. There are no further incidences of missed or late assignments.

The hypothetical example presented at the end of this chapter also considers the impact of positive and negative factors on student success.

Organizing Student Data

Organizing the data gleaned from the admission and selective criteria and student self-assessments as illustrated in Table 4.1 allows faculty to determine individual characteristics of each student as well as general characteristics for the entire class of students. Many elements of the Student Success Program are built based on this data. Some of the data can be collected prior to the student starting the nursing program, and other data will be collected after the student is admitted into the program. This emphasizes the need for ongoing data collection and evaluation as noted in the beginning of this chapter.

How to Use the Collected Data

Although sorting through all the data may appear to be an overwhelming task, it is helpful to have a planned approach for this process. One suggestion is to look for recurring themes and issues. Then pertinent data are extrapolated and used to develop a Student Success Program. Following are examples of how to extrapolate data and use it in a Student Success Program.

Example #1

During a self-assessment, a student cites difficulty with being able to balance personal, work, and school commitments. This student may benefit from attending a study skills course or an individualized counseling session to address ways to study more efficiently and to manage time. Faculty can implement a pre-nursing course that explains the specific demands of their program, and ask currently enrolled nursing students to speak to the incoming students to offer suggestions about how to anticipate and meet the demands that will be placed on them. Faculty discuss with students alternative ways to finance a college education than perhaps previously considered to lessen the number of hours worked each

Chapter 4: Planning a Student Success Program

week. Students may need help to evaluate realistically the number of hours they can work and attend school.

Example #2

Several students report problems with obtaining child care. Faculty talk with their early childhood education department to explore ways to offer on-campus child care at a discounted rate for students registered at their institution.

Example #3

Faculty learn 32% of the students have a commute of more than one hour. Faculty agree to podcast lectures so students may listen to lectures during their commute. Faculty also explore class scheduling options to address the most efficient use of time and reduce the number of days a student would need to commute to campus for class.

Example #4

Students are frustrated by lack of available space to meet and work in study groups or on group assignments. To help meet this need, four rooms are reserved in the library for student use for three two-hour time blocks every Monday and Wednesday, when students are on campus.

Example #5

A student reports strong support from significant others and little financial concern because scholarship money has been obtained and the student will not need to work more than 10 hours per week. The student does not anticipate worrying about how to pay for tuition or books and is not the supporter of the family. The student anticipates having ample time to study and meet family demands. If necessary, work hours could be decreased or eliminated. At present, this student appears positioned for success; however, this situation could change. Faculty will need to monitor the student for any signs of stress.

Preferred Learning Styles

"Learning styles refer to individuals' modes of making meaning of and dealing with knowledge and not merely reacting to external forces" (Colucciello, 1999, p. 295). Learning styles are highly individualized. Learners differ in the amount of structure and autonomy they want. To illustrate, consider one section of the Center for Innovative Teaching Experiences (CITE) Learning Style Instrument developed by Babich, Burdine, Albright, & Randol (1976), which focuses on work conditions. Students may identify that they work better in groups versus working alone. According to this instrument, this preference would be labeled social-group. The student with this preference studies with at least one other student, and would not accomplish as much when studying alone as when studying with a group. With this learning style preference, socialization is important to the learning process and group interaction serves to enhance learning and fact recognition for the learner. If students have a good sense of the learning styles used by others with whom studying will occur, such as a study partner or teacher, they are better positioned to learn well (Hopper, 2004).

Learning modalities measured by learning style inventories include visual, auditory, and kinesthetic. Visual learners learn from seeing, auditory learners from hearing, and kinesthetic learners from touching, doing, and moving.

There are many learning style inventories that faculty and students might select. You and your students may wish to complete the 45 item CITE Learning Styles Instrument that appears on the CD accompanying this book.

Knowledge of learning styles is important not only to the individual student but to faculty as well. Faculty should consider all facets of student learning, and knowledge of learning styles is one facet. Teachers who are aware of their students' learning styles can tailor instructional strategies to best match their students' learning styles. Offering a variety of instructional strategies is important to accommodate learning preferences for all students in the class. There must be a balance when designing instruction so all students benefit (Thompson and Crutchlow, 1993).

An individual's preferred learning style can change as that person goes through life, but does not change from semester to semester. A student may use one learning style for a particular course but prefer a different learning style for another course. Additionally, a student may adapt a different learning style in response to the way learning is presented.

Several interventions related to learning styles help students study more effectively. For example, if a student's preferred learning style fits into one of the auditory categories, a few suggestions include:
- read aloud when studying
- tape class sessions and later transcribe the information
- study with another student and discuss information together

If a student's preferred learning style fits into one of the visual categories, faculty might suggest the student:
- read the text before listening to the lecture in class
- write words that are given orally, to learn better by seeing them on paper
- make charts, graphs, or tables of the information being studied
- take notes in brief, outline-type formats, not narrative style

Faculty must realize no one learning style is preferable over another, and all have merit (Casady, 2002). In addition, certain class content may lend itself to one type of learning style. Faculty should employ creative teaching strategies to meet a variety of learning styles.

Research Study – How Faculty Assess and Make Use of Learning Styles

The authors designed a two-phase study to learn more about how faculty use information about learning styles of their students. Phase I is presented below, and entails a survey to gain a sense of the percentage of nursing educators who assess learning styles and how such information is used to plan teaching. The second phase, presented in Chapter 7, is an in-depth case study conducted to explore how one college consortium implemented a student success program, of which one component was assessing and teaching to student learning styles. Phase I of this research is presented in this chapter. There were three purposes for the Phase I survey:
1. Determine the percent of the sample population who assess students' learning styles.
2. Determine how faculty use the information they collect about students' learning styles.
3. Determine changes in students' learning that occurred as a result of assessment of students' learning styles.

The authors administered the survey via a blind mailing to faculty of 201 randomly selected nursing programs from all levels of undergraduate, pre-licensure, registered nursing programs. A total of 35 faculty completed the survey for a response rate of 17%. The details of how the survey was written and administered, the total survey, and the complete results can be found on the CD-ROM accompanying this book.

Faculty were asked the following three questions about assessing student learning styles:

1. Is the learning style of each of your nursing students formally assessed using a learning styles inventory at some point in your nursing curriculum? Results: 26% of the 35 respondents formally assess student learning styles.
2. At what point in the curriculum is the learning style of your students assessed? See Table 4.2 for a summary of this data.
3. What learning style inventory do you use? Select all that apply:
    Canfield's Learning Styles Inventory
    Center for Innovative Teaching Experiences (CITE) Learning Styles Instrument
    Dunn, Dunn, and Price's Productivity Environmental Preference Survey (PEPS)
    Gardner's Multiple Intelligences
    Grasha-Riechmann's Student Learning Style Scales
    Gregoric's Style Delineator
    Honey and Mumford's Learning Styles Questionnaire
    Kolb's Learning Style Inventory
    Myers-Briggs Type Indicator
    Educational Resources Inc., Nurse Entrance Test (NET)
    Other _____

Table 4.2 contains the learning style inventory tools respondents report using.

Faculty were asked the following three questions about their own learning style:

1. Have you assessed your own learning style? Results: 69% of the 35 respondents indicated they had assessed their own learning style.
2. Do you use knowledge of your own learning style when planning teaching/learning strategies? Results: 54% of the 35 respondents said yes, they

Chapter 4: Planning a Student Success Program

Table 4.2 – Student Learning Styles Assessment Survey Responses

Type of program and total number responding	Number of programs that formally assess using a learning styles inventory	Point in curriculum when learning styles are assessed	Learning Style Inventory Tool Used
Associate Degree 11	2 A third program noted that beginning students are often directed by advisors to a website that has a link to a learning style inventory.	First semester (both programs)	1 uses Assessments Technology Institute 1 does not know which tool is used Third program uses Diablo Valley College Learning Style Survey
Baccalaureate Degree 18	4	First nursing school semester (3 programs) Freshman year (1 program)	1 uses Myers-Briggs Type Indicator 1 uses Health Education Systems Incorporated A^2 1 uses independent learning styles inventory * Myers-Briggs
Diploma 1	1	Prior to beginning the program	Myers-Briggs Type Indicator and Nurses Entrance Test
Baccalaureate and Masters Degree 2	0	0	0
RN to BSN with no generic program 1	1	First class	Solomon and Felder-Index of Learning Styles
Degree completion 1	1	Second module	Kolb's Learning Style Inventory
Associate and Baccalaureate 1	0		

*Note: respondent indicated use of an independent learning styles inventory but no comment was provided about this tool.

did use knowledge of their own learning style when planning teaching/learning strategies.
3. Describe how you have used knowledge of your own learning style in your teaching/learning strategies. Table 4.3 presents a summary of comments shared by faculty regarding use of knowledge of their own learning styles to develop teaching/learning strategies.

Table 4.3 – Faculty Learning Styles Assessment

How Knowledge of Own Learning Style is Used in Teaching/Learning Strategies.

Have incorporated different teaching aides such as play-doh and legos, music, aromatic candles, and visual aides.

Simple to complex, understanding rationales helps to see the whole picture.

Use a lot of visuals, also use quizzes to review info from previous lectures.

I am a visual learner. I talk with students about the many learning styles of students. I try to use visual, auditory, and emotional/feelings type of format. For example: lecture, videos for auditory. PowerPoint, skill demonstration, conceptual care maps, videos for visual learners and interactive papers, questionnaires etc. for the emotional/feelings learner.

I make a reasonable attempt to include teaching strategies that are not in my personal style, but may be prevalent in students. Without this deliberate thought, I would probably only teach to my type of learner.

I am a see-er, do-er learner rather than a reader learner. I teach in lab...I make sure that in addition to reading assignments and having demonstration/return demonstration activities, the students have situation assignments requiring them to apply content in a virtual environment (and later defend their actions/decisions to classmates). We have a web-based virtual hospital populated with virtual patients who pose many interesting situations for beginning nursing students to ponder. Much better to make judgment mistakes and learn on virtual patients (who are hard to kill) than the flesh and blood kind!

I am an auditory/visual learner so I use many different methods to relay content: graphs, flow diagrams, case studies, role playing.

I plan activities that actively involve the students in the class content, getting them up out of their chairs and interacting with me and one another.

Because I have learned that (1) my preferred style of learning is read-write; (2) that teachers usually teach the way they like to learn; AND (3) that most of my nursing students are kinesthetic learners, I have to be very careful to gear my teaching to all styles of learning. I use lots of word pictures and body language in my teaching to enhance the visual memory. I try to get the students to visualize concepts, use non-nursing examples to contrast to nursing use of the same concepts. I just wanted to comment on one of your questions above: We don't evaluate learning styles at any point during the program. However in my class (nursing research) I have the students go to the VARK website to discover their preferred learning style during the first week of class and report to me.

I am a visual learner and I try very hard to add visual components to my classes.

I have used my style to enhance my lectures and presentations in the classroom as well as not to use my style of choice too much.

sequential visual; I highlight lecture material; use PowerPoint and algorithms to fishbone diagrams, also

I learn better with hands-on and discussion, in my classroom I use more interactive learning teaching strategies rather than just lecture.

Try to include a variety of styles in teaching.

In determining which learning activities will best suit the material, i.e. using auditory/visual materials.

I use more interactive techniques with the students.

I try to make sure that I address as many styles as possible, not just my own preference. Recognize introverts and extraverts. Try to include a variety of teaching strategies to meet the needs of a variety of students. Switch styles every 30 minutes or sooner.

Use of examples, illustrations.

(All text in the above table is drawn from a survey and is presented verbatim.)

The responses noted in Table 4.3 suggest faculty use knowledge of their own learning style when designing instruction. While the ways in which faculty learn best influence the style of teaching they use, faculty believe it is important to teach to a variety of learning styles. The particular learning outcome faculty hope to achieve, the learning style of the individual teaching, and the learning style of the students should be considered collectively when determining an approach to teaching and learning. Just as faculty prepare for class with a thorough understanding of the topic they present, they should plan instruction based on their knowledge of learning styles to facilitate student learning.

The results of this survey may be typical; however, with the small number responding, the sample may or may not be representative of how faculty assess or use learning styles. Additional research is needed to explore faculty assessment and use of learning styles.

Curriculum Choke Points

In most nursing curricula there is what can be described as curriculum choke points. Choke points are areas of the curriculum traditionally difficult for students to master and may include specific content, clinical experiences, or entire courses. Examples of traditionally difficult content areas include theory on fluid and electrolytes, care of the client with alterations in the nervous system, and high-risk pregnancy. Clinical areas that present particular challenges may include critical care environments, very busy medical units, and nursing leadership rotations, all of which require students to apply several concepts to complex areas of practice.

Faculty should examine past experiences to identify their own particular areas of concern. Data about these choke points can be gathered from places such as grade sheets, which indicate areas of weakness for individual students as well as overall course grades, clinical evaluation tools, faculty discussions about student progress, and student course evaluations. Faculty should consider purchasing and reviewing their *NCLEX Program Report*, to review their NCLEX results as broken down by the test plan. Faculty may set specific outcome criteria for each course to determine which ones represent difficulty for students. An example outcome criteria may be "95% of students will pass the exam on alterations of the nervous system with a B⁻ or higher." Choke points can then be validated with correlation to this specific measure of success.

If the school has a testing policy for progression using proprietary tests such as those from Health Education Systems, Incorporated (HESI), those tests can provide valuable, specific information about difficult content areas. Knowledge of predictable choke points, in combination with assessment of an individual student's at-risk status and learning needs, helps faculty know when to implement particular interventions to enhance student retention.

Research Study – Student Success Programs

To gain a sense of the percentage of nursing education programs that offer a student success program and what the components of those programs might be, the authors conducted a survey. The survey was administered via a blind mailing to 198 randomly selected nursing faculty from all levels of undergraduate, pre-licensure, registered nursing programs. Faculty from 26 schools completed the survey for a response rate of 13%. The details about the way the survey was written and administered, the total survey, and the complete research results can be found on the CD-ROM accompanying this book. The text in Tables 4.4 through 4.6 is verbatim as reported by the survey respondents. Faculty were asked the following seven questions about success programs:

1. Is there an established student success program open to all students within your college or university? Results: 16 (62%) of the 26 respondents have an established program within their institution.
2. What components comprise the student success program? Of the 16 respondents who have an established success program, 15 described the components of the student success program. See Table 4.4 for a summary of these responses.
3. How are students notified about the services provided by the student success program? Respondents checked all that applied. Results are indicated by percentages:
    o General advising session (44%)
    o General orientation program (69%)
    o Institutional publications (69%)
    o Other: announcements on web-based bulletin boards and in class; required to meet with advisor.
4. Does your school have a student success plan specifically for your nursing students? Results: Ten of the 26 respondents have a success plan for their nursing students.

5. Describe the student success plan that is specifically for your nursing students. See Table 4.5.
6. At what point in your curriculum is your student success plan for nursing students offered? See Table 4.6.
7. Which students participate in your student success program for nursing? Eight of the ten respondents said their program was open to all students. Two of the ten respondents said their program is open only to those students "at-risk" for not passing nursing courses. One program described "at-risk" as a C in at least one nursing course or below 850 on a required examination from HESI.

Table 4.4 – Success Program Components

Developmental studies are offered for all students in reading, math, and English. The college offers a new student orientation session to help students learn how to navigate the campus, registration, and various services on campus. A course is offered called orientation that is a 1-hour course that teaches study skills and library skills. This course is required for students who fail 2 sections of the required college placement test (THEA, Accuplacer, or other Texas Higher Education Coordinating Board approved test).

Tutoring, counselors.

Placement testing, orientation program, courses on study skills, tutoring...etc. Availability of mentor-tutor. Success strategies for nursing elective course. Open Skills Lab for practice and media and computer resources. Early intervention with students with clinical or academic difficulty.

Study skills, open access counseling, NCLEX review, tutoring.

Freshman seminar, tutors, study hall and academic advising by counselors.

Early identification of at risk students, use of a risk appraisal inventory, use of student test failures to generate counseling and follow-up services in nursing classes. All senior level students are assigned an advisor at the beginning of the year to help guide them in being successful on state boards, identifying areas of needed improvement, using standardized testing (ATI, HESI) to assess student abilities and provide remediation as needed.

Chapter 4: Planning a Student Success Program

> Student counseling.
>
> Grades, MOSBY test scores, clinical performance.
>
> Learning Resource Center.
>
> Workshops, group and individual tutoring, writing center.
>
> Reading lab. Math lab study skills.
>
> I have no idea.
>
> We do HESI reviews as well as the Lippincott study guides. Each student must meet a certain criteria on the HESI Exam or will do 3500 review questions. We have an excellent pass rate.
>
> Free weekly tutoring.

(All text in the above table is drawn from a survey and is presented verbatim.)

Table 4.5 – Success Plan Specific to Nursing Students

> The nursing program has a full-time nursing counselor who is a regular nursing faculty member. The nursing counselor offers focus sessions weekly for students at-risk and any others are also welcome to attend. She covers test-taking strategies, gives sample questions, guides students in study skills, and helps students focus on the important points of nursing content. A college counselor offers stress management sessions for nursing students about six times/semester. At risk students are encouraged to attend and the sessions are open to all nursing students. Tutoring is provided by the Career Development Office that is free to students.
>
> Identify potential problems, counsel, talk with every student at beginning of program; summer workshop; workshops for reading, test-taking during year; Peer-led team learning workshops every week; instructors refer students as are having difficulty with tests, etc…
>
> General advising session.
>
> General orientation program.

Our college is a single purpose institution so the answer was given in #6: required to meet with advisor.

Remediation in preparation for NCLEX

Course designed especially for students that score low on the MOSBY'S ASSESS TEST. Mandatory tutoring involving review of NCLEX Style questions.

Though the College of Nursing and Health Sciences Learning Resource Center we offer workshops, group and individual tutoring, skills practice sessions and skills testing. The Director of the LRC meets with all students who are placed on probation to develop a plan for success. Students are notified of the resources in orientation and via flyers, e-mails and class announcements.

We have definite benchmarks that students must meet. If they fall short they are refereed to individual counselors who assign particular units of supplementary materials to assist the student learn the concepts. They are assigned review questions if they are absent or late and if they do not achieve a 90% or better on the HESI Exam.

Free tutoring.

(All text in the above table is drawn from a survey and is presented verbatim.)

Table 4.6 – Point in Curriculum Success Plan Offered

From the first nursing course on.

Summer before start nursing program.

Multiple points - every course.

First term.

From the first nursing class which is the second semester of the freshman year.

Junior level.

Senior level.

Begins when they begin nursing courses 1st semester 2nd year.

Chapter 4: Planning a Student Success Program

> It is offered throughout but the bulk is offered toward the end of the program.
>
> From the beginning.

(All text in the above table is drawn from a survey and is presented verbatim.)

The responses to these seven survey items indicate that over half of all those who responded to the survey have a student success program within their college or university and 38% have a plan specifically for their nursing students.

This survey data suggest that programs of nursing are addressing student success. A success program may begin as early as the summer prior to the student beginning the nursing program to as late as the senior level of study. Success program components include a variety of interventions to help students which may include advising, counseling, tutoring, testing, remediation, help with study and test-taking skills, and benchmarks that students must meet.

The results of this survey may be typical; however, with the small number responding, the sample may or may not be representative of how faculty design and implement success programs for their students or the percent of schools with a student success program. Additional research is needed to explore faculty use of success programs.

Indicators of Success

Once admission and selective criteria are established, student characteristics identified, and available resources noted, faculty use this information to define outcome criteria to measure effectiveness of their Student Success Program. Typical outcomes include a specified retention rate and NCLEX pass rate. Additional outcomes might include:
- students earn a minimum of a C grade in all nursing courses
- students who retest on material identified as choke points will attain a minimum of 85% on the second test
- 75% persistence rate – 75% of those students who were delayed in their graduation date will return and successfully complete the program
- 85% graduation rate
- 15% graduation rate with one stop-out

Faculty establish indicators of success and data are analyzed to evaluate the extent to which these outcomes are met. Faculty attempt to determine factors impacting each particular outcome. If established outcomes are not realized, revision to components of the Student Success Program may be indicated. Sufficient time must be allowed to realize desired outcomes. Student data should be collected for a minimum of 3 years for reliable trends to be noted.

A Hypothetical Nursing School Example

Chapter 3 discussed how faculty at Hypothetical Nursing School (HNS) applied the model depicted in Figure 3.1 to develop their admission and selective criteria. Now the information will be used to plan a Student Success Program. The faculty at HNS determined a means of organizing and evaluating the data collected from former students during the admission and self-assessment processes. The faculty followed the steps listed in the model in Figure 4.1 to aggregate the data as a basis for a Student Success Program and then established indicators of success to measure program outcomes.

Admission and Selective Criteria

The first step in using the model was to organize and analyze data collected during the admission process to identify areas to address in a Student Success Program. The faculty of HNS examined the admission data of 40 students who were admitted to their program. All students admitted met the general requirements for admission to the college. In addition to the general requirements, students met the following criteria specific to the nursing program:
- minimum GPA of 2.5
- college level reading score on reading test
- middle to high range math score on mathematics computation test
- attendance at a mandatory advising session prior to submission of application
- completion of prerequisite courses of one semester each of biology, chemistry, and anatomy and physiology with a grade of C or higher in each course

Selective criteria scores were calculated and noted in each student's file. Selective criteria addressed: GPA, math tests scores, previous college experience, and grades in anatomy and physiology, biology, and chemistry courses as shown in Table 4.7.

Table 4.7– Point System for HNS

Selective Criteria	Points Earned
GPA 3.7 – 4.0 4 points 3.3 – 3.6 3 points 2.9 – 3.2 2 points 2.5 – 2.8 1 point	
Math Test Score High score 1 point Middle range score 0 points	
Previous College Experience College degree earned 2 points Some college courses 1 point No previous college experience 0 points	
Anatomy and Physiology Grade A 2 points B 1 point C 0 points Repeat course 0 points	
Biology Grade A 2 points B 1 point C 0 points Repeat course 0 points	
Chemistry Grade A 2 points B 1 point C 0 points Repeat course 0 points	
Total Points (Selective Criteria Score)	

The greater the GPA, math score, course grades and college experience the candidate attained, the higher the selective criteria score. Currently, the faculty do not have a minimum selective criteria score established. The faculty plan to collect data about the relationship of selective criteria scores to student success when making decisions about future admission practice.

The faculty decided to arrange the data according to academic/school related, personal, and environmental factors, and added two columns to note sources where the data were obtained. Table 4.1 was slightly modified and the numbers of students for each factor were entered as shown in Table 4.8. While some data can be collected prior to the student's entrance, other data will be collected as it becomes available. For example, faculty will not be able to assess how a student manages time until the student is faced with balancing the demands of the nursing program with other personal factors.

Admission and Selective Criteria - Positive Factors

Entering the numbers in the table provided an organized presentation of data that was easily studied. The data in Table 4.8 were analyzed to indicate positive academic and school related factors ascertained from admission data for this group of students in this specific nursing program. Analysis of the data for this class revealed:
- 50% had a GPA of 2.9 or higher
- 62.5% had As or Bs in prerequisite science courses
- 37.5% had high range math scores on the mathematical computation test
- 100% read at college level
- 100% received pre-entrance nursing advising prior to admission

While HNS faculty believed these variables positioned many students for success, other factors may influence the extent to which students with strong academic standing succeed. For example, if the student also works 20 or more hours per week, maintaining a strong GPA, or even the requisite passing percentage, may be difficult. Faculty anticipated that while the academic variables looked mostly positive, several students would need some intervention to succeed. Particular emphasis was accorded during communication with nursing students about the rigors of nursing school, so students had a realistic view of the process, knew what to expect, knew what resources were available, and could plan accordingly.

Chapter 4: Planning a Student Success Program

Table 4.8 – Student Data

Column A Classification of Factors	Column B Factors	Column C Available from Admission Data	Column D Available from Self-Assessment	Column E Data Unavailable or Not Used
Academic/School-Related Factors	Academically well prepared – acceptable pre-nursing GPA	20- GPA 2.5-2.8 2- GPA 2.9-3.2 10- GPA 3.3-3.6 8- GPA 3.7-4.0		
	Acceptable science scores Note: these grades were used to compute the selective criteria points.	10- A's 15- B's 15- C's		
	Acceptable math scores	15- high range 25- middle range		
	Reading at college level minimum	13- above college reading level (1 non-English language background (NELB) student is included in this subset.) 27- at college reading level (4 NELB students included in this subset.)		
	Attendance at mandatory nursing advising session	40- attended mandatory session		
	Selective Criteria Score	12- score of (7) 16- score of (8) 10- score of (10) 2- score of (13)		
	Studies at least 3 hours per credit hour per week		8 study 5 or more hours per credit hour per week; 12 study 3 or more hours per credit hour per week; 20 study sporadically, often less than 3 hours per credit hour per week.	
	Positive attitude toward educators		8 indicated a negative attitude toward educators. 32 indicated a positive attitude toward educators.	
	Previous college degree		15 have earned a previous college degree.	

103

	Pre-entrance counseling	12 received no pre-entrance counseling. 28 received pre-entrance counseling.		
	Good test-taking skills		16 report they have good test-taking skills. 24 report their testing skills could be improved.	
	Critical thinker			Difficult to assess. No test administered at this time. Faculty plan to evaluate critical thinking as students progress through the program
	Good time management skills		10 report they manage time well. 15 report that most of the time they feel okay with time management, but could use some help. 15 report they have trouble balancing needs and demands.	
	< 20 minute travel to school		11 report < 20 minute travel to school. 29 report > 20 minute travel to school.	
Personal Factors	Very motivated			Difficult to assess with accuracy. Faculty will consider this aspect as they interact with students.
	Strong social support		9 report strong base of support. 9 report little to no support. 22 report that most of the time they have support.	
	Manages stress well		8 report high degree of stress and being overwhelmed. 17 report that most of the time they can manage stress. 15 report ability to mange stress well.	

Chapter 4: Planning a Student Success Program

	Age on entry		10 were 18 - 25 years of age. 15 were 26 - 35 years of age. 10 were 36 - 45 years of age. 5 were 46 - 55 years of age.	Data obtained and recorded, but only for demographic purposes.
	High self-efficacy			Difficult to measure. More evident as student/faculty interact.
	Self-confident			Difficult to measure. More evident as student/faculty interact.
	No health problems			Difficult to obtain data.
Environmental Factors	Minimal church, community commitments		10 report monthly community commitments. 15 report minimal commitments. 15 report no commitments.	
	No family responsibilities		31 have family responsibilities. 9 have no family responsibilities.	
	No issues with child care		15 report concerns with child care. 25 report no difficulty with child care.	
	No family problems		4 report grave family concerns. 22 report some family concerns, which they feel are under control. 14 report no family problems.	
	Works <20 hours per week		4 work 0 hours per week. 14 work 5 - 10 hours per week. 12 work 11- 20 hours per week. 10 work 21- 40 hours per week.	

105

Admission and Selective Criteria - Factors Needing Improvement

The data in Table 4.8 also indicated those academic and school related factors which needed improvement. Analysis of the data for this group of students revealed:
- 50% had a GPA of 2.5 to 2.8.
- 37.5% had Cs in prerequisite science courses.
- 30% had no pre-entrance counseling.
- 62.5% had middle range math scores on the mathematical computation test.

The faculty considered these findings to project needs to address in the Student Success Program. Since minimal competencies were met, faculty believed that students might not be at high risk, but there were still concerns. Faculty planned to monitor how those students with a GPA between 2.5 and 2.8 and with Cs in their prerequisite science courses perform in the program. The faculty will provide counseling for those who had no pre-entrance counseling related to stress reduction, support systems, and other counseling issues. To maintain or enhance math computational abilities, faculty will administer weekly quizzes in clinical. Students will also be asked to bring a sample math problem to post-conference. All students will work to solve the problem. Individual math deficiencies will be addressed by peer tutors.

Self-Assessment

For the purpose of student self-assessment, the faculty decided to use *Start Right in Nursing School: A Self-Assessment Tool* by College of DuPage. The *Start Right in Nursing School* program offers the student an opportunity to look at academic and non-academic dimensions of success. The tool includes student demographics, assesses individual learning styles, concentration, and reading skills, and provides a measure of student skills in note-taking, test preparation, and test-taking. It also provides basic data on time management skills and the impact of family commitments on learning. With this tool, students receive suggestions immediately with their assessment results. From this tool, faculty were able to determine positive and negative factors for each student.

Chapter 4: Planning a Student Success Program

Self-Assessment: Positive Factors

Student responses on the self-assessment tool indicated positive positioning for several academic, personal, and environmental factors. These factors included:
- study time: 50% of the students studied at least 3 hours per credit hour per week.
- attitude toward educators: 80% indicated a positive attitude toward educators.
- previous degree: 37.5% reported having earned a previous degree.
- test-taking skills: 40% indicated good testing skills.
- time management skills: 25% reported they manage time well.

Faculty decided to take advantage of the skill set and positive attitude these students presented. They plan to select peer tutors from the cadre of students who reported good test-taking and time management skills, to help those students who reported difficulties with these areas.

Self-Assessment: Factors Needing Improvement

Several areas of concern presented as a result of administering the *Start Right in Nursing School* program. Some of these concerns included:
- study time: 50% studied sporadically, often less than 3 hours per credit hour per week.
- attitude toward educators: 20% indicated a negative attitude toward educators.
- test-taking skills: 60% indicated their testing skills could be improved.
- time management skills: 37.5% reported they have trouble balancing needs and demands.
- travel time: 72.5% reported travel time of more than 20 minutes to school.
- social support: 22.5% reported little to no social support.
- community commitments: 25% reported monthly community commitments.

The faculty evaluated this data and decided they will mandate a study skills course for those students who indicated a need. The course will include test-taking skills and time management. Faculty plan to monitor students in the study skills course to track their progress. Data collected will be reviewed and used to inform future decisions.

The faculty are concerned that some students will be overextended as they try to balance school and community commitments. The HNS faculty would like to offer some support for those students who are stressed and have little to no social support. Faculty decided to hold monthly forums with students to discuss any concerns the students might wish to express. Faculty recognized some students might not be comfortable sharing concerns with them. To provide support and enhance student comfort with the process, faculty will offer students the option to attend forums led by the liaison from counseling. Through these forums, faculty hope to discover student needs and design necessary support. Class time on campus and faculty office hours are reviewed to determine if they can provide more convenient class offerings and faculty availability. A convenient place to meet and study is part of their goal, especially for the students who commute to campus. Faculty will consider these elements when they develop their Student Success Program.

Faculty noted that a large percentage of the students had no previous college degree. While attainment of a previous degree was part of the computation for the selective criteria score, faculty do not know the significance of this factor. Attainment of a previous degree will be tracked along with each of the selective admission criteria to determine the impact on successful completion of the nursing program.

Learning Styles

Results from the learning style inventory administered as part of the self-assessment tool helped the HNS faculty identify several factors that will impact their teaching. They found that 65% of the incoming students learn best with visual cues. About 25% of the students indicated kinesthetic approaches help them relate to material. The HNS faculty considered the results of the learning style inventory relative to their teaching methods, and realized they do little to incorporate instruction with an emphasis on kinesthetic or tactile teaching techniques. They concluded they do not know how to address these learning needs. Faculty development programs were planned to target instructional strategies employing a variety of learning styles.

Faculty also decided they would like to know how they learn best, to gain insights for their teaching. All plan to complete the CITE Learning Style Inventory and set aside time in their faculty meeting to discuss their findings.

Curriculum Choke Points

HNS faculty decided to gather data about curriculum choke points. This information will be used to address the identified areas in advance of future presentation of that particular content. Data on test items from all exams for currently enrolled students were reviewed for lowest number of correct responses to identify problematic content. The faculty also wanted to determine if knowledge of particularly difficult content areas pointed to similar needs, such as the need to apply information to a clinical situation. To do this, faculty reviewed how problem content was taught to determine if other approaches would be more productive. Two content areas stood out as difficult for students:
- study of the pediatric client with alterations in cardiac function
- study of the client with neuromuscular dysfunction

Faculty determined they would look for clinical experiences to compliment these two content areas and enhance lecture presentations with case studies that specifically address this pathophysiology. Test results from the previous year's class will be compared with the current class to determine any differences. Surveys of students will be used to ascertain their perceptions of their learning of the material. Classroom assessment techniques, such as asking "what was the muddiest point in class today?" will be implemented to gather ongoing assessment data and provide an opportunity for immediate intervention (Angelo & Cross, 1993).

Areas to Address in the Student Success Program

Using the information from the admission and selective criteria, student data depicted in Table 4.8, the learning style inventory as measured by the self-assessment tool, and the identified curriculum choke points, the HNS faculty outlined individual student and class needs to address for the incoming class:

- study skills course (mandatory) for those who indicate difficulty with test-taking or score a C or lower on an exam
- focus group with students and faculty or liaison from counseling to discuss student concerns and help reduce student stress
- optional review of anatomy and physiology for those students who obtained a C in the course, and/or took it more than 3 years ago
- math and reading skills assistance developed in conjunction with the study skills course for nursing students to include dimensional analysis and a special emphasis on reading nursing textbooks for main points and comprehension of content. This assistance will be open to all students and mandatory for students not scoring a passing grade on either their first dosage calculation test or first nursing exam
- discussion of the learning styles inventory results, with a specific focus on instructional strategies to enhance visual modes of learning to compliment the 65% of students who learn best with visual cues. Kinesthetic modes of learning will be addressed to a lesser extent, to compliment the 25% who learn best with tactile cues.
- general test-taking skills relative to answering items that will be typical of nursing exams
- discussion of time management skills to address how students can manage the demands of nursing school, work, and other environmental factors
- peer-tutoring for assistance to learn especially difficult or challenging content identified as choke points in the curriculum

Establish Indicators of Success for the Student Success Program

HNS faculty established indicators of success for their program founded on a thorough review of admission and selective criteria, the students' self-assessments and learning style inventories, identified curriculum choke points, and general program outcomes faculty believe exemplify excellence. Established indicators for success include:
- attain 85% retention rate.
- improve grades by 10% on exams which test the two content areas identified as curriculum choke points:
    o pediatric client with alterations in cardiac function.
    o client with neuromuscular dysfunction.

- expand teaching skill set and establish expectation that all faculty teach using visual learning cues and add at least one learning strategy to address the needs of the kinesthetic learner. Faculty will document the learning strategies related to specific learning styles they implement and the teaching strategies they use to address that learning style.
- improve exam scores by at least 5% for all students who engage in at least one of the following interventions:
  o study skills course.
  o optional review of anatomy and physiology.
  o math and reading assistance.
  o peer tutoring.
  o general test-taking skills.
  o time management seminar.
  o focus group to address student concerns and reduce stress.
- attain 85% student satisfaction rate with the program.
- increase NCLEX pass rate by 5%. NCLEX pass rate average over last three years is 84%.

Faculty established a three-year time frame in which these outcomes will be met and plan continued surveillance of student needs.

Closing Thoughts

Effecting retention requires a variety of strategies and mechanisms to foster student success in programs of nursing. Retention strategies flow from the carefully constructed assessment process, where data is collected and evaluated from the first point of contact with the student and continues throughout the student's tenure in the nursing program.

Faculty are responsible for determining the strategies that best meet the needs of students who enroll in their programs. These needs are not static, and may change for each class. Faculty must evaluate student needs with each new class on an ongoing basis. Ideally, the support students receive to complete a nursing program sets the stage for future success – success on the licensure exam and success in the role of professional nurse.

Learning Activities

1. Plan a method to track and evaluate data that you gather during your admission and selection process, the students' self-assessments, and the results from the students' learning style inventory. Modify Table 4.8 to meet your individual needs.
2. Determine how best to meet identified needs. Consider available resources, such as counseling, study skills center, and financial aid, then identify other resources that would be necessary to establish a Student Success Program. Present this data to administration for necessary infrastructure and support.
3. Assess your own learning style. Use the learning styles inventory on the CD accompanying this book. List three instructional strategies you use that compliment your style of learning.
4. Talk with your class about their learning styles and yours, then compare and contrast different ways of learning. Encourage students to discuss approaches to learning that have been beneficial to them. Offer suggestions for students to better deal with a variety of instructional approaches.

References

Abdur-Rahman, V., & Gaines, C. (1999). Retaining ethnic minority nursing students (REMNS): A multidimensional approach. *Association of Black Nursing Faculty Journal, 10*(2), 33-36.

Allen S., & Pappas, A. (1999). Enhancing math competency of baccalaureate students. *Journal of Professional Nursing, 15*(2), 123-129.

Allen, G. D., Rubenfield, M.G., & Scheffer, B. K. (2004). Reliability assessment of critical thinking. *Journal of Professional Nursing, 20*(1), 15-22.

American Association of Colleges of Nursing (2003). Faculty shortages in baccalaureate and graduate nursing programs: Scope of the problem and strategies for expanding the supply, White Paper. Retrieved December 23, 2006, from http://www.aacn.nche.edu/Publications/WhitePapers/FacultyShortages.htm.

Angelo, T.A., & Cross, P.K. (1993). *Classroom assessment techniques: A handbook for college teachers.* San Francisco: Jossey-Bass.

Babich, A. M., Burdine, P., Albright, L., & Randol, P. (1976). *Center for Innovative Teaching Experiences (CITE) Learning Style Instrument.* Wichita, KS: Murdoch Teacher Center.

Casady, M. J. (2002). *Getting the college edge.* Boston: Houghton Mifflin.

Colucciello, M. (1999). Relationships between critical thinking dispositions and learning styles. *Journal of Professional Nursing, 15*(5), 294-301.

Fox, O. H., & Broome, B. S. (2001). Mentoring: A supporting act for African-American students and faculty. *Association of Black Nursing Faculty Journal, 12*(1), 9–14.

Hopper, C.H. (2004). *Practicing college learning strategies* (3rd ed.). Boston: Houghton Mifflin.

Ironside, P. (1999). Thinking in nursing education. Part I: A student's experience in learning to think. Part II: A teacher's experience. *Nursing and Health Care Perspectives, 20*(5), 238-247.

Jeffreys, M. (2004). *Nursing student retention: Understanding the process and making a difference.* New York: Springer.

Lockie, N. M., & Burke, L. J. (1999). Partnership in learning for utmost success (PLUS): Evaluation of a retention program for at-risk nursing students. *Journal of Nursing Education, 38*(4), 188–196.

Matteson-Kane, M., & Clarren, D.S. (2003). Recruiting students is one thing; Keeping them is another. *Nurse Educator, 28*(6), 281-283.

Mississipi Council of Deans and Directors of Schools of Nursing (2004). Nursing education opportunities in Mississippi. Retrieved December 28, 2004 at http://www.monw.org/images/stories/pdf/nursinghandbookforwebtouse2004.pdf.

Sandiford, J., & Jackson, K. (2003). *Predictors of first semester attrition and their relation to retention of generic associate degree nursing students.* East Lansing, MI: National Center for Research on Teacher Learning. (ERIC Document Reproduction Service No. ED481947).

Stone, C. A., Davidson, L. J., Evans, J. L., & Hansen, M. A. (2001). Validity evidence for using a general critical thinking test to measure nursing students' critical thinking. *Holistic Nursing Practice, 15*(4), 65-74.

Thompson, C., & Crutchlow, E. (1993). Learning style research: A critical review of the literature and implications for nursing education. *Journal of Professional Nursing, 9*(1), 34-40.

Thompson, C., & Rebeschi, L. (1999). Critical thinking skills of baccalaureate nursing students at program entry and exit. *Nursing and Health Care Perspectives, 20*(5), 248-255.

Chapter 5:
Elements of a Student Success Program Prior to Entering a Nursing Program

Chapter 4 discussed the sources of information that can provide the framework for developing a Student Success Program. As shown in Figure 5.1 these sources include the admission criteria, selective criteria, student self-assessment, learning style, and curriculum choke points. The information gleaned from these sources is analyzed, studied, categorized, and arranged into the components of a Student Success Program. Faculty delineate the scope of their Student Success Program based on the specific needs of their students. The Student Success Program, as well as an individualized Student Success Plan, can be introduced to students prior to entering a nursing program then extended throughout the program.

Figure 5.1 - Data Flow for Planning Your Student Success Program

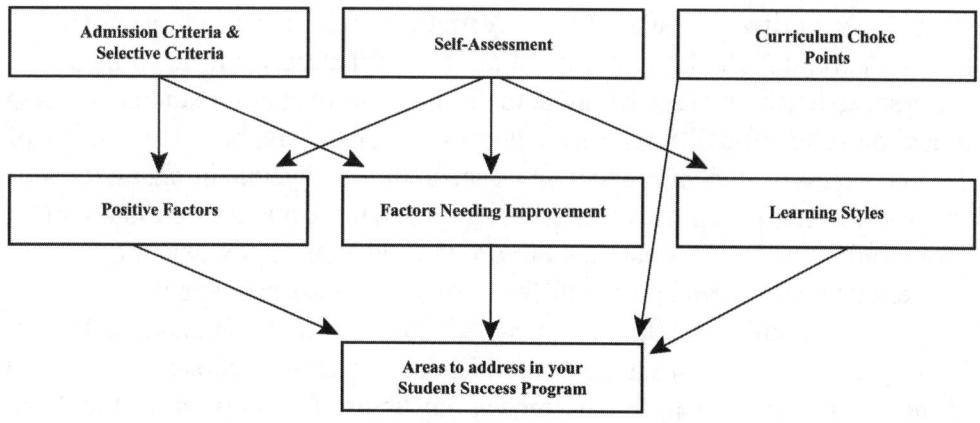

This chapter offers ideas about what to include in a pre-nursing course as part of a Student Success Program. This course is offered prior to the student entering the nursing program or before enrolling in the first nursing course. This chapter presents a discussion of various mechanisms for offering such a pre-nursing course and the content to include in the course.

Identifying the Data

Data are extrapolated from various sources as shown in Figure 5.1. The first step in planning the elements of a Student Success Program is to study the data from the students' files regarding the admission criteria and selective criteria to gain a better understanding of the characteristics of the students who will be entering the nursing program. Although all students admitted have met the admission criteria, a closer analysis can provide important details. The data are analyzed for recurring themes or issues. For example, one admission criterion may be that the student must have a minimum cumulative GPA of 2.5 for all previous course work. Are the students' GPAs clustered around 2.5 or are they clustered around 4.0? Or, are they evenly distributed from 2.5 to 4.0? A class with a GPA range from 2.5 to 2.9 may be quite a different group of students than those entering with a GPA range from 3.5 to 4.0.

Selective criteria are also studied. Variations exist in each class depending on the degree to which these criteria are met. What may appear to be subtle differences between classes may actually have an impact on student success unless these specific differences are addressed. Therefore, prior to the entry of each new class of students, faculty must spend time analyzing the characteristics specific for that group of students. What problems are identified that can be addressed in the Student Success Program? Revisions of any existing Student Success Program should be considered to address these problems.

Prior to planning the Student Success Program pre-nursing course, faculty identify any curriculum choke points. These curriculum choke points were discussed in Chapter 4 and are defined as any areas of the curriculum that have proven to be particularly difficult for past students. Once these areas are identified, faculty should plan activities to help students prepare. For example, if students have a difficult time processing content on caring for clients with fluid and electrolyte imbalances, perhaps a review of the basics may help. Of course, another approach for dealing with curriculum choke points is for faculty to restructure the teaching/learning experiences so the material is more manageable by the entering class of students.

Scheduling a Pre-Nursing Success Course

There are a variety of ways to offer a pre-nursing course. Keeping in mind that at-risk students in a retention program are more likely to graduate than at-risk students not in such a program (Lockie & Burke, 1999), the course may be recommended, or even required, for students who meet "at-risk" criteria. See Chapter 2 for a full discussion of the assessment and definition of the "at-risk" student. If the course is required for students who meet the "at-risk" criteria, faculty and advisers must explain the importance of the course in relation to the goals of the students. Students may express anger and frustration for taking a course that requires additional time (Symes, Tart, Travis, & Toombs, 2002); therefore, the value of the course must be emphasized. On the other hand, students may be grateful for the intervention aimed at helping them succeed.

If students are required to take the pre-nursing course, it is wise to select students based on pre-established criteria. An impartial approach for selecting students minimizes student objections to participating in the pre-nursing course (Symes, Tart, Travis, & Toombs, 2002).

The course may be required for identified "at-risk" students, but also open to any nursing student requesting to enroll. Depending on available resources, the course may be restricted to only students who meet certain criteria and unavailable for students who do not meet that criteria. Another option is to require the course for all nursing students. Requiring the course for all students is ideal, but often impractical because of limited resources and mandates limiting the number of credit hours of a nursing program. If the course is a requirement for all nursing students, or if all nursing students take the course even if not required, then the number of credit hours is usually included in the total hours of the nursing program for accreditation purposes.

The faculty must also consider how the course will be scheduled. There are several approaches that can be considered. Offering the course throughout the semester preceding the first nursing course is most helpful. Each class session meets weekly for two or three hours. Another approach is to offer the class for lengthy sessions over the course of a few days. For example, the course is offered during an interim session or immediately prior to the start of the fall semester over four 8-hour days. This provides an immersion experience for the student immediately prior to the start of the nursing courses.

There are both positive and negatives to each type of scheduling. For the full-semester course, the positive is that students have time to develop a plan of action and address areas that need strengthening. It also provides greater opportunity for the faculty to interact with the students. However, a full semester course may interfere with scheduling other courses or may not be available for students who are accepted into the nursing courses on short notice, such as off a waiting list. Scheduling the course for a short, but intense immersion experience may better accommodate the adult learner. Because the course is primarily informational, interactive, and self-reflective, time to study the material and prepare for testing is not needed. Therefore, a course offered over several days is ideal.

Putting Together the Course Content

The purpose of a pre-nursing success course is to bring awareness to students as they identify the strengths that have brought them to this point in their education and to prepare a plan of action for helping them address factors that may interfere with continued success. The course is a diagnostic-prescriptive approach to helping students succeed (Jeffreys, 2004). Another purpose of a pre-nursing course is to prepare students on all fronts to academically, psychologically, and practically handle the demands of a nursing program (Jeffreys, 2004). When planning the overall pre-nursing course, the faculty select areas identified from the student data. The pre-nursing course focuses on helping students be successful by highlighting skills students use to succeed. When students improve skills such as study skills, test-taking skills, time management, mathematical computation, reading, and stress management, retention is enhanced (Symes, Tart, Travis, & Toombs, 2002). Therefore, topics for a pre-nursing course might include:
- self-assessment
- overview of nursing school
- connecting with faculty
- preparing for class
- reading/math
- time management
- stress management

Chapter 5: Elements of a Student Success Program Prior to Entering a Nursing Program

- addressing curriculum choke points
- example NCLEX style questions

Class Session 1: Overview of Nursing School

A general program overview provides the framework for understanding all the components of the nursing program. It is helpful for students to invite a family member, friend, or support person to this session so these significant people will understand what being a nursing student involves (Jeffreys, 2004). This general program overview includes the following:
- mission, purpose, philosophy, and educational outcomes of the program
- standards of conduct expected of the student while in the nursing program
- types of assignments and grading scale
- program costs
- class and clinical schedule
- travel to and from sites used for both clinical and community experiences

A Sample Syllabus and the Student Handbook

Nursing syllabi can be very intimidating. They are lengthy, contain many rules and regulations, and incorporate information about a myriad of learning experiences. Explaining the different sections of the syllabus and their meaning is helpful.

Because the syllabus reflects what is in the student handbook, a good understanding of the student handbook is a requirement. Typically the handbook delineates the policies, procedures, grading scale, attendance requirements, academic dishonesty, progression policy, readmission policy, and any other information pertinent to the nursing program.

Prerequisites and Nursing Courses

Provide a discussion about how the prerequisite courses fit into the nursing curriculum and how the content relates to nursing. Discuss the nursing curriculum and how the nursing courses relate to each other. For example, advanced medical nursing may be taught prior to a course on high-risk pregnancy so the student can better relate pathophysiology such as diabetes mellitus or hypertension to possible complications during pregnancy. Understanding these relationships helps students see the bigger picture and appreciate how important every course in the curriculum is to the overall program outcomes. If students understand how each course builds on a previous course, they gain a sense of the whole. Adult learners need to know the practical application of what they are learning. Explicating this from the onset serves to meet this need and makes for a smooth transition.

Progression through the Nursing Program and Graduation Requirements

Ways to progress through the program are explained so students can plan their course of study. Many nursing programs employ a fast-track where students move through the program quickly. Some programs use flexible scheduling that allows students to customize somewhat their path through the nursing courses. In these types of programs, the student may choose to take a longer period of time than the traditional route.

Learning Environments

Students often state that nursing courses are very different than other courses they take. Nursing education takes place in many environments. During this class session, students can tour the nursing lab. The faculty can talk about the didactic portion of the course as well as the clinical. Finally, the relationship among these three learning environments and how they each impact the other is discussed. It is important for students to realize each learning environment is not a separate entity but part of the larger whole.

Also included in this class session is an overview of the various types of learning experiences the students may encounter. Explore what is meant by cognitive, affective, and psychomotor domains. Explain and provide examples of teaching strategies using case studies, lecture, small group discussion, skill demonstrations, and clinical experiences. Ask nursing faculty to "guest lecture" during the course to provide students experience with different teaching styles, as well as to get to know some of the faculty (Keane, DiMattio, & Gaudet, 2002). If available, demonstrate the use of a human patient simulator or other simulation equipment in the nursing laboratory. Discuss the use of this equipment to help students feel more comfortable in the clinical area.

An important part of nursing education is to teach students critical thinking. Concept maps can foster higher-order thinking skills such as critical thinking. This is an ideal time to provide basic information on concept mapping and to

Chapter 5: Elements of a Student Success Program Prior to Entering a Nursing Program

talk about its use in developing thinking skills. Prior to the authors making this recommendation about concept maps, an integrative review was conducted to provide an evidence-base for this recommendation. In the integrative review, three questions were posed:
1. What guidelines for using concept maps have been reported in the current literature?
2. What evidence is available that describes the effectiveness of using concept maps to foster thinking?
3. What are the problems identified with the use of concept maps?

The integrative review considered all studies addressing some aspect of using concept maps to develop thinking skills. A search of the literature revealed 48 articles. Of these 48 articles, 7 were included in the integrative review (Castellino & Schuster, 2002; Daley, Shaw, Balistrieri, Glasenapp, & Piacentine, 1999; Daley, 1996; Farrand, Hussain, & Hennessey, 2002; Rooda, 1994; Wheeler & Collins, 2003; Wilkes, Cooper, Lewin & Batt, 1999). The remaining 41 articles were not research articles. Following are the findings related to the specific research questions:

1. What guidelines for using concept maps have been reported in the current literature? Findings include the following:
    - introduce concept maps early in the curriculum. This is the basis for the recommendation to have students in the pre-nursing success course learn about concept maps.
    - to get started, demonstrate the technique to students and then have students map a concept individually; use these samples for discussion. Assign students to create a concept map of something familiar to them such as planning for holiday activities.
    - encourage creativity when constructing concept maps.

2. What evidence is available that describes the effectiveness of using concept maps to foster critical thinking? Findings include the following:
    - self-evaluation by students and faculty indicate that using concepts maps helped students develop critical thinking skills.
    - faculty reported concept maps were beneficial in demonstrating the knowledge that students gained over the course of a semester.
    - faculty believed they were able to see the development of students' thinking processes when using concept maps.

- faculty reported that concept maps helped them assess student competency in providing safe care.
- faculty reported that concept maps were a means for correcting student misperceptions when discussed in postconferences.

3. What are the problems identified with the use of concept maps? Findings include the following:
   - concept maps are time consuming. Faculty can promote their use by providing in-class time for map construction and encouraging variation in map appearance to meet individual creativity.
   - before recommending concept maps as a study technique, a way of providing effective training is needed to encourage and motivate students about adopting this approach to study.
   - grading concept maps can be difficult; it may be difficult to assess the concept map for accuracy.

 Refer to the CD-ROM accompanying this book for a complete discussion on the process used to conduct this integrative review.

Throughout all types of learning experiences, students should be encouraged to participate. Herrera-Shepard (2006), a retention specialist, states that participation is the most important factor for success in all nursing classes. Ways students can participate include:
- attend classes regularly
- bring all necessary materials to class
- use a calendar for time management
- ask questions
- take effective notes
- form study groups; talk about what they are learning
- meet and talk with faculty
- participate in college activities
- use college resources

College Resources

Students who seek support are more successful (Ofori & Charlton, 2002). Introduce students to all resources the college or nursing program has to offer. Ask representatives of each of these resource areas to talk with students and

Chapter 5: Elements of a Student Success Program Prior to Entering a Nursing Program

answer questions. Include both academic and nonacademic resources. Examples of academic resources include the learning resource center and tutoring services. Nonacademic resource examples include financial aid and child care.

Class Session 2: Self-Assessment

If not previously completed, students work through a self-assessment. An example of a self-assessment is the *Start Right in Nursing School: A Self-Assessment Tool TM* from College of DuPage, specifically designed by nursing faculty for nursing students. This tool was described in Chapter 4 and provides students with information and feedback in the areas of:
- personal demographics
- study skills
- personal learning style
- time management
- concentration
- reading
- note-taking
- family issues
- test-taking strategies

The *Start Right in Nursing School* program provides a starting framework for students to identify their strengths and weaknesses. It also helps them become aware of strategies that best help them learn. This awareness is necessary for becoming a self-directed learner (Symes, Tart, Travis, & Toombs, 2002). The *Start Right in Nursing School* program generates an individualized report for each student. A sample of a student report is on the CD accompanying this book.

After completing the self-assessment, students take an in-depth look at their individualized report. The faculty help students interpret and use the information contained in the report to develop an approach for success. Together, the student and faculty outline an individualized Student Success Plan.

Students are then introduced to other factors that may influence their success. These include additional factors, extrapolated from Table 2.6, that are not part of the students' self-assessment. Those factors are listed in Table 5.1.

It is important for students to be aware of these factors and to self-monitor for them. If any of the negative factors are present, the student should talk with faculty or counselors about resolution.

Table 5.1 – Additional Factors that May Influence Success

Classification of Factors	Positive Factors	Negative Factors
Academic/School-Related	Positive attitude toward educators	Negative attitude toward educators
	Critical thinker	Difficulty with critical thinking
	< 20 minute travel to school	> 20 minute travel to school
Personal Factors	Very motivated	Lacks motivation
	Strong social support	Lack of social support
	Manages stress well	Difficulty dealing with stress
	High self-efficacy	Low self-efficacy
	Self-confident	Low self-esteem
	No health problems	Health problems
Environmental Factors	Minimal church, community commitments	Many church, community commitments
	No family problems	Family problems

Class Session #3: Math/Reading

Math

If a preadmission math test was given, the students review their results. If a math test was not given as a preadmission criterion, administer one at this session to evaluate the students' math abilities and possible need for remediation. Review the type of math needed to perform dosage calculations and demonstrate application of this math using simple dosage calculations.

Reading

Frequently, many pages of reading are assigned in a nursing course. Completing the reading is one thing – understanding its importance, or relevance to practice (the application piece that students find so challenging), is another. Assist students to learn to scan the text, use objectives at the beginning of chapters, and review end-of chapter summaries. A clear expectation for knowledge of topics to be tested helps students focus their study and read with purpose. This means that if a student is assigned to read 600 pages, the student needs to know how these pages relate to expectations on the part of the faculty teaching the content and designing the exam. Only those pages essential to the intent of the instruction should be assigned. This is an important consideration because it takes more time for students to read the assignment than for faculty to read the assignments, particularly students with English as a second-language (ESL).

During this session, the teacher provides guidance on how to use the textbooks. The teacher goes through a chapter in each book and helps students understand the organization of the content, the introductory material such as objectives and key words, the format of examples such as nursing care plans or concept maps, and end-of-the-chapter questions. Students also need to learn about glossaries, the table of contents, and the index, and how these components of a book can be used to understand and locate information. Any additional materials provided by the textbooks' publishers can be discussed with demonstrations on how to use these resources, such as materials that are located online or contained on a CD-ROM.

Class Session #4: Connecting with Faculty

One of the primary factors that promotes student success is a supportive faculty-student relationship. Faculty play an integral role in the success of nursing students and are reported to be a major contributor to student success (Wells, 2003). Students need to know and to trust their faculty. Tracey (2003) found that when asked what students do to cope, students listed "Consult with instructor" as fourth on their list of interventions. The first three options selected over talking with faculty were engaging in physical exercise, consulting with family, and praying or meditating.

Advise students to make appointments to talk with faculty when they are having difficulties with coursework. Include when it is important for students to make appointments and discuss what students can and cannot expect faculty to do for them. Discuss how to make the most of their relationship with nursing faculty.

Class Session #5: Preparing for Class

Discuss what students can do to prepare for each type of learning experience: lecture, case studies, skills laboratory, clinical, and any other learning experiences. Suggest ways to cope with the large amount of homework, such as enhancing reading skills, note-taking, and studying.

Class Session #6: Time Management

The diverse student population in nursing education includes students who have many responsibilities unrelated to nursing school. These responsibilities often compete with school responsibilities for the student's time. Time management is critical to success. Important content to cover about time management includes:
- how to deal with not having enough time
- how much job-related work is too much
- how to get the most out of study time

Part of time management is setting priorities. Students learn to identify the important factors in their lives and how to prioritize these factors. Identifying priorities and knowing what's important to them helps students organize their lives in a meaningful way and to cope when unexpected events occur.

For students to plan and manage time effectively, they need to know the tasks and responsibilities before them. Faculty should provide a comprehensive and realistic overview of course expectations and time required to complete assignments. Faculty may want to complete all student reading assignments and calculate the time necessary to manage projects, so they have realistic expectations for student workload. Creating meaningful, doable assignments that augment the learning experience is important.

Once workload is determined, students can put into place the components of time management: planning, organizing, and implementing actions to control the use of time. Activities such as setting priorities, scheduling activities, and creating a "to do" list all contribute to a plan for studying. Managing personal space and organizing the environment so they are conducive to studying help students avoid distractions. These are just some of the topics that can be covered under time management.

Class Session #7: Stress Management

Many nursing students indicate they are stressed. Some stress can facilitate learning, but a high degree of stress can interfere with academic performance (Bolan & Grainger, 2003). A major stressor for nursing students is a heavier or more difficult workload than expected (Bolan & Grainger, 2003). A class session devoted to the concept of stress is helpful. Areas to address include:

- what stress is
- what causes stress
- the effects of stress
- how to deal with stress

There are a variety of sources of stress related to the educational environment for nursing students. Some of these include fear of poor evaluations, excessive academic load, test anxiety, and concerns about safe practice (Bolan & Grainger, 2003).

Heavy work schedules and family commitments also add to the stress. Many nursing students arrive for clinical sessions after working many hours in their place of employment or caring for family members. The physical demands of clinical nursing may add to the student's physical stress.

Students may also experience emotional stress as a direct result of nursing school. Many students fear causing harm to clients or they often voice concern that they are disturbing clients because it takes them longer to carry out a procedure or gather data than it takes for a licensed nurse to perform the same task.

Engaging in discussion with students about these common concerns reassures students these concerns are real, acceptable, and manageable. Currently enrolled students can be invited to talk with incoming students about how to deal with these concerns. Shadowing a nurse is helpful, especially if students have no healthcare experience. Students who have spent a few hours with a nurse before starting clinical courses report this has been very helpful in decreasing their stress of the unknown (Symes, Tart, Travis, & Toombs, 2002). A shadowing experience will also provide students with no healthcare experience a realistic picture of what a nurse does. One non-academic factor associated with attrition is a change in student perception of nursing as a career (Bolan & Grainger, 2003). Even a few hours observing the reality of nursing may prove helpful for these students.

Students are encouraged to share how they currently deal with stress and if those interventions are working. A psychologist may attend class and teach stress reduction techniques including relaxation techniques (Symes, Tart, Travis, & Toombs, 2002). Students are provided contact information for school counselors who are experienced with helping with many stressful situations.

Class #8: Curriculum Choke Points

Academic failure is the most commonly cited reason for students failing from a nursing program (Ofori & Charlton, 2002). Therefore, it is extremely important that any curriculum choke points are addressed. Faculty who have previously identified curriculum choke points may choose to use a class session reviewing foundational material so the difficult material will be easier for students to understand when encountered in the curriculum. The content of this class session varies according to the identified areas of difficulty and the needs of the students.

Indicators of Success

Help students identify indicators they can use to determine if they are succeeding or need help in their nursing courses. Students use this information to self-monitor their need for intervention. Students need to learn to be self-directed, especially with the current learning environment that embraces the benefits of student-centered, active learning. In these learning environments, students are active in their learning and in their evaluation. To be successful in these environments, students must be guided in the acquisition of self-directed skills (Lunyk-Child, et al., 2001). Because early intervention is so important for student success, students need to know what factors indicate they need help. Types of indicators include clinical weaknesses that require additional practice with skills or dosage calculations and test scores that indicate a downward trend. A grid that students can fill out on a weekly basis evaluating their performance is helpful for early identification of needs.

Retention Specialist

An effective Student Success Program, starting with a pre-nursing course, takes faculty time and energy. This diverts time and energy from other teaching functions; and, with the nursing faculty shortage, may interfere with a successful Student Success Program (Symes, Tart, & Travis, 2005). Many nursing programs are adopting the idea of hiring a specific person to help students be successful. This position is not a faculty position and may or may not be a nurse. Each school must assess student needs and the organizational culture, then determine if this position is best filled with a nurse, nursing faculty, or non-nurse professional. This person must understand the needs of nursing students and be able to develop strategies for dealing with areas that are challenging for students. Some titles for this type of position are Retention Specialist and Achievement Coach. In this book, the term Retention Specialist is used.

The Retention Specialist is introduced to the students during the pre-nursing course. When designing the pre-nursing course, provide time for this person to be introduced, give an overview of the position, and answer questions. It is helpful for students to understand how the Retention Specialist can help them succeed.

Dr. Jennifer Bissett is a Retention Specialist for College of the Mainland in Texas City, Texas. In the following section, Dr. Bissett shares what her role as Retention Specialist entails and provides insight regarding this type of position.

The Retention Specialist: Role, Philosophy, and Effectiveness
Dr. Jennifer Bissett

The nursing shortage has been thoroughly documented as a national crisis in great need of immediate attention. For years this attention has focused on recruitment efforts, and has successfully resulted in an increase of applications to nursing education programs. However, many programs are turning away qualified candidates due to issues related to space and a concurrent nursing faculty shortage. Additionally, though programs are functioning at capacity and enrolling the maximum number of new students prudently possible, there is a nationwide problem with nursing student attrition rates. Consequently, the increased enrollment has not resulted in a substantial increase in graduation rates.

Development and maintenance of effective retention programs in nursing education can bring hope for more efficient output of qualified nurse candidates. A principal factor toward meeting the goals of increased retention is the implementation of a Retention Specialist in nursing education programs. This section explains the scope of the Retention Specialist role, defines the goals of employing a Retention Specialist, delineates the related duties and responsibilities of such a position, and highlights the results relative to actual student retention and graduation.

Scope of the Retention Specialist Role

The focus of the Retention Specialist is on the academic preparedness and persistence of nursing students. Through the design and implementation of a comprehensive consultation model, the Retention Specialist acts as an expert consultant to administration, faculty, and students regarding the variety of complex issues that impact student retention and persistence in nursing school. By design, retention is approached as a complex and holistic process whereby to be retained students need much more than the traditional support of tutoring and mentoring. The effective candidate for this position will be versed in systematic evaluation, assessment, survey development and research, academic support, personal counseling, learning disabilities assessment, admissions knowledge, and experience with the workings and resources of college campuses.

The roles of the Retention Specialist consist of consultant, counselor, liaison, and advocate. To be effective in these multiple roles, it is my opinion (Dr. Bissett's), that the Retention Specialist not be a nurse. While nursing faculty are very knowledgeable and skilled in nursing content, many faculty members do not have the time and/or specialized skills to address the breadth of specific student needs that impact retention. Poor academic performance is caused by a plethora of factors including study skills, test-taking skills, motivation, interpersonal difficulties, anxiety, limited support networks, psychological strains, and other life stressors.

Many students feel intimidated by and uncomfortable talking with their faculty about the issues that impact their performance. Some students fear being labeled problematic, others fear their grades will suffer based on disclosure of personal problems, and still others fear a lack of confidentiality. While nursing faculty are certainly able to maintain appropriate objectivity in grading and professional boundaries, students are often unconvinced that negative consequences will not result from their disclosures to faculty. By employing a non-faculty Retention Specialist, this threat is essentially eliminated. Students often comment that a major reason they seek the services of the Retention Specialist is because they know this person is not currently, and never will be, in a position to grade the student. They also comment that confidentiality is of the utmost importance.

Goals and Objectives of the Retention Specialist

The ultimate goal of the Retention Specialist's activities is to increase the overall rate of students who successfully complete the nursing program. While on-time completion is the primary goal, persistence in the nursing program following a set-back (e.g. need for a repeated course due to unsuccessful progress, absenteeism, illness, etc.) is also considered an important focus. A sample of appropriate objectives would be:

1. Obtain an on-time retention rate of 75%; meaning that of those students who initially enroll, a minimum of 75% will graduate in the prescribed period of time. Depending on the levels of on-time retention prior to hiring a Retention Specialist, an appropriate objective may be to improve the on-time retention rate of basic nursing students by 5 to 10% over the pre-hire rate each semester until at least the 75% goal is reached.
2. Obtain a persistence rate of 75%; meaning that of those students who were delayed in their graduation date (due to failure, illness, etc.) **and are eligible to continue**, a minimum of 75% will return and successfully complete the program. Depending on the persistence rate prior to hiring a Retention Specialist, an appropriate objective may be to improve the persistence rate of basic nursing students by 5 to 10% over the pre-hire rate each semester until the 75% goal is reached.
3. Similarly track and improve the retention and persistence rates of transition, transfer, and any other types of nursing students.

Retention Specialist Activities

Integral to the effectiveness of a Retention Specialist is a clear and comprehensive understanding of the academic program, including knowledge of the academic, clinical, administrative, and social demands of the nursing program. With this knowledge, the Retention Specialist becomes the appropriate individual to provide informational support to pre-nursing students and continued support to enrolled students throughout the nursing educational program, in addition to being a resource of information for faculty and administration.

Support to Administration

The effective Retention Specialist is constantly gathering and analyzing data related to student satisfaction and success factors that can be readily used for data-driven decision making. These data can be used to inform nursing program administrators about potential areas needing improvement, as well as program strengths. Likewise, these data often will support systematic evaluation efforts of the program.

The Retention Specialist is also in a position to advocate for students and faculty with administration, based on the data collected in daily activities. The Retention Specialist can help to communicate student and faculty needs to the administration, and likewise communicate administration needs to the faculty and students. One important administrative area where the Retention Specialist has the potential to make a strong impact is in the development of admissions criteria. In many ways, admissions decisions have a strong influence on retention. The goal of admissions decision making is to maximize the positive hit rate. That is, the goal is to increase the probability that students capable of completing the program are selected, and to minimize the likelihood that these same students are rejected. A 100% retention rate from admission to graduation is unrealistic. However, the more predictive the admissions formula, the better prepared the students are for successful completion.

Support to Faculty

Faculty retention is as important as student retention. While the primary goals of the Retention Specialist are related to the direct improvement of student retention, there is no doubt that the milieu set by the faculty plays an important role in student success and student personal choices to remain enrolled. As students feel more supported by their faculty, the learning environment is improved. As faculty feel more supported by administration, their ability to maintain a positive and constructive learning environment is also improved. The Retention Specialist can enhance the faculty experience by serving as a liaison between the faculty and administration, as well as between the faculty and students. Furthermore, just as a non-faculty Retention Specialist will not be in a position to grade students in the present or future, this person will also not be in a position to evaluate faculty in either the present or the future. With this barrier eliminated, the Retention Specialist becomes a resource for faculty to vent their stress and concerns. The Retention Specialist also serves as a consultant to the faculty regarding such issues as dealing with difficult students, identifying and addressing different learning needs of students, helping with team development on teaching teams, and identifying and addressing student success needs.

When a Retention Specialist is newly added to a nursing program team, one of the major concerns of faculty tends to be that the Retention Specialist will want to lower standards such that all students are passed irrespective of their actual abilities. Open communication and collaborative goal setting can alleviate these faculty concerns. The goal is to increase the number of students who successfully complete the program, graduate, pass the licensure examination, and enter the nursing workforce. This overarching goal cannot be met by reducing standards.

Pre-Nursing Student Support

For most programs, it is unreasonable to assume that the Retention Specialist can perform all recruiting and pre-nursing advising that is needed. It is helpful, however, for the Retention Specialist to collaborate with other individuals who are responsible for these functions to insure that all information distributed about the program is consistent and accurate. In addition, it is important for the Retention Specialist to host periodically informational sessions about the nursing program to assist pre-nursing students in making informed decisions about their pursuit (or not) of a career in nursing. Students need assistance with making decisions about if, when, and where to seek admission to nursing schools. Thus, the impact of the Retention Specialist begins upon initial contact to the nursing program. This includes a conversation about the academic details of a nursing program, such as credit hours and prerequisites, as well as answers to questions about the personal demands of nursing school such as time demands, academic rigor, and real-life scenarios of what is involved in nursing. Ensuring that the personal demand piece is covered is especially essential so that students are not lost due to the realizations that they will actually have to touch people, see people naked, and be present for or implement many unpleasant procedures.

Proactive Efforts with Nursing Students

Many activities can be implemented by the Retention Specialist in an effort proactively to prevent retention difficulties. A typical proactive effort is involvement in New Nursing Student Orientation. The Retention Specialist can help in the planning of success initiatives to be included in the orientation session, and the role of the Retention Specialist should be explained to the students at this time. Again, a realistic discussion of academic and personal demands can aid in students' proactive preparation for the rigors of the nursing program. When possible, it is helpful for the Retention Specialist to speak with new nursing students' family members to educate them about the demands on the student.

Another proactive retention effort is to teach the topics of the pre-nursing success course; or, if such a course is not offered, conduct a series of workshops. A common list of topics to be covered in separate sessions are time management, stress management, coping with test anxiety, test-taking strategies, reading nursing/science textbooks, note-taking, study strategies, how to study efficiently in a group, and critical thinking.

Group test reviews can also serve as proactive retention efforts despite the fact that they occur after an examination is taken. Using test reviews as a retention activity requires that the Retention Specialist approach the test content from a different strategy than a faculty might review the test. The non-faculty Retention Specialist will be unable to re-teach the content or explain nursing concepts that were difficult for a large number of the students to comprehend. The test review session is instead used as a time to teach students how to read and respond to actual test questions, to assist the students through the critical thinking process required to answer the application level questions necessary in nursing education, and to model peer tutoring. The Retention Specialist utilizes the knowledge of the students present at the review to work through the test items. This is an opportunity to model for students how best to approach test questions, how to support one another in study sessions, and how to apply their knowledge.

Reactive Efforts with Nursing Students

Despite our best efforts for successful proactive retention endeavors, there are always students who continue to struggle academically and personally. For these students, one-on-one, individualized support is necessary. Assessment of individual deficiencies of these struggling students by the Retention Specialist is important. It is very important in the assessment phase for the Retention Specialist to ask for very specific details to help determine the potential problems the student is having. For example, students often report that they are studying "all of the time," or "so much more than I have ever studied for any class before." With specific probing, the student may reveal that "all of the time" is a single eight hour study session one day per week, or that "more than I have every studied before" might translate into two hours the night before a test rather than their previous habit of 30 minutes the day of the test. Individualized assistance may then take the form of short-term academic counseling, short-term personal counseling, skills development, or referral to community resources for more long-term support. Table 5.2 summaries the activities of the Retention Specialist.

Results of Retention Specialist Efforts

Ultimately, the effectiveness of the Retention Specialist's performance is reflected in the measurable impact on the retention and persistence rates of all nursing students. Tracking of student success by cohort and by identified student characteristics is crucial. Statistical analyses of increases in retention are important, as are the qualitative reports of students regarding their perceptions of the assistance provided by the Retention Specialist.

Statistical Results

Quantitative success is measured by statistically significant increases in the number of students who persist in nursing school as well as in the number of students who complete the program on time. While different programs have seen different levels of success with the institution of a Retention Specialist, most programs find it is not uncommon to realize statistically significant differences between pre-hire and post-hire data.

In one program that received a grant to hire a Retention Specialist, the success was overwhelming. A 20% increase in the number of students who progressed from the first semester to the second resulted in the program needing to scramble for additional clinical rotation sites and adjunct faculty to cover the increase in the number of students who progressed. This increase in the number of students

Table 5.2 – Summary of Retention Specialist Activities

Supported Group	Activity	Description
Administration	Self-Study Activities	The effective Retention Specialist is constantly gathering and analyzing data related to student satisfaction and success factors that can be readily used for data-driven decision making.
	Orientation Programming	The Orientation session is an important tool in preparing students for nursing school. It is an opportunity to proactively prepare students for the rigors of nursing school and provide primary prevention workshops (e.g. pre-entry discussion of study and test-taking strategies specific for nursing school, diagnostic testing, etc.).
	Admissions Review	Analysis of current admissions practices helps in efforts to make improvements in the positive hit rate of admissions decisions.
	Campus Consultant Regarding Nursing	Collaboration with Recruitment, Foundation, Admissions, Financial Aid, Registrar, Advisement, Student Support Services, and other similar offices on campus who interact with nursing and pre-nursing students to insure that information about the nursing program is presented in a consistent and accurate manner.
Faculty	Liaison	Liaison between students and faculty to inform faculty of student concerns and to support the faculty voice to both students and the administration.
	Consultation	Act as a consultant to faculty on issues related to student performance (e.g. language barriers, students with disabilities, behavioral difficulties, testing strategies, etc.).
	Remediation Activities	Facilitate group remediation activities held after each examination for all students regardless of academic performance. (Consider mandatory participation requirements for students who fail the examination).
	Mini-Research Endeavors	Data analysis for faculty regarding student performance questions (e.g. comparison of students across multiple sections of the same course, or comparison of test performance for specific content areas), as well as regarding faculty grading practices (i.e. consistency of grades for each faculty member teaching a section of the same course), and various other short-term projects.
	Faculty Workshops	Offer a series of workshops to the nursing faculty regarding issues related to student retention. Potential topics include Addressing the needs of an Adult Learner, Students of the 21st Century, Dealing with Difficult Students, Student and Faculty Rights, Developing Learning Communities, and Mentoring Students.
Students	Liaison	Act in support of student voice to both faculty and administration and attempt to increase student awareness of faculty expectations and supportive intentions.

Chapter 5: Elements of a Student Success Program Prior to Entering a Nursing Program

Students	Orientation Activities	*Pre-nursing Student Information Sessions*—Students seek a career in nursing for many different reasons, and often their decision is not based on grounded and realistic information about nursing school. Pre-nursing information sessions can provide individuals with the information they need to make informed decisions about when, where, and whether to enter a nursing educational program. *New Student Orientation*—The Orientation session is an important tool in preparing students for nursing school. It is an opportunity proactively to prepare students for the rigors of nursing school and provide primary prevention workshops (e.g. a pre-nursing course covering study and test-taking strategies specific for nursing school, diagnostic testing, etc.).
	First-Level Test Reviews	For first semester freshmen nursing students, conduct an item-by-item review of all nursing examinations to facilitate the development of excellent test-taking strategies. The Retention Specialist walks students through how to read test items, identify key words, interpret the question, and apply their knowledge to result in the selection of a correct answer. During this time, student support and teaching of one another is also fostered.
	Remediation Activities	Facilitate group remediation sessions following each examination. Facilitate individual remediation sessions with students needing additional assistance and/or specific feedback regarding study techniques and test-taking strategies.
	Individualized Support	Maintain an open-door policy allowing students to make walk-in and future appointments to meet with the Retention Specialist to discuss issues related to academic success, persistence, and retention. Students tend to seek assistance regarding study skills, test-taking strategies, time management, stress management, transition to nursing, vocational choice issues, anxiety management, financial issues, personal crises, psychological difficulties, learning difficulties, etc.
	Students with Disabilities	Interview screening of individuals struggling with academic success for learning difficulties and/or psychological difficulties. Students are referred to campus support personnel (e.g. Disabilities Services, Psychological Services) and/or community resources when appropriate.
	Check-Off Support	Present during many clinical skills check-off sessions to help manage student anxiety.
	Financial Resources	Facilitate the student securing appropriate financial assistance by collaborating with campus offices that coordinate financial aid, scholarships, and grants.
	Student Organization Support	Provide support to the nursing student organizations through promotion of membership and events, supporting leadership development, and collaborating on events that enhance student learning and professional development.

persisted to the second year, and was replicated in the following class (again comparing pre-hire retention and persistence rates to post-hire rates).

Another program was able to show a 100% increase in the number of students who graduated from one year to the next. In this program, students also achieved NCLEX pass rates well above the national average, which was a significant improvement over the pass rates of a few years earlier.

Qualitative Results

While it is certainly important to realize a significant positive impact in the overall numbers of students who are retained in nursing programs and who eventually graduate and pass licensure exams to successfully enter the workforce, it is equally important to consider the students' qualitative experience. Though there will always be a handful of students who continue to see the services of the Retention Specialist as punitive or as acceptance of a "handicap," most students report very positive outcomes from one-on-one assistance provided. Many students make statements such as, "I would have never made it through this program without the Retention Specialist." Following vignettes highlight the personal success of a few students who received individualized attention.

- JB suffered from severe test anxiety. He reported difficulty sleeping for three nights prior to an exam and stated he had extreme difficulty concentrating during examinations due to time pressures. JB tutored many fellow students who consistently passed exams, but JB continued to perform marginally or even fail exams despite clear knowledge attainment. Upon meeting with the Retention Specialist and learning specific relaxation strategies and anxiety management as well as developing a calm-producing rather than anxiety-provoking test day routine, JB saw his test scores improve by 20 points.
- ER struggled with studying the massive volumes of material that a nursing student is responsible to learn for a single test. She reported she tried all the standard study strategies of studying in a group, color coding her notes, and making flashcards, but to no avail. ER continually made low Cs on tests, despite her tremendous efforts to do better. Upon assessment of the student's predominant learning style, the Retention Specialist encouraged the student to use study strategies that complemented her auditory learning style. The student reported her children thought she was "crazy" as she began reading nursing material out loud during her

study time and talked through her learning outcomes as if there were an audience listening. Her efforts paid off; and, by using more appropriately matched study strategies, this student began consistently to make A's on her tests.
- AW struggled with the transition to the role of the nurse. After the freshman lecture on legal and ethical responsibilities, this student was excessively worried about her personal liability. She was so concerned about not making a mistake in caring for the client, that she was almost paralyzed during her clinical rotations. Though her theory performance was stellar, she was at risk of failing her clinical course due to her inability to meet the clinical objectives based on her fear. After addressing her concerns with the Retention Specialist over a series of short-term counseling sessions, the student was able to manage her anxiety and meet successfully her clinical objectives.

The highest compliment paid by the students is when they urge and encourage underclassmen and classmates to seek the services of the Retention Specialist because they personally found that "it works."

Summary of Dr. Bissett's Contribution

Current demand for nursing education is high, but without heightened awareness and action to ensure student retention, considerable waste of student and faculty resources can occur. Timely completion of nursing education is a winning situation for all. Students complete their course of study in the published time frame; college, faculty, and student resources are most efficiently used; and more graduates are prepared for introduction into the workforce. While recruitment efforts increase the number of nurse candidates on admission, retention efforts are needed to increase the number of nurse graduates ready for employment. The implementation of a Retention Specialist in nursing education programs is one important step toward improvement. Data regarding the effectiveness of a non-nursing Retention Specialist is compelling, and the position needs to be clearly dedicated to the nursing department, rather than a general position across campus, due to the unique difficulties faced by students of nursing. It is likely that both direct and indirect actions of the Retention Specialist contribute to the success that has been seen in programs employing this position.

Direct efforts are obvious in the explicit activities and contacts of the Retention Specialist.

Also of note are the indirect impacts of the presence of a Retention Specialist on the nursing team. The simple establishment of the position signifies commitment of administration to improvement of the nursing program for the benefit of students. Inherent in the retention dilemma is the need to make changes toward solutions, thus the willingness to bring a Retention Specialist to staff also suggests the readiness of a department for positive change. The presence of an active and focused Retention Specialist amid this implied commitment and readiness for change elicits a heightened level of awareness of each individual member of the faculty and staff regarding issues of retention. Additionally, knowledge of the availability of thoughtful retention services validates the students' experiences and sense of importance.

Hypothetical Nursing School Example

The faculty at the Hypothetical Nursing School (HNS) decided that an important addition to any Student Success Program is a Retention Specialist. The faculty agreed a Retention Specialist would be required if they were to increase their retention rate. The retention rate over the previous five years had not been above 75%. Because one of the goals the HNS faculty established was a retention rate of 85% on-time graduation and 15% graduation with one step-out, an attrition rate of 25% is no longer acceptable. The faculty believe this position is justified because retaining more students will maintain a higher enrollment which will support the cost of the position.

Pre-Nursing Success Course

Once the decision to hire a Retention Specialist was made, the faculty worked on a plan for a pre-nursing success course. The elements of that course follow.

Scheduling

The course will be two credit hours, indicating a total of 32 clock hours of class time. The course will be offered during the two weeks prior to the beginning of the first nursing course. It will be scheduled for two 8-hour days for two weeks. The faculty believe this scheduling best accommodates students who are admitted off the "wait list." The course will be co-taught by one nursing faculty and the Retention Specialist.

Requirements for Taking the Course

After a lengthy discussion, the faculty decided that not all nursing students will be required to take the course. The enrollment will be limited to students who meet a specific requirement. Any student who fits HNS's definition of "at-risk" will be required to take the course. HNS's definition of an at-risk student is as follows:

A student entering the Hypothetical Nursing School is considered at-risk for failing a nursing course if one or more of the following factors apply to that student:

1. Low GPA
2. Low science grades
3. Reading score below college level
4. No prior college experience
5. Difficulty with critical thinking
6. Difficulty with time management
7. Multiple family responsibilities
8. Works 20 or more hours per week

Currently, the admission policy for the HNS states that students must have a GPA or 2.5 or higher, read at the college level, score in the middle range or higher on a mathematical computation test, and earn a grade of C or higher in prerequisite courses of biology, chemistry, and anatomy and physiology. Based on the "at-risk" criteria and the admission policy guidelines, the faculty decided that students meeting one or more of the following criteria will be required to take the pre-nursing success course:

1. GPA between 2.5 and 3.4
2. A grade of C in any of the prerequisite science courses
3. Prior college experience limited to courses that are prerequisites for the nursing program

The faculty also decided to include in this group all students who scored at the middle range on the mathematical computation test.

Because all students must read at the college level for acceptance into the nursing program, reading level was not a factor. The other four factors (difficulty with critical thinking, difficulty with time management, multiple family responsibilities, and works 20 or more hours per week) represent data that is not available prior to admission. These factors will be assessed in the pre-nursing success course for those who enroll in that course and in the first nursing courses for all other entering students.

Curriculum Choke Points

HNS faculty had previously identified content areas that stood out as difficult for students over the last several years. These two areas were:
- study of the pediatric client with alterations in cardiac function
- study of the client with neuromuscular dysfunction

The faculty determined a review of cardiac and neuromuscular anatomy and physiology would be part of the pre-nursing success course. Very simple case studies will be used to demonstrate application of this content to nursing. The material related to these curriculum choke points will be tested in the program course where it applies. To determine if the pre-nursing course helped in these areas, students who completed the pre-nursing success course will be tracked and their scores compared to those students who were not enrolled in the pre-nursing course.

Course Outline

The HNS faculty agreed to use the topics presented in this chapter as the basis for their pre-nursing success course. In addition, faculty will spend time reviewing cardiac and neuromuscular anatomy and physiology. To determine the effectiveness of the pre-nursing course, students' grades will be tracked throughout the nursing program as well as their performance on the NCLEX. The faculty will use this information to determine if any changes in the pre-nursing course are warranted.

Chapter 5: Elements of a Student Success Program Prior to Entering a Nursing Program

Closing Thoughts

For a nursing student, a pre-nursing course can raise awareness of what a nursing program entails. Such a course prepares the student for the rigors of nursing school. Students can then plan their approach for success in a way that is realistic and practical. The concept that early intervention is the best intervention holds true for a pre-nursing course; in fact, a pre-nursing course is a proactive intervention that sets the stage for success in a nursing program. Students who are aware of what a program of nursing involves are empowered for success.

Learning Activities

1. Consider your school's definition of an at-risk nursing student. Structure a pre-nursing success course that you can offer for these students as a proactive intervention for their success.
2. Identify curriculum choke points. How can these choke points be addressed in a pre-nursing success course?
3. If your school does not currently employ a Retention Specialist consider how one might be used in your nursing program. Develop a job description including goals for the position, responsibilities, and measures of effectiveness.

References

Bolan, C. M., & Grainger, P. (2003). High school to nursing. *Canadian Nurse, 99*(3), 18-22.

Castellino A. R., & Schuster, P. M. (2002). Outcomes management. Evaluation of outcomes in nursing students using clinical concept map care plans. *Nurse Educator*, 27(4), 149-150.

Daley, B. J. (1996). Concept maps: Linking nursing theory to clinical practice. *Journal of Continuing Education in Nursing*, 27(1), 17-27.

Daley, B., Shaw, C., Balistieri, T., Glasenapp, K., & Piacentine, L. (1999). Concept maps: a strategy to teach and evaluate critical thinking. *Journal of Nursing Education*, 38(1), 42-47

Farrand, P., Hussain, F., & Hennessey, E. (2002). The efficacy of the mind map study technique. *Medical Education, 36*(5), 426-431.

Herrera-Shepard, D. (2006). *Student strategies to promote student success.* Paper presented at the Nurse Educator Institute, April 19, 2006.

Keane, K., DiMattio, N., & Gaudet, C. (2002). Education news. *Nursing Education Perspectives, 23*(3), 110-111.

Jeffreys, M. R. (2004). *Nursing student retention: Understanding the process and making a difference.* New York: Springer.

Lockie, N. M., & Burke, L. (1999). Partnership in learning for utmost success (PLUS): Evaluation of a retention program for at-risk nursing students. *Journal of Nursing Education, 38*(4), 188-192.

Lunyk-Child, O. I., Crooks, D., Ellis, P. J., Ofosu, C., O'Mara, L., & Rideout, E. (2001). Self-directed learning: Faculty and student perceptions. *Journal of Nursing Education, 40*(3), 116-123.

Ofori, R., & Charlton, J. P. (2002). A path model of factors influencing the academic performance of nursing students. *Journal of Advanced Nursing, 38*(5), 507-515.

Rooda, L. A. (1994). Effects of minds mapping on student achievement in a nursing research course. *Nurse Educator,* 19(6), 25-27.

Symes, L., Tart, K., & Travis, L. (2005). An evaluation of the nursing success program. *Nurse Educator, 30*(5), 217-220.

Symes, L., Tart, K., Travis, L., & Toombs, M. S. (2002). Developing and retaining expert learners: The student success program. *Nurse Educator, 27*(5), 227-231.

Tracey, G. (2003). A national study of support programs (efforts) in baccalaureate and associate degree programs to enhance retention and success of students. (Doctoral dissertation, University of Central Florida, 2003). *Dissertation Abstracts International, 64*(2598).

Wells, M. (2003). An epidemiologic approach to addressing student attrition in nursing programs. *Journal of Professional Nursing, 19*(3), 230-236.

Wheeler, L.A., & Collins, S.R. (2003). The influence of concept mapping on critical thinking in baccalaureate nursing students. *Journal of Professional Nursing, 19*(6), 339-346.

Wilkes, L., Cooper, K., Lewein, J., & Batts, J. (1999). Concept mapping: Promoting science learning in BN learners in Australia. *The Journal of Continuing Education in Nursing, 30*(1), 37-44.

Chapter 6: A Student Success Program for Currently Enrolled Students

Chapters 2, 3, and 4 discuss the data needed to develop a Student Success Program. Such data includes assessment of the at-risk student, formulation of an admissions policy that positions a student for success in a nursing program, and student assessment to frame the challenges students face.

Once this data is collected what do you do with it? Remember, data is a means, not the end! It is important to use data to formulate academic and nonacademic support that impacts student learning. The end result should be a Student Success Program with positive outcomes. Chapter 5 discussed essential elements of a Student Success Program before students enter nursing courses. This chapter presents the next phase of the Student Success Program, support for students once they have entered nursing courses. The chapter provides an in-depth look at three major elements essential to the development of a Student Success Program: academic support, non-academic support, and cultural considerations. A discussion of the implementation, evaluation, and revision of a Student Success Program concludes the chapter.

Overview of a Student Success Program

The task at hand is to develop a Student Success Program for the entire class with individualized interventions for those students characterized as "at-risk." The class Student Success Program includes interventions that benefit all students. Examples include instruction on basic math for dosage calculations, test-taking related to nursing exams, how to use critical thinking skills, and resources available for financial need. Interventions of a Student Success Program for individual students considered at-risk may include mandatory enrollment in a pre-nursing course, individual tutoring, or special courses planned throughout the nursing program. Such courses might be tailored to review material presented in regularly scheduled classes to ensure that students comprehend concepts and learn how to apply information presented in program courses.

The overall process for using a Student Success Program is to identify, inform, and intervene.

First, identify student needs. Identification begins upon admission to the institution using admission data or a pre-nursing course that prepares students for the nursing program.

Second, inform the students of the results of the assessment data from the Checklist of Positive and Negative Factors (see Table 2.6) and the *Start Right in Nursing School: A Self-Assessment Tool* ™ from College of DuPage by the start of the first course in the nursing program.

Third, intervene early for increased success for students. Interventions are proactive. Some interventions are designed to anticipate and meet needs of the student population at large. For example, the entire class might benefit from an overview of math as it applies to medication administration. In contrast, interventions established for the individual, at-risk student are by necessity highly individualized, depending on identified needs or concerns.

Essential Elements for a Student Success Program

The essential elements of a Student Success Program are discussed in this chapter. These elements are grouped into three main categories: academic support, non-academic support, and cultural considerations. Figure 6.1 provides an overview of the essential elements that comprise a Student Success Program.

Academic Support

Figure 6.1 lists the many components that comprise academic support for students. These components are implemented immediately when students begin the nursing program and conclude when they graduate. Each component is important when designing academic support for the Student Success Program.

Creative Class Scheduling

Consider current class offerings and clinical sessions. Determine if the best approach is used to meet student needs and facilitate learning. Look at time

Chapter 6: A Student Success Program for Currently Enrolled Students

Figure 6.1 – Elements of a Student Success Program

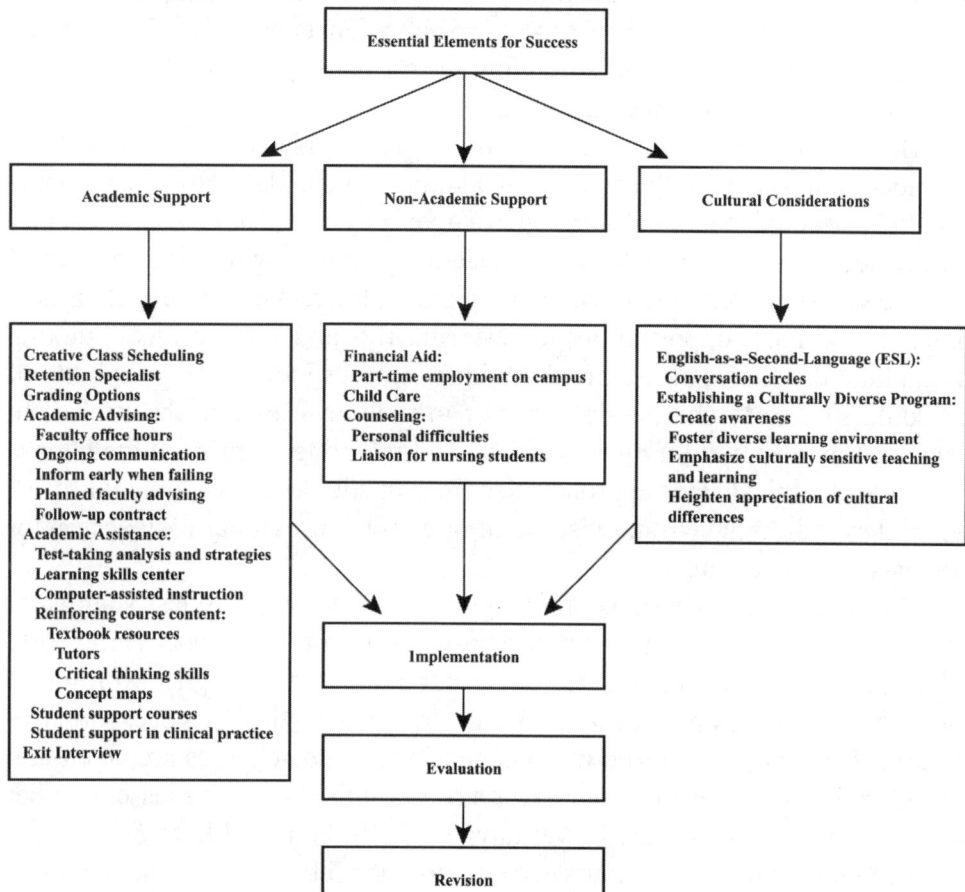

spent for both clinical and classroom instruction. Weigh the pros and cons of instructional strategies in light of ways in which to schedule classes. For example, students may be required to go to the clinical site the day before a clinical class to gather data to develop a care plan for assigned clients. Students spend travel time the day before and may be up late into the night to prepare the required assignment. The next day, the students are expected to perform at an optimal level. However, students may be tired, a less than favorable state for the necessary cognitive function required for safe practice. Also, clients may have been discharged or transferred prior to students having an opportunity to provide care the subsequent day. Consider the benefit of this practice. Would a reasonable alternative be to allow students time to learn about clients during the clinical day or to arrive a few hours early to gather data? Might expectations be tempered to allow for this learning on site, with an instructor present who can focus students and still meet expected outcomes?

The number of hours spent in a clinical session also deserves thoughtful consideration. What are the benefits of a longer clinical day? How many hours should be devoted to clinical learning in a given day: 6, 8, 10, 12 hours? Faculty may believe longer clinical days provide less days traveling to and from clinical sites, fewer days spent at clinical while yielding the requisite hours of clinical practice, and more opportunities to perform skills and apply critical thinking throughout the course of the day. Additional benefits include the possibility of scheduling days off when students do not go to clinical sessions the week of an exam, essentially building in study days and relieving them from the intense demands of clinical. This approach also frees faculty to be available for office hours they would have otherwise spent in clinical, providing easy access for students prior to testing.

The negative implications of a longer clinical day may be less stamina to contend with longer days and limited exposure to a variety of clients, particularly when census is low and specific client populations are sought. More days, rather than fewer, may provide more chances to encounter the types of experiences desired. This may not be true when admissions and discharges are taken into consideration. Perhaps a 10-hour day is a compromise between a lesser number of hours and a 12-hour day. Fewer days may still be possible to provide the required number of clinical hours and eliminate the fatigue of a 12-hour clinical session. Each approach offers potential advantages and disadvantages. Consider which approach best meets your learning objectives.

Rethinking past approaches to scheduling classes can result in better use of time. Whatever your approach, share the rationale for that approach during course orientation. Relate the class scheduling to time management. For example, when clinical scheduling permits fewer days in clinical, suggest students not build in more work time, but that they take advantage of this time to study. Sharing the rationale and suggestions for use of the time further serves to educate students about success strategies.

Chapter 6: A Student Success Program for Currently Enrolled Students

Retention Specialist

The role of the Retention Specialist was discussed in Chapter 5. This professional is an important part of a Student Success Program. Refer to Chapter 5 for a full discussion of this position.

Grading Options

Communicate clearly from the onset how individual assignments are graded, such as pass/fail, satisfactory/unsatisfactory, or letter grade, as well as the overall means of grading for the course. Any rubrics used to determine grades should be provided at the onset of the assignment. Sample papers, examination questions, and resources are useful to students in gaining a clear understanding of expectations and possible approaches to the content they are learning to master.

Academic Advising

The faculty teaching the course or a Retention Specialist may serve as an academic advisor. The academic advisor provides students with information about what to expect in the course, how to meet these expectations, and the best way to communicate with their advisor, such as when office hours are held or when e-mail communications are answered. Academic advising is most effective when implemented early. If the intent of academic advising is to provide timely counsel for students to circumvent or address a concern, the academic advisor establishes clear communication pathways with students to meet this goal.

Faculty office hours. Establish and maintain office hours that allow students to avail themselves of faculty help. It may be possible to hold office hours at the clinical site so students do not have to return to campus to meet with faculty. Online synchronous chat times or virtual office hours present additional options. Discuss with students which options best meet their needs to determine how and when to conduct office hours. Post or communicate office hours so students will know how to reach faculty.

Ongoing communication. Open lines of communication between students and faculty are important for information exchange in a timely, pertinent fashion. Important or especially complex information should be in writing, so students can refer to this information throughout the term. Whatever method of communication is selected, and how and what to communicate, should be determined at the beginning of the term so students know what to expect. For example, faculty may opt to post information online, or send communications via phone-tree or e-mail. Students also need to feel comfortable communicating with faculty and believe the environment is conducive to such exchanges. When students perceive the lines of communication are open, they feel what they have to say is valued. An open, inviting line of communication forms the basis of a helping relationship, contributing to student success.

Inform early when failing. The sooner a student is aware of an academic problem, the sooner interventions may be planned and realized. Without faculty intervention, students may believe they have a handle on the problem when in fact they do not. When the student realizes a problem exits, a time crunch may negate implementation of interventions to enable the student to pass the course. Consider the student who fails the first exam in a nursing program that requires a C average in all nursing coursework. The student does not seek help and gets a better grade on the second exam, but still has a D average. If the student waits until the third or fourth test of the term to seek help, the student may not be able to pass the course. The student realizes this situation when the course is three-quarters over and has not mastered material that may be revisited in some shape or form – a cumulative exam or carry through of a concept. In addition, there is now a great deal of stress due to the need to do well with little or no margin for error. Early faculty contact to discuss a problem can circumvent problems in the long run.

Planned faculty advising. Determine when and under what circumstances faculty advise students. There may be set points throughout a term during which contact occurs for students and faculty to evaluate student progress within the course. Faculty may track individual student progress in clinical and classroom environments and meet with each student on a predetermined schedule. During these sessions, faculty and students can together design interventions to address identified needs.

Follow-up contract. Students who experience difficulty in their clinical performance or with their classroom testing may benefit from a structured contract that delineates specific behaviors to help them succeed in the course. The purpose of the contract is to identify the area of concern and establish a means to overcome deficiencies or lapses in performance. For example, a student displaying unprofessional behavior would be expected to change the behaviors of concern. An example of unprofessional behavior is tardiness. The contract might include arriving on time for class.

Opportunities to discuss the concern often provide insights that faculty can use either to design interventions with the student or obtain help they might otherwise not have known the student needed. The student's progress in meeting the terms of the contract is assessed periodically throughout the term. The frequency of such assessments can be part of the contract. Attainment of established goals is noted and further revision or extension of the contract is implemented as necessary or feasible.

Academic Assistance

Faculty may perceive that academic assistance occurs after the fact, when a student is in grave difficulty in the course, perhaps already failing. Examine the concept of academic assistance from a different vantage, a proactive strategy employed to assist students to achieve the highest level possible. Ideally, this assistance is provided when the student first enters the nursing program. This approach encourages students to avail themselves of faculty and institutional resources.

In particular, testing has been a major concern among nurse educators, as they strive for ways to position their students effectively for success on tests within their program and on NCLEX. The next sections discuss several approaches to assist students to achieve academic success.

Test-taking analysis and strategies. Ideally, exam reviews occur after each exam with the class at-large followed by individual exam reviews. Such reviews provide an opportunity for immediate feedback, when the exam is fresh in the student's mind.

Exam Analysis Program

The Exam Analysis Program developed by the Loma Linda University School of Nursing (LLUSN) Learning Assistance Program (LAP) provides an avenue for the student and faculty to discuss test results in detail, identify problem areas, and offer techniques for successful testing. Objective data that students and faculty review together provides insights that may lend to better testing on subsequent tests. The Exam Analysis Program consists of six components:

- exam analysis
- summary of exam techniques for multiple choice questions
- the exam analysis procedure
- objective exam analysis worksheet
- assessment and intervention protocol
- suggestions to improve exam performance.

Figures 6.2 through 6.7 provide an overview of each of the above components of the Exam Analysis Program.

College of DuPage Press and Drs. Linda Caputi and Lynn Engelmann wish to thank the author, Vaneta M. Condon PhD, RN, Associate Professor, for her assistance and Loma Linda University for permission to include their Exam Analysis Program in *Teaching Nursing: The Art and Science – It's All About Student Success.*

Figure 6.2 – Exam Analysis

LOMA LINDA UNIVERSITY SCHOOL OF NURSING LEARNING ASSISTANCE PROGRAM EXAM ANALYSIS

The exam analysis was developed by the LLUSN LAP staff to help students who perform poorly on examinations to identify problem areas. Using the student's exam paper, the student and instructor/learning facilitator discuss each question that was answered incorrectly. The purpose of doing this is to identify the reason why the student chose the incorrect answer.

In this way it is possible to identify how many questions were answered incorrectly due to lack of knowledge (retention or application) of the subject matter as compared to the number of questions missed due to use of poor exam techniques (failure to identify key words, failure to consider each option carefully, changing answers etc.) Exam anxiety, English language and other problems interfering with success on examinations are also identified. Weak understandings of specific concepts and content areas can

Chapter 6: A Student Success Program for Currently Enrolled Students

also be noted as areas requiring remediation.

The instructor/learning facilitator and the student then plan interventions that will assist the student to strengthen specific exam skills, study habits, concepts or content areas.

Loma Linda University grants permission for other schools to use the Exam Analysis method to assist individual students to improve examination performance. However, use of this method for profit, publication or research requires permission for use from Loma Linda University.
Vaneta M. Condon, PhD, RN.
Coordinator, Learning Assistance Program
Associate Professor, Undergraduate Nursing
vcondon@llu.edu

Copyright 2006, Loma Linda University

Figure 6.3 – Summary of Exam Techniques for Multiple Choice Questions

LOMA LINDA UNIVERSITY SCHOOL OF NURSING LEARNING ASSISTANCE PROGRAM SUMMARY OF EXAM TECHNIQUES FOR MULTIPLE CHOICE QUESTIONS

A. <u>Be Sure You Know What The Question is Asking</u>
- Read question carefully.
- <u>Underline</u> important words.
- Try to answer the questions yourself <u>before</u> you look at the answer options.
- Create a pool of possible answers (jot down key word(s) for each)

B. <u>Consider Each Option Carefully</u>
- Compare answer options given on exam with your own pool of possible answers.
- Re-read the question carefully.
- Read the answer options carefully underlining key words.

- Mark each answer option as either true, false, T?, F?, or ?.
C. <u>Use Your Knowledge When Choosing the Best Answer</u>
    - Choose your answer based on what you have learned in the course. Example: Choose answer marked true above one marked?
    - Do not choose an answer just because "it sounds good" if you have not heard of it before (in lecture or textbook) – it may be a cleverly worded distractor.
D. <u>Use Your Time Wisely</u>
    - Do not spend too long on any one question.
    - Read the question and answer options carefully (twice if necessary).
    - If you are not sure which choice is correct, guess and mark the question number so you can come back to it if you have time.
    - Do not be in a hurry to leave. Check your paper to be sure you have answered all questions.
    - Check carefully for clerical errors (marking wrong answer by mistake).
    - Read each stem with the answer you have marked to be sure it makes sense.
E. <u>If You Do Not Understand The Question or Answer Option Ask For Help</u>
    - Ask the instructor to clarify what is not clear.
    - Ask the instructor to "restate" a confusing question or option.
F. <u>Do Not Change Your Answers</u>
    - The only time you should change an answer is when you know <u>why</u> the first answer is wrong and/or <u>why</u> the second answer is right.
    - Never change an answer just because you feel uncertain.

Copyright 2006, Loma Linda University

Figure 6.4 – Exam Analysis Procedure

> **LOMA LINDA UNIVERSITY SCHOOL OF NURSING**
> **LEARNING ASSISTANCE PROGRAM**
> **THE EXAM ANALYSIS PROCEDURE**
>
> 1. The student and instructor/learning facilitator become aware that the student has a problem with taking exams.
> 2. The student requests an exam analysis.
> 3. The student and instructor/learning facilitator, who are doing the analysis, discuss the LAP Summary of Exam techniques.
> 4. The student and instructor/learning facilitator go over each question which the student missed on the exam. The student uses the exam techniques to answer these questions. (The student does not look at the former answer or at the correct answer on the answer key).
> 5. The student and instructor/learning facilitator identify the main category and specific problem or contributing factor for why the student missed each question.
> 6. The instructor/learning facilitator records why each item was missed on the exam analysis worksheet.
> 7. The instructor/learning facilitator totals the number of items missed and the percentages for each specific problem and each main category.
> 8. Suggested interventions are developed with input from the student and recorded on the Suggestions to Improve Exam Performance checklist.
> 9. A copy of the exam analysis is given to the student, and another is retained in the student's record.
> 10. Follow-up appointments (or referrals) for help with exam skills, tutoring, counseling, and evaluation of progress are made.

Copyright 2006, Loma Linda University

Teaching Nursing: The Art and Science

Figure 6.5 – Learning Assistance Program Objective Exam Analysis Worksheet

Test Item Missed	INSUFFICIENT INFORMATION					TEST ANXIETY				LACK OF TEST SKILLS							OTHER		
	I did not read the text thoroughly.	The information was not in my notes.	I studied the information but could not remember it.	I knew the information, but could not apply it.	I studied the wrong information.	I experienced a mental block.	I spent too much time daydreaming.	I was so tired I could not concentrate.	I panicked.	I carelessly marked a wrong choice.	I changed a correct answer to a wrong one.	I did not choose the best choice.	I did not notice qualifiers.	I did not notice a negative.	I misread the question.	I made poor use of the time provided.			
Number of Items Missed																			

Copyright 2006, Loma Linda University

Figure 6.6 – LLUSN Learning Assistance Program Exam Analysis: Assessment and Intervention Protocol

PROBLEM AREA	POTENTIALLY RELATED FACTORS	ASSESSMENT NEEDED	POSSIBLE INTERVENTIONS
I. Lack of Knowledge of Subject Matter	Poor retention of information	Determine whether or not student spends adequate time in study and/or review.	• Help student set up schedule using the PLRS cycle. (Preview lecture, review, and intensive study). • Set up a pre-exam schedule. • Encourage student to make flash cards, summary sheets, etc. for drilling on important information.
	Inadequate lecture notes	Determine whether information needed to answer the questions the student missed was given in lecture or taken from textbook. If it was given in lecture, check to see if the information is in the student's notes. Is the information adequately recorded?	• Set up note-sharing with a peer tutor. • Encourage student to share notes with others in a study group. • Encourage student to get help in improving note-taking skills. • Encourage student to record lectures with a tape recorder and then complete notes from the tape after class.
	Failure to understand concept well enough to apply knowledge correctly	Attempt to pinpoint what the student does not understand.	• Encourage student to study with the goal of understanding – not memorizing. • Encourage student to compare textbook with other sources in order to clarify concept. • Encourage student to seek help from instructors. • Set up tutoring for the student with goal of discussing important concepts including possible applications. • Encourage student to discuss concepts with other students in a study group setting.

PROBLEM AREA	POTENTIALLY RELATED FACTORS	ASSESSMENT NEEDED	POSSIBLE INTERVENTIONS
II. Inadequate English Language Skills			
Reading Comprehension	Failure to understand the meaning of the question(s) and/or the answer option(s)	Ask the student to restate or explain the question or option.	• Encourage the student to seek clarification from the instructor to be sure the question or answer option is understood correctly. • Encourage student to seek help with reading comprehension skills.
Vocabulary	Inadequate vocabulary to understand the meaning of question(s) or answer option(s)	Ask the student to restate or explain the meaning of the word(s) causing the difficulty. Determine whether difficulty is with medical or general vocabulary terms.	• Encourage student to look up unfamiliar words in a dictionary when studying. • Encourage student to make a list of all new vocabulary encountered. • Encourage student to make flash cards of unfamiliar words with their meanings. Drill with these flash cards. Use these words in sentences. Practice pronouncing these words. • Encourage student to work on vocabulary programs. Several levels of general vocabulary and medical programs are available in L.A.P.
Reading Speed	Lack of time to complete all items on examination(s) or unwise use of time	Determine whether or not student answered all items. Determine whether or not items left undone were unfinished due to lack of time.	• Encourage student not to spend too long on any one item. • Encourage student to read question carefully (twice if necessary), then guess if not sure of correct answer and mark the question to come back to it if time permits. • Discuss with instructor(s) whether or not it is possible for ESL student to have extra time to complete exam. • Encourage student to get help to improve reading speed.

Chapter 6: A Student Success Program for Currently Enrolled Students

PROBLEM AREA	POTENTIALLY RELATED FACTORS	ASSESSMENT NEEDED	POSSIBLE INTERVENTIONS
III. Exam Anxiety			

Unable to concentrate during the exam	Does not read questions or answer options carefully enough	Determine whether or not the student is able to answer the questions correctly during the exam analysis (when student is not under the stress of taking an exam).	• Practice good exam techniques with student to develop a specific routine to follow in answering every exam question.
			A. Concentrate on what the question is asking:
			  o Underline key words.
			  o Jot down own answer before looking at answer options.
			B. Consider each option carefully:
			  o Underline key words.
			  o Make each option as true, false, true? or false?
			C. Choose answer using information you have learned during the course.
			• Practice using above techniques – A,B,C before each exam quiz, or when answering review questions, etc.

Student gets "easy" questions wrong	Student does not bother to use the steps involved in good exam techniques on "easy" questions		• Encourage student to use these techniques on <u>every</u> question – not just those that are difficult.
Mental Block – (can't remember what has been learned during the exam due to anxiety)	Did not learn material thoroughly enough Lacks confidence in ability to do well on exam Unable to break exam anxiety cycle (can't relax)		• Over-learning may help. • Drill with flash cards on important concepts and related materials. This will build confidence in knowledge of materials. • Practice relaxation techniques frequently so student can use them to break panic cycle during exam. • If problem persists, refer student for psychological counseling.

PROBLEM AREA	POTENTIALLY RELATED FACTORS	ASSESSMENT NEEDED	POSSIBLE INTERVENTIONS
IV. Poor Exam Skills	Read questions carelessly or too quickly. Fail to note key words	Have student answer the question without looking at the former answer or the correct answer. Then ask the student why the wrong answer was chosen on the exam.	Teach student to: • Read each question carefully. • Underline key words. • Attempt to answer question (jot down "pool of answers" before looking at answer options). This ensures that student understands <u>what</u> is being asked.
	Did not consider each option carefully		• Underline key words in options. • Compare you "pool" of possible answers with answer options on exam. • Mark each option as true, false,? true?, or false?
	Chose attractively worded distractor		• Choose answer you have marked true above one marked? • Use knowledge you have learned in course – do not choose something unfamiliar just because it "sounds good."
Changed answer from right to wrong	"Read too much into the question"	Note how many answers student changed. Calculate the percentage of questions changed that the student got wrong.	• Never change an answer unless you know <u>why</u> the first choice was wrong and/or <u>why</u> the second choice is right. Never change an answer just because of uncertainty or lack of confidence in your knowledge. First impressions are usually right. Later on you may "read too much into the questions."
Difficulty with "<u>except</u>" questions		Note whether or not student has frequent difficulty with "<u>except</u>" or negatively worded questions.	• Disregard the word "<u>except</u>"/ negative word. • Mark each option as true, false or ? • Choose answer that is different from the others. • Re-read step including "<u>except</u>" with answer option chosen to be sure your answer makes sense.

Chapter 6: A Student Success Program for Currently Enrolled Students

PROBLEM AREA	POTENTIALLY RELATED FACTORS	ASSESSMENT NEEDED	POSSIBLE INTERVENTIONS
IV. Poor Exam Skills (cont.)			**Teach student to:**
Failure to use time wisely • Did not answer all of the questions • Failed to answer a question even though student knew correct answer	Spent too long on difficult question(s). Did not have enough time left to answer all of the "easy" questions		• Don't spend too long on one question. • Read question carefully twice if necessary. • Guess if you don't know. • Mark question number and come back if time permits.
Did not answer essay question adequately	Did not note difference in number of points given for each question	Determine whether or not the student knew other key factors and failed to include them in the answer.	• Give more time to questions worth more points. • Make outline (include all key points) before writing answer for each essay question.
"Forgot" to answer question(s)	Carelessness or lack of concentration		• Do not be in a hurry to leave. • Take time to recheck paper to be sure all questions have been answered.
Marked wrong answer "by mistake" on the scantron card	Carelessness or lack of concentration		• Take time to check paper for clerical errors. • Re-read each question with the option you have chosen to be sure you have marked the answer you intended.
V. Other (Please specify)			

Copyright 2006, Loma Linda University

Figure 6.7 – Suggestions to Improve Exam Performance

Name: _____ Date: _____ Class: _____

Priority # _____ Lack of Knowledge of Subject Matter

_____ 1. Use study guide/objectives/specific class guidelines to identify important content while reading textbook.
_____ 2. Write out key points from #1 and use for later review.
_____ 3. Take careful notes during class.
_____ 4. As soon as possible <u>after class</u> and at <u>the end of each week</u> review #2 and #3 from above.
_____ 5. Participate in study group each week.
_____ 6. Use NCLEX-RN review books to review important content and to practice application on review questions.
_____ 7. Predict exam questions. Use these for group review.
_____ 8. Schedule time to review each lecture carefully before each exam.
_____ 9. Note weak areas such as pathophysiology, medication side effects, lab values, etc.
_____ 10. Other: _____

Priority # _____ Exam-taking skills

_____ 1. Read each question carefully and <u>underline or circle key words</u>.
_____ 2. Give your <u>own answer</u> (write down a few words BEFORE looking at choices given on exam).
_____ 3. Mark each answer choice as T, F, ?, T?, or F?.
_____ 4. Choose the best answer based on what you learned in this class.
_____ 5. Don't change an answer unless you <u>know why</u> the first answer is wrong. (<u>Never</u> change an answer just because you <u>feel uncertain</u>).

Chapter 6: A Student Success Program for Currently Enrolled Students

_____ 6. <u>Practice application</u> of knowledge using <u>case studies and NCLEX-RN review questions</u>.
_____ 7. Other: _____

Priority # _____ English Language/Vocabulary

_____ 1. Look up vocabulary terms/new words identified in reading assignment, lecture, and study groups, etc.
_____ 2. Write out the meanings of these words, note pronunciation and use them in a sentence, make flash cards or write them in a notebook.
_____ 3. Drill on these words several times each week.
_____ 4. If you don't understand an exam question or answer choice, ask the instructor for clarification.
_____ 5. Other: _____

Priority # _____ Exam Anxiety

_____ 1. <u>Over-prepare for exams</u> so that you feel <u>confident</u> about your knowledge.
_____ 2. Use recommended exam skills on every question. This helps you think logically.
_____ 3. Use positive self-talk- i.e. "I know these concepts," "I am going to do well on this exam."
_____ 4. Don't spend too long on a difficult question. This lowers your confidence and increases anxiety. Read it carefully 2 times, guess and move on to easier questions. Come back later if you have time.
_____ 5. Pray that God will help you feel calm, remember what you have learned and apply knowledge and exam skills. *
_____ 6. Practice relaxation techniques (deep breathing, etc.) so you can use them p.r.n.
_____ 7. Other: _____
Priority # _____ Other (Please Specify Below):

* Loma Linda University, as a basic philosophy, stresses the unity of spiritual life and wholeness.

Copyright 2006, Loma Linda University

A copy of the Exam Analysis Program (Figures 6.2 though 6.7) may be accessed on the CD-ROM accompanying this book.

Condon and Drew (1995) surveyed 105 nursing students who had completed the Exam Analysis at Loma Linda University. The purpose of the survey was to collect student opinions pertaining to the effectiveness of the Exam Analysis in improving student examination performance. Students in their study ranged from 20 to 54 years of age. Of these, 49% were over 25 years old. The population surveyed was 11% male, 33% Asian, 30% White/Anglo, 19% African American/Black, 13% Hispanic, and 5% other/missing data. While 65% of the population surveyed spoke English as a primary language, 51% had at least one parent whose primary language was not English.

Students in this study ranked from most to least important the following exam-taking techniques:
- identifying key words in the questions
- formulating an answer to a multiple choice question before reading the answer options
- considering each answer option carefully
- marking each option true or false
- using "test-wise" guessing strategies

Overall, a large majority of students surveyed expressed a positive opinion of the Exam Analysis Program. While this study provides perspective from the students' viewpoint, limitations of the study include not measuring examination scores before and after exam analysis. The authors recommend repeating the study using a qualitative approach to validate the Exam Analysis as an accepted method to enhance exam performance (Condon & Drew, 1995).

Integrative Review – Collaborative Testing

Another test-taking strategy that faculty might employ is collaborative testing. Prior to recommending this educational strategy, the authors performed an integrative review to explore how collaborative testing has been used to enhance learning for nursing students. In this integrative review, three questions were posed:
1. What guidelines for collaborative testing have been reported in the current literature?

2. What evidence is available that describes the effectiveness of collaborative testing to enhance learning for nursing students?
3. What are the problems identified with the use of collaborative testing?

The integrative review considered all studies between 1995 and 2006 that addressed collaborative testing to enhance learning for nursing students. A search of the literature revealed 10 articles that addressed collaborative testing. Of these, seven research studies were included in the integrative review (Hickey, 2006; Ligeikis-Clayton, 1996; Lusk, 2003; Mitchell & Melton, 2003; Rossignol, 2004; Vinten & Ellett, 2000; Wink, 2004).

Following is a summary of findings related to the three research questions: Question 1: What guidelines for collaborative testing have been reported in the current literature?

- random or assigned pairs for dyad testing may be used. Consider the pros and cons of allowing students to self-select their groups versus faculty assigning the groups. For example, if faculty assign the groups for dyad testing it is possible to establish more equality within the group, balancing the number of students who achieve A, B, or C grades. In contrast, if students self-select their group members, they may choose to work with others who earn similar grades. Student learning may be impacted by variables such as the student's knowledge of the content and the student's willingness to share that knowledge with other group members. Totally random assignment may promote collaboration skills that would not have been realized if an assigned-pairs approach is used. Faculty may be in a better position to evaluate the best method to use to establish dyad pairs once they gain a sense of group dynamics. Whatever method is selected should be based on the objectives the faculty hope to achieve.
- determine which types of tests lend best to collaborative testing. Literature revealed researchers used both multiple choice and short answer tests for collaborative testing.
- if time for testing is limited, use tests with fewer number of items. Allow enough time for both individual and collaborative testing. In general, the collaborative testing does not require as much time as the individual testing. Do not rush students through individual testing.
- determine how points will be awarded. How many points would be an acceptable gain for students on the collaborative test? It is possible to

structure test percentages so students earn most of their points on their individual tests and the remaining points on the collaborative test?
- determine the mechanics for giving the tests. Decide whether the group will submit one answer sheet or if each individual student will submit their own answer sheet for the collaborative test. Students might take the test individually, then discuss items; or, they might take the test collectively, with no individual testing.

Question 2: What evidence is available that describes the effectiveness of collaborative testing to enhance learning for nursing students? Findings include:
- typically, students increased their test scores on the test they took collaboratively. Studies suggested students learned during collaboration by processing test items and their rationales. All students may not learn something new if their responses were correct on individual testing; however, knowledge for these students was validated during the process of group discussion.
- studies suggested the following benefits of collaborative testing: better critical thinking and problem solving skills, increased confidence in personal abilities, decreased test anxiety, and enhanced communication skills, which are necessary to discuss effectively rationales for selected responses. These findings were derived from surveys conducted by researchers. They represent opinions of students and faculty as opposed to quantitative data.

Question 3: What are the problems identified with the use of collaborative testing? Findings include:
- insufficient time for testing frustrates students. Faculty must provide sufficient time for individual and collaborative testing periods.
- students experience anxiety with some aspects of collaborative testing. Anxiety is precipitated by not knowing group members, or being confident that all students in the group will prepare for tests and not simply rely on other students to study and provide the answers for them.
- students may be frustrated by the ability of others potentially to persuade a student to change a right answer to a wrong answer. At times, students disagree. If the group submits one answer sheet, consensus must be reached. If students are allowed to select their own answer after group

- discussion and submit individual answer sheets, this may be less of an issue.
- depending on how the two tests are processed and scored, students may or may not fully engage in the process of collaborative testing. For example, if students are allowed to submit an individual answer sheet, they may decide to hold back in the collaborative testing session, especially if they feel others have not done their part to contribute to the group.

This integrative review is limited in scope by the paucity of research articles that discuss collaborative testing in nursing education. Nonetheless, evidence suggests several benefits from this practice. The following is offered as an evidence base for the use and application of collaborative testing in nursing education:

- communication and negotiation skills: students engaged in the process of collaborative testing must demonstrate sound rationales for their answers and the ability to communicate these rationales to their testing partners. Communication skills are essential to practice as a licensed nurse.
- critical thinking and comprehension of material: students are challenged to identify and explain why an answer is either correct or incorrect. They must apply information to a situation and demonstrate knowledge of the content. Critical thinking skills are also essential to practice as a licensed nurse.
- test-taking skills: students learn how others process and synthesize information as they discuss how answers were derived. Better understanding of rationales for test items and learning how to navigate tests are facilitated through collaborative testing. Enhanced test-taking skills serve students in future test situations.
- enhanced confidence: students gain confidence through the process of collaboration. Their testing process is either validated or they learn new ways to approach testing and improve their test-taking ability. This builds confidence for future testing.
- decreased test-taking anxiety: in all but one of the studies, students reported a decrease in test-taking anxiety. If students are able to decrease anxiety, a more realistic view of student performance may be realized.

To enact collaborative testing faculty should:
- determine which objectives will be met with use of collaborative testing and how these objectives will be measured. For example, determine guidelines for participation in collaborative testing and provide these guidelines to students in advance of the test date. Observe students during the collaborative testing for their ability to meet the objectives, which might include:
    o demonstrate negotiation and collaboration skills
    o explain rationale for test items
    o verbalize the critical thinking skill used to respond to test items
- consider the following when designing a test using the collaborative testing approach:
    o level of difficulty
    o number of items
    o amount of time for testing
    o total points for the course
    o percentage collaborative test comprises of total course grade
- establish procedure for testing:
    o number of students per group
    o use of group answer sheet or individual answer sheet
    o guidelines for discussion and selection of answer
- establish procedure for grading the collaborative test. Options include:
    o calculate the individual and group test grades
    o record the grade that is higher
    o limit the total number of additional points possible based on objectives of the course and level of difficulty of the test

The use of collaborative testing in nursing education appears to provide several benefits relative to student learning and merits further study. Future studies are needed to identify learner characteristics that most benefit from participating in collaborative testing.

Refer to the CD-ROM accompanying this book for a complete discussion of the process used to conduct this integrative review.

Learning skills center. Many educational settings establish a skills center where students may obtain help with academic needs related to successful course completion. For example, students may need assistance to hone their reading, math, or language abilities. The student's self-assessment, as discussed in Chapter 4, identifies particular needs, which may be addressed by the skills center.

If a skills center is not formally established within the institution, nursing faculty may establish liaisons with faculty in English, math, and English-as-a-second-language (ESL) divisions to help design instruction to meet student needs. Remediation or instruction might be offered through independent study or small group sessions.

Faculty may also document the need for a skills center and seek administrative support. Proposals may be written for grant funds to establish a skills center or provide other means to meet student learning needs that a skills center might provide. Schools may wish to consider grant procurement individually, or in conjunction with another facility that would share the resource.

Websites, such as mathhomework.com, which provides instruction and tutoring in basic math concepts, offer another avenue to meet specific needs in the absence of a learning skills center.

Computer-assisted instruction. Content needs may be addressed via computer-assisted instruction. Faculty may evaluate and recommend purchase of instructional media accessed via computer. Computer labs offer students an opportunity to take advantage of a multitude of resources that are specific to particular course content, which are purchased and networked by the institution. Computer labs located at multiple sites allow students greater flexibility in utilization of resources if the programs are not available via the internet.

Students are made aware of the availability of these resources and contact names and hours of operation. Provide students with guidelines about how to use the instructional media. It is essential to have support staff in place should students have questions or difficulty accessing materials.

Reinforcing course content – textbook resources. Textbooks, dense with information, often intimidate students. Students experience difficulty distinguishing important from not so important content. They get lost in the pages. Depending on the structure, organization, and reading level of the text, students may be frustrated in using it for effective study. For these reasons teachers encourage the use of textbook resources and devote some time explaining to students how to use these resources.

Typically, publishers include a variety of organizing schemes to augment the text, which include objectives, a review of physiology, highlighted text boxes with special topics, concept maps, care plans, critical thinking challenges, and case studies. Additional learning aides include CD-ROMs with a variety of tools and a website that offers an expanded discussion of a topic presented in the text. Additional websites for further study of a topic may be provided. Many texts have accompanying workbooks or study guides that focus students on key concepts, which may prove beneficial to class preparation.

Reinforcing course content – tutors. Students may not fully comprehend concepts or relationships presented in class or in their textbook. Another person's perspective might focus their view of the content they are attempting to learn. Tutoring sessions can provide additional support. Some nursing programs establish mandatory review sessions with a tutor for students who are not obtaining a minimum score on course tests.

Tutors should possess a special skill set, which includes knowledge of the subject matter, well-developed interpersonal skills, and an ability to identify problems areas the student being tutored is experiencing (Higgins, 2004). Tutors are able to engage with the material and shape it into schemes that make sense to them personally (Blowers, Ramsey, Merriman, & Grooms, 2003). As a result of these abilities, tutors are able to explain difficult material to tutorees.

Tutors serve to clarify material, discuss assigned readings, and help students identify what they need to learn. Tutors help facilitate learning. Ultimately, their task is to interact with the student being tutored to convey ways to organize information into personal schemata that can be internalized.

Tutors may be peer tutors, nursing faculty, or faculty from other disciplines. Peer tutors generally undergo training and may tutor one-on-one or in small group sessions. This may be a heavy load for a peer tutor, so it is essential to monitor how the peer tutor is faring in the process.

Graduates or alumni tutors offer a viable means to provide tutoring for students. This practice is particularly advantageous because graduates are familiar with the nursing program and can provide valuable insights for currently enrolled students. Alumni tutors have perspective and knowledge to share.

Integrative Review – Peer Tutors

This section discusses an integrative review addressing peer tutoring conducted by the authors. The study considers the definition and ways in which peer tutoring may be used.

Chapter 6: A Student Success Program for Currently Enrolled Students

The literature in nursing education discusses peer tutoring as a process to produce academic success for the student being tutored. Jeffreys (2004) describes peer tutoring as a process that focuses on learning cognitive and psychomotor skills. While the concept of tutoring is relatively straight forward -- to teach or instruct someone (Dictionary.com, 2006) -- the ways in which peer tutoring is enacted are varied and impact the extent to which tutoring is successful. The peer tutoring process may involve a variety of patterns, such as one-on-one, small-group, or large-group relationships (Blowers, Ramsey, Merriman, & Grooms, 2003).

For the purposes of this integrative review, peer tutoring is defined as a relationship between at least one peer tutor and one student in academic difficulty with the goal of active involvement between the two parties to promote academic success. This process involves recognizing individual learning needs for instruction, setting goals, and measuring outcomes of success. Peer tutoring may address academic needs in any academic setting: clinical, classroom, or nursing skills laboratory.

In this integrative review, three questions were posed:
1. What student problems are addressed by use of peer tutors?
2. What are the benefits of peer tutoring?
3. What mechanisms must be in place to implement peer tutoring?

The integrative review considered studies between the years 1995 and 2005 addressing use of peer tutoring to promote academic success for nursing students. A search of the literature revealed 20 articles. Of these, five articles were research focused on the topic of peer tutoring (Blowers, Ramsey, Merriman, & Grooms, 2003; Higgins, 2004; Owens & Walden, 2001; Ramsey, Blowers, Merriman, Glenn, & Terry, 2000; Valencia-Go, 2005).

Following is a summary of findings related to the three research questions:
Question 1: What student problems are addressed by use of peer tutors?
- inadequate academic preparation for nursing coursework
- inadequate support systems to successfully complete a program of nursing
- anxiety in the performance of psychomotor skills
- anxiety in test-taking
- inadequate knowledge base
- inability to identify important concepts or make associations among concepts

Question 2: What are the benefits of peer tutoring?
- self-evaluation by students and faculty suggest that using peer tutoring helped students develop study skills.
- self-evaluation by students and faculty suggest that using peer tutoring helped increase self-confidence.
- faculty reported that students experienced learning gains to the extent that retention rates were increased in a medical-surgical nursing course.
- faculty believed students developed the ability to learn content rather than memorize content.
- faculty believed students who were tutored benefited from hearing content explained in lay language.
- in most of the studies students who participated in peer tutoring were academically successful.

Question 3: What mechanisms must be in place to implement peer tutoring?
- before recommending peer tutoring, a way of providing effective training is needed so both tutor and student understand their roles.
- peer tutors and students need a contract to ensure compliance with tutoring.
- peer tutors should be paid for their tutoring. This helps recognize their value and time for tutoring, and establishes accountability.
- collaboration with faculty may be necessary to ensure interpersonal compatibility between peer tutor and student.

Discussion of peer tutoring is greatly limited in the nursing literature. While five research articles comprise this integrative review, they may not represent a complete synopsis of the benefits or draw backs to peer tutoring. Despite this fact, there is evidence to suggest several benefits from the practice of peer tutoring. The following is offered as an evidence base for the use and application of peer tutoring as an intervention for nursing students.
- knowledge acquisition: students engaged in a peer tutor relationship must be able to demonstrate or articulate knowledge of psychomotor or cognitive skills. This is true for both the tutor and the tutoree. Through application of the tutor's knowledge, the tutor helps the tutoree gain an understanding of psychomotor, study, and test-taking skills, and the cognitive processes of making associations and meaning of content. Knowledge gains are measured by evaluation tools faculty design.

Chapter 6: A Student Success Program for Currently Enrolled Students

- a way to think: Both tutor and tutoree learn about their thinking process in a peer tutor relationship. Tutors revisit material already processed, reinforcing their own knowledge. Tutorees explore ways to process and learn information based on successful strategies shared by the tutor. Strategies for time management and prioritization of goals and tasks are often part of the discussions that occur between tutor and tutoree.
- compliment to diversity: Students of similar background, such as two students who are both ESL students, may find commonalities that lend to discussion about how to meet certain challenges. In their relationship, the peer tutor provides a personal frame of reference to which the tutoree can relate.
- opportunity to discuss issues: Tutorees may avail themselves of tutor expertise to discuss issues which adversely impact their academic success. Tutors give students a means to solve problems.

To establish peer tutoring, faculty should:
- determine the selection process they will use to choose peer tutors.
- define the role of the peer tutor:
    o consider a contract which delineates role and responsibilities.
    o outline payment.
- define the role of the tutoree:
    o establish consequences for noncompliance.
    o establish timeline for goal achievement.
- establish the structure for peer tutoring:
    o one-on-one
    o small group
    o large group

In summary, peer tutoring in nursing education needs further exploration. Refer to the CD-ROM accompanying this book for a complete discussion of the process used to conduct this integrative review.

Reinforcing course content – critical thinking skills. Teaching students to think using critical thinking strategies prepares them for academic success. Knowledge is crystallized when there is an opportunity to apply the information in a particular context, such as the clinical setting or when discussing a case study. Faculty must model how to think using critical thinking skills (Caputi,

173

2004). Students unaware of critical thinking skills may miss important distinctions between distracters on test items, or experience difficulty determining nursing interventions based on clinical findings and client needs.

Prior to teaching or evaluating a student's ability to think critically, educators must have a good idea of what critical thinking actually is. While little consensus about the definition of critical thinking exists, the Delphi study conducted by Scheffer & Rubenfeld (2000) offers a consensus statement summarized as follows:

> Critical thinking in nursing is an essential component of professional accountability and quality nursing care. Critical thinkers in nursing exhibit these habits of mind: confidence, contextual perspective, creativity, flexibility, inquisitiveness, intellectual integrity, intuition, open-mindedness, perseverance, and reflection. Critical thinkers in nursing practice the cognitive skills of analyzing, applying standards, discriminating, information seeking, logical reasoning, predicting and transforming knowledge (p. 357).

Nurse experts who participated in this study identified creativity and intuition as additional affective components of critical thinking (Scheffer & Rubenfeld, 2000).

If faculty are to encourage and embrace critical thinking in nursing education, the first step is to create an awareness for students of what critical thinking is. When planning orientation content, include a discussion of elements and modes of critical thinking so students gain familiarity with the tenets and uses of critical thinking as it applies to nursing. When teaching critical thinking in the practice setting, choose instructional methods that highlight the importance of critical thinking and its relevance to clinical practice. Students must have opportunities actively to practice critical thinking. Figure 6.8 provides an example of identifying learning needs and guiding the critical thinking process in nursing students. Faculty may use this as an example of guided critical thinking for the student caring for a client with congestive heart failure. Similar applications may be made with any number of topics. Demonstrating to students what they know, as well as what they need to know, helps students apply knowledge and information to client situations.

Figure 6.8 – Relating Theory to Practice — Encouraging Cognitive Leaps

Consider the student who is caring for a client with congestive heart failure (CHF). The student administers the prescribed diuretic at 0900, and by afternoon, the client is complaining of blurred vision and a headache. He has a blood pressure of 80/54. The physician is notified and the client is prescribed an intravenous bolus of saline and oral potassium.

Pertinent facts: at the time the diuretic was given, the client's lung sounds were clear, there was slight peripheral edema, and the potassium level was within normal limits. The client was no longer using oxygen and was breathing comfortably with minimal activity. The blood pressure was 130/85, which was within recent range for the client.

What was the student missing when putting all the pieces of the puzzle together?

To facilitate critical thinking, the faculty should guide the student to:
- apply normal manifestations of CHF to this situation to determine what, if anything, might have predicted this outcome (moist lung sounds, dyspnea, difficulty with ADLs, weight gain, edema)
- highlight the role of the nurse in monitoring treatment and nursing interventions for the client with CHF. Questions to consider:
    o what is the usual treatment? (bedrest, oxygen, diuretic, potassium, cardiac glycoside)
    o what are pertinent nursing interventions? (record intake and output and daily weights, assess lung sounds, assess for signs of peripheral edema, assess ability to perform activities without dyspnea, assess breathing for rate, depth, and rhythm, and assess heart tones)

What do faculty know about CHF and nursing care that students don't know?
- that it is important to have an understanding of baseline data to understand the client's overall cardiac health status. This includes: weights over period of time, hydration status, lung sounds, and response to pharmacologic agents.
- that CHF is a complex disease, and varying degrees of decompensation are possible. Considerations include: extent of cardiac compromise, cardiac reserve, and ejection fraction.
- that the client with CHF is mercurial and conditions can change in a matter of seconds

> While students are still developing their practice base, how can faculty teach students to make cognitive leaps? The following ideas are offered:
> - bring examples to light. Encourage students to compile data with which they are familiar and review it with peers and faculty to get a sense of the overall client condition.
> - encourage students to discuss aspects of cardiac conditions with other healthcare providers to broaden their knowledge base.

Research Study – Critical Thinking

To gain a sense of the percentage of nursing educators who assess, teach, and evaluate critical thinking and how such information is used, the authors conducted a survey. The survey was administered via a blind mailing to 205 randomly selected nursing faculty from all levels of undergraduate, pre-licensure, registered nursing programs. A total of 34 faculty completed the survey for a response rate of 17%. The details of how the survey was written and administered, the total survey, and the complete results can be found on the CD-ROM accompanying this book.

Faculty were asked the following three questions about assessing critical thinking in nursing students:

1. Do you assess critical thinking in your nursing students? Results: 91% of the 34 respondents assess critical thinking.
2. At what point in the curriculum do you assess critical thinking in your nursing students? See Table 6.1 for a summary of comments shared by faculty reporting when critical thinking is assessed.
3. Describe how you assess critical thinking in your nursing students. See Table 6.1 for a summary of comments shared by faculty regarding assessment of critical thinking.

Chapter 6: A Student Success Program for Currently Enrolled Students

Table 6.1 – Student Critical Thinking Assessment Survey Responses

Type of program and total number responding	Number of programs that assess critical thinking in their nursing students	Point in curriculum when critical thinking is assessed and number responding	How critical thinking is assessed
Associate Degree 12	12	<ul><li>Day one of the program-2</li><li>At each level, throughout the program-2</li><li>Ongoing-2 (one program stated assessed in care plans in clinical every week)</li><li>Freshmen and sophomore years-1</li><li>Second semester and fourth semester (formally) and informally throughout all four semesters-1</li><li>Critical thinking assessment tests are given to students upon entering and exiting the program-1</li><li>Throughout the curriculum-1</li><li>First semester-1</li><li>All semesters in clinical-1</li></ul>	<ul><li>Class discussions, care plans, quizzes, multiple choice tests, class assignments, games, group assignments.</li><li>Observation, journals, written care planning activities, multiple choice questions (NCLEX- type questions).</li><li>Clinically.</li><li>With a standardized test and better written questions on the tests. We try to emphasize critical thinking when it is recognized in the clinical setting.</li><li>Care plans, case studies, in class exercises, occasionally a paper assignment.</li><li>Formally with the ATI exam, informally with use of the nursing process in caring for patients demonstrated in clinical preparation and paperwork.</li><li>Computerized assessment tests.</li><li>Reflective journaling, testing, clinical performance, writing assignments, case studies.</li><li>Exam questions.</li><li>Give clinical scenarios, critique how students move forward in problem solving, finding multiple answers to a problem, looking at problems from more than one perspective.</li><li>Instruction, exercises, clinical evaluation.</li></ul>

177

Baccalaureate Degree 17	14	• Upon entry, exit and during the program-1 • With the first nursing course in the sophomore yr. No nursing courses freshman year-1 • First semester junior year-1 • Sophomore, junior, and senior years-1 • Sophomore level and up-1 • Ongoing -1 • From the very beginning-1 • Each semester of the upper division major (Jr & Sr year)-1 • We use no specific test, but try to assess throughout the curriculum through our courses-1 • Beginning in the first semester of nursing school-1 • From the beginning-1 • In exams throughout the curriculum-1 • Sophomore year-1 • At the start of the upper division courses, a CT assessment test is given. Beginning in the first year nursing course, CT is discussed. Assessment for CT is utilized for all courses, but is stressed and expected more as the students begin the upper level courses junior year-1	• Used to administer the CCTST & the CCTDI but now use HESI. • Written and verbal assignments and testing. • All students take a critical thinking test on entrance, critical thinking is evaluated on clinical sites and in the format of test questions throughout the curriculum. • Written work, thinking during clinical experiences, objective and subjective testing, standardized testing (although we have not been pleased with the quality of the standardized tests). • Incorporated into the class and clinical with use of case studies, clinical logs, care plans, and written assignments. • Through coursework papers and clinical paper responses. Had been doing formal critical thinking assessments, using critical thinking assessment tools, but not at the present. • The students are given an Assessment Test immediately after acceptance into the program. A specialty exam is given at the end of every semester and an exit exam is given prior to graduation. • This is mostly assessed in practicum courses through an objective. However, it is also assessed in a strategies course that I teach through having the students give rationale for their answers for five multiple choice questions on every exam. • Through essay exams, and by evaluating decision-making in clinical situations. • Throughout the course with assignments and ATI testing. • Application questions on

Chapter 6: A Student Success Program for Currently Enrolled Students

Diploma 1		1	Begin with nursing I and assess again prior to graduation.	Arnett standardized test.
Baccalaureate and Masters Degree 2		2	At entry into the upper division Note: only one school responded to this question.	Multifaceted....standardized tests and teacher generated exams, care plans and papers. Note: only one school responded to this question.
RN to BSN and Masters Degree 1		1	RN to BSN: Critical thinking (CT) is a course objective for every core RN to BSN course. It is also a program and college graduation competency. We begin to assess CT at entry to the RN to BSN program, over the course of the program, and at the end of the program. Graduate level: We begin to assess CT at the time of application to the graduate program, over time in the program, and at the end of the program.	We assess evidence of CT in writing assignments, oral communications, and technology assignments. RN to BSN program: We use initial (return-to-college) assignments, oral presentations, and online assignments. A culminating senior project is a community assessment. The rubric grading for this assignment is used to assess CT. The CT premises are based on work by Case and Watson & Glaser, and reflect a definition, composite of abilities, and components. We also administer a standardized NLN baccalaureate achievement test. Additionally, we use standardized IDEA evaluation forms that provide student feedback about the extent to which they view themselves as exhibiting characteristics of CT. Graduate level: We use the same strategies as stated in sentence one. We use a culminating capstone (thesis, project, practicum) to assess CT. At both levels: We use various alumni surveys with elements that reflect CT.
Baccalaureate Masters, and Doctoral Degree 1		1	Across the curriculum — in each course.	Papers, tests, and discussions.

(All text in the above table is drawn from a survey and is presented verbatim.)

The responses noted in Table 6.1 suggest faculty believe in the importance of assessing critical thinking and establishing a structured time during which the assessment is made. Critical thinking is assessed in a variety of ways, in both clinical and classroom settings, using formal and informal measures.

Faculty were asked the following five questions about teaching and evaluating critical thinking:

1. Do you teach critical thinking skills in your nursing courses? Results:

88% of the 34 respondents said they do teach critical thinking skills in their nursing courses.
2. How do you teach critical thinking in your nursing courses? See Table 6.2 for a listing of comments shared by faculty regarding teaching critical thinking.

Table 6.2 – How Faculty Teach Critical Thinking

How Faculty Teach Critical Thinking in Nursing Courses

First I would like to say that my whole college is committed to critical thinking in all courses. I am on a collegewide committee to promote critical thinking. As far as nursing goes, we start with information on critical thinking found in our fundamentals text. Of course, we begin teaching the nursing process in the first semester. This of course is critical thinking. One thing I now do on a regular basis is use the words "Critical Thinking" in class when we are doing an exercise in class.
Discussion, case studies, clinical practice.

In lecture and clinical.

It is a lecture format with various teaching methods selected by the instructor.
Care plans, clinical, theory with application exercises, and case studies. Individual help depending on what part of the process is the problem – sometimes means coming in with more information to process before making the decision.

Through problem solving techniques, role modeling, and use of process for higher order thinking.

Review and practice various methods for thinking used to assess, plan, and evaluate practice; learn about learning; reflect on experiences.

Lecture/study guides/case studies.

Discuss what it is (components as defined by Richard Paul and Facione). Do exercises to think through scenarios (clinical and other).

Lecture and exercises.

Various ways including discussions of text descriptions of CT e.g., definitions of CT; questioning e.g., Socratic; various assignments & projects requiring reflection etc.

Chapter 6: A Student Success Program for Currently Enrolled Students

We also give students a copy of *The Miniature Guide to Critical Thinking: Concepts & Tools* by Paul & Elder. We could certainly make better use of it.

First the concepts are introduced/taught then emphasized in various situations.

Introduce the concepts of critical thinking. Follow with exercises. Use situations that require application for classroom discussions and activities. Case studies, scenarios, nursing care plan development, build on critical thinking introduced in required two freshman English courses (gen. eds.), synthesis paper at end of senior year, pre- and post-conference clinical discussions, examples and discussions during classroom teaching, computer-assisted instruction programs, etc.

I present case studies for critical care and then we discuss patients in clinical. I also have the students read and complete assignments in a book that teaches critical thinking and critical judgment. It involves some self-evaluation. It teaches 10 steps in critical thinking.

Reading, didactic application through discussions and papers.

Critical thinking and the nursing process. Various case studies throughout necessitating the use of critical thinking in class and in clinical.

Lecture – describing what critical thinking is. Exercises – practical application of critical thinking. Practicum – one-to-one discussions with students about patient/family care.

Integrated throughout the course.

Using case studies, role playing and hands-on practicums.

Case studies, self care plans, skits, application questions, journaling, and clinical experience.

Through clinical situations/simulations and in discussions/postconferences.

Deductive and inductive thinking exercises.

Begin in NI with general exercises then progress to clinical situations in the following courses.

The faculty are very cognizant of the importance and expected evidential outcomes of CT in our students at all levels of study. We openly discuss the concept in curriculum

> meetings and general division faculty meetings. We strive to incorporate learning activities and evaluative methods that consistently and accurately assess CT. We continuously explore course content that either addresses CT or alludes to ways that one can develop CT. The faculty share current literature on CT. We discuss rubric grading and evaluation methods that reflect CT. We guide students to explore ways to meet the CT expectations. We discuss ways of knowing, thinking, and application in various courses.
>
> Presented in the first nursing course then is an expected behavior in the courses and clinicals. Faculty employ teaching methods that encourage and assist students with CT.
>
> Using texts that address critical thinking.
>
> Processing case studies.
>
> Continually asking them to apply material...role modeling processes.

(All text in the above table is drawn from a survey and is presented verbatim.)

The responses noted in Table 6.2 suggest faculty teach critical thinking using a variety of methods. Case studies, clinical applications, deductive and inductive reasoning exercises, role-playing, hands-on practicum, study guides, and discussions in lecture and clinical are examples of the types of methodologies used to foster critical thinking. More research is needed to determine specific learning activities using these teaching methodologies and the outcomes of their use.

3. How are students expected to apply what they learn about critical thinking?
4. How do you determine if students are using critical thinking in their work as nursing students?
5. How do you evaluate the growth of critical thinking abilities in your students as they progress through your nursing program?

See Table 6.3 for a listing of comments shared by faculty addressing questions 3, 4, and 5: application, measurement, and evaluation of critical thinking.

Chapter 6: A Student Success Program for Currently Enrolled Students

Table 6.3 – How Faculty Apply, Measure, and Evaluate Critical Thinking in Nursing Students

How students apply critical thinking	How faculty determine use of critical thinking	How growth of critical thinking is evaluated
First and foremost, in their planning and care of patients.	We check to see if they can plan and implement safe and appropriate care individualized to their patients.	We grade care plans to see if they are appropriate. We give written exams. We ask questions in class. We give written assignments. I play "games" with the students. I make sure they know that these are critical thinking exercises. For example, the other day I divided my class into three groups. I stated, "You have a three year old patient that just came back from surgery. She cannot understand how to use the incentive spirometer. What could you do with a three year old to accomplish the same thing?" They thought of blowing bubbles, pin wheels, etc. The team with the most answers wins, but I make sure that all teams win.
Written care plans, journals, clinical practicum experiences.	Observation, discussion with students, questioning of students.	As noted previously in application and use of critical thinking.
In clinical and in written work.	Questioning.	As noted previously in application and use of critical thinking.
On the test and then as it is observed or experienced in the clinical setting.	Behavior in the clinical setting and correct answers on the tests to case study questions.	Standardized tests given both years to compare and contrast results.
Clinical, case studies and application exercises in class, some community projects.	Care plans, clinical setting.	Care plans, clinical setting.
In the preparation and care of patients in the clinical arena.	Use of process and problem solving is demonstrated in clinical preparation paperwork and discussion.	Scores on ATI are compared. Clinical preparation and paperwork requirements are leveled throughout the program requiring more complex thinking as students progress.
Writing: formal and reflective journaling, clinical problem solving: solo and collaborative, performance on higher order test questions: application and analysis level test questions.	Bench marks are set for performance levels, criteria shared with students.	Ability to move from simple to complex problem solving; utilize thinking skills individually and in groups; utilize thinking skills in a variety of classroom, community, and clinical settings.
Exams, postconference after clinicals, case study presentations.	Observation during clinicals, exam questions.	Increased level of difficulty.
Clinical, discussions, case studies.	Mostly by their problem solving and discussions.	Difficult to assess growth, we pretty much just monitor continuation.

Yes.	It is part of our student performance evaluations (subjective and objective measures).	Each semester it is evaluated and compared to previous semesters.
CT is one of our seven curricular competencies. Students are expected to demonstrate critical thinking through application of the nursing process with various patients including populations.	We have a rubric for evaluating CT that we use with samples of student work e.g., integration paper describing care of a medical-surgical patient.	We use the same rubric which requires progressively higher scores. We are working to refine the teaching and assessment of CT as well as the other six competencies in the program.
Ability to answer or not answer questions.	Response to various questions, situations, and papers presented.	Not sure.
In course testing and clinical performance.	By the quality of their decision making. Are they accurate? Are they thorough?	I would say that 75% of the students show SIGNIFICANT growth in critical thinking.
During clinical care of patients and families, in written work, in discussion, when working through case studies, and computer programs.	Journal entries specifically asking for the thinking process related to clinical experiences, individual conferences, group conferences, reflection assignments, results of problem-solving exercises, and in some of the ways described in question 6.	Is evaluated at different points in the program. University has initiated course imbedded assessment. Thinking is one of the core abilities all students in the university are expected to develop. Certain courses are designated to teach the ability and certain courses are designated to assess the ability during the four years at the university.
I have them take the 10 steps of critical thinking and apply them on one identified problem of their patient assignment for the day. They are completing two per week.	We discuss patient problems in the clinical setting as they come up, and I try not to give answers, just direction. I try to get them to come up with solutions themselves and guide them to resources.	Measured in their clinical evaluations for each course. Goals set for each grade level.
Class and clinical assignments.	Criteria for assignments include critical thinking assessment components.	At one time, did a pre-and post- (beginning and end) of nursing program assessments. Discussion around whether critical thinking is a state or trait. Cost of assessments has led us away from that approach.
In case studies, patient situations.	Level of understanding regarding specific patient situations.	Ability to apply didactic knowledge to clinical situations.
By being able to talk about situations in clinical, work through case studies in class, etc.	In practicum, can they answer my questions about their patients and the nursing process they are using to care for them? In testing, can they give rationale for the answer they chose (or for those they did not choose) on a multiple choice test?	We track their scores on the critical thinking objective throughout the practicum courses each semester.

Chapter 6: A Student Success Program for Currently Enrolled Students

Examples: Challenged in various clinical situations. Essay exams that are application-based (view a video and base exam questions on what was seen).	My observations and questioning of students.	Not specifically done.
Orally and in writing.	By the writings, assessments, and plans they develop for their patients.	By the ATI testing and more advanced assignments.
Tests, written work with case studies, journals, care plans on self and patients, role playing, and skits.	Graded on all the above.	More difficult questions, case studies, leadership roles, and assignments. Clinical experience, journaling on experience from the beginning of curriculum to the end.
In clinical experiences and conferences.	Testing with formal feedback.	Periodic comparisons.
Case study analysis, exam questions, and discussion groups.	Analysis of above.	At senior year, comprehensive case analysis exercise that includes all the areas of critical thinking to include data identification, analysis of data, evaluation of data, priority setting in patient care, etc.
They are expected to apply it in testing and in clinical practice.	We have a very detailed clinical evaluation which identifies these points.	We follow them with the clinical evaluation tool and through our pre- and post-test in critical thinking.
We expect to see evidence of CT in students' work across their program of study. We review the expectation that is printed on course syllabi, in college catalogs, and other sources. We also expect students to locate, peruse, and integrate current literature about CT and related concepts. We expect students to exhibit characteristics of CT (i.e., work that reflects thoughtful, current, in depth, curious, creative, pertinent, valid, scientific, conclusive, systematic approaches).	We have common interests and understanding about CT among our faculty. When we compare our thoughts, we usually arrive at similar conclusions re: our students' evidence and progress in the area of CT. We have formal grading mechanisms that are based on our philosophy, literature, experience, expected outcomes, and national organizations. In all, we use a variety of ways to examine students' use of CT in their work.	We have competency maps that tie course syllabi, program competencies, and college graduation competencies (along with professional and accreditation guidelines). We match selected evaluation methods (assignments, etc.) from selected courses to those expected competencies (outcomes). Over students' program of study, we use designated grading tools to evaluate those selected assignments. We record those data in templates that the Institutional Research Office then analyzes to produce tangible outcomes information at course, section, campus location, and program levels. These data are communicated to appropriate stakeholders who then examine and use the outcomes data to make decision about specific courses, programs, etc.
In assignments, testing, and clinical discussion/performance.	Through evaluation of their performance and assignments.	The last semester, students again take a CT test and the results are assessed with the incoming scores. Each nursing course assesses for CT and the expectations increase as the student progresses through the curriculum.

(All text in the above table is drawn from a survey and is presented verbatim.)

The responses noted in Table 6.3 suggest faculty apply, evaluate, and measure critical thinking via several avenues: case study, testing, class discussions, clinical performance, journaling, written work (care plans), formal writing, role-play, and skits. Additional research is needed to further explore the issue of teaching and assessing critical thinking. Results of this study may be typical; however, with the small number responding, the sample may or may not be representative of how faculty assess or students use critical thinking.

Reinforcing course content — concept maps. One way to bring course content to life is via the use of concept maps. Concept maps encourage identification of key concepts, graphically illustrating their relationship (Caputi & Blach, 2007). In the process of constructing a concept map, students think through ideas and construct knowledge frameworks resulting in deeper learning of the content (Gaines, 1999). Concept mapping necessitates that the student have a "grasp of the entire situation rather than rely on fragmentary facts from rote memory" (Hsu, 2004, p. 510). With this method, students move into the realm of discovery learning, as compared with knowledge-based learning (Hsu, 2004). See Chapter 5 for discussion of an integrative review using concept maps to teach critical thinking.

Faculty may use concept maps to highlight or reinforce course material. For example, students may be assigned to create a concept map for subject matter discussed in class. The concept map provides a vehicle for faculty and students to discuss the topic and provides a visual representation that allows the faculty to identify gaps in the student's knowledge (Engelmann & Caputi, 2005). This active learning strategy facilitates encoding of information into long-term memory, which enables successful recall of data at a later date (Gaines, 1996). As an instructional strategy, concept mapping helps students relate the nursing process to the client care situation and encourages linkages between theory and practice.

Student support courses. As students move through the nursing program, additional courses can be designed to support all students (Tracey, 2003). For example, once students have completed a set number of nursing courses, a seminar-type workshop can be offered to help students with testing at the application and analysis cognitive levels and understanding the NCLEX test plan.

Other courses can be designed to help special populations of students. For example, faculty may wish to establish an interdisciplinary course that addresses

Chapter 6: A Student Success Program for Currently Enrolled Students

the special needs for English-as-a second-language students (Caputi, Engelmann, & Stasinopoulos, 2006).

Student support in clinical practice. Faculty can employ several proactive strategies to enhance student learning in the clinical practice setting. Faculty can provide guidance to help students create meaning from their clinical experiences. Tools and exercises designed to meet specific learning needs assist in the process. For example, critical thinking tools (Caputi, 2004; Engelmann and Caputi, 2005) provide direction and focus and encourage reflective practice.

Tracking student progress and discussing student performance with the student is important. Use of a clinical experience assessment and documentation tool, such as that depicted in Table 6.4 provides an objective view of what the student has actually accomplished, or has yet to accomplish. Students and faculty together can establish personal goals for the student and highlight those goals that were obtained or have yet to be obtained. This tracking mechanism can be used in conjunction with clinical evaluation tools and maintained in clinical portfolios.

A copy of this Clinical Experience Assessment and Documentation Tool may be accessed on the CD-ROM accompanying this book.

Exit Interview

Talking with students as they exit the program, whether prior to or upon graduation, offers insight for both faculty development and program enhancement. Faculty may choose to interview graduates individually or as a group. The interviews may be conducted face-to-face or via phone. All students may be interviewed or only those students exiting prior to graduation.

If a structured interview is not feasible, a written or on-line program evaluation can be administered. Once this information is collected, it may be reviewed and analyzed by the appropriate committee and shared with full faculty.

If a student exits a course prior to completion of that course, it is important to track the reason for exit. Was the reason academic or personal? This helps pinpoint where the highest rate of attrition occurs and why. Faculty can investigate the reasons students leave and design interventions to increase retention in the future.

Table 6.4 – Clinical Experience Assessment and Documentation Tool

Clinical Experience	Dates/Comments
Medication administration	
Topical	
Eye/ear gtts	
Suppository	
Rectal	
Vaginal	
PO	
IM	
Sub Q	
IV	
NG	
Enema	
Inhaler	
Nose gtts/nasal spray	
IV Skills	
IV	
Flush	
Saline lock	
Central/PICC line	
Primary	
Secondary	
Infusion pump	
Patient Controlled Analgesia	
Insertion	
Removal	
GI Skills	
NG	
Feeding	
Insertion	
Removal	
Check for residual	
Rectal tube	
Stool specimen	
Obtainment	
Testing	
Colostomy/ileostomy care	
Skin Assessment	
Central/PICC line	
Wound	
Surgical	
Trauma	
Pressure ulcer	
Turgor	
Drain type and management	
Equipment maintenance	
Bed type	

Chapter 6: A Student Success Program for Currently Enrolled Students

Neurological Assessment	
Pain/PCA management	
LOC	
Pupil response	
Special scale	
Glasgow coma	
Trauma score	
Respiratory Assessment	
Breath sounds	
Specimen obtained	
Oxygen administered	
Pulse oximetry	
Tracheostomy care	
Tracheostomy suction	
Oral suction	
Oral airway placement	
Chest tube management	
Assist with procedure	
Incentive spirometry	
Thoracentesis	
Chest tube insertion/removal	
Other _____	
Cardiovascular Assessment	
Heart rate (apical)	
Heart sounds	
Peripheral pulses	
Radial	
Femoral	
Posterior tibial	
Dorsalis pedis	
Doppler	
Applications	
TED hose	
Compression device	
Urinary Assessment	
Maintenance	
Foley catheter	
Urostomy	
Leg bag	
Suprapubic catheter	
Irrigation	
Continuous bladder irrigation	
Musculoskeletal	
Transfer techniques	
Bed to chair	
Bed to cart	
Use of lifts/transfer devices	
Use of ambulatory aides	

	Crutches	
	Cane	
	Walker	
Range of motion		
Continuous passive motion device		
Cast care		
Thinking Sills		
Goal setting		
Charting		
	Plan of care	
	Client education	
Completion of critical thinking tools for specific objectives		
Critical monitoring		
	Pre-procedural care	
	Post-procedural care	
Communication skills		
	Obtaining report	
	Giving report	
Calling a physician		
Contacting members of healthcare team		
Delegating to members of healthcare team		
Admitting a client		
Transferring a client		
Discharging a client		

Non-Academic Support

Students may have personal needs or considerations that impact their ability to complete a nursing program. Resources to provide students with support of a non-academic nature must be available. Consider the following variables and their impact on student success.

Financial Aid

Students who must work while going to school, to support their household and finance their education, may be at risk for failure. Financial assistance may be available that would reduce or offset student workload and stress. Determine the resources students might access to apply for financial assistance. Counselors, or knowledgeable faculty, may help evaluate a student's particular situation and recommend help from a variety of sources. Such assistance may be available in the form of scholarships, grants, work-study, and loans.

Part-time employment on campus. Students should be apprised of employment opportunities on campus. Student aide positions may be available that would help offset monetary demands. Frequently, such positions are somewhat flexible in their hours, so students may work their time around their class schedule. Added benefits of working on campus include connection with the institution, familiarity with institutional policies and workings which can expedite tasks that need to be accomplished, and access to resources otherwise not readily apparent or available.

Child Care

Students often need child care. Obtaining reputable child care can be a major concern impacting a student's ability to progress through a program of nursing. In addition, child care adds another expense that some students have difficulty meeting. In some instances, child care may be offered on campus at rates less expensive than those in other settings. If child care is not offered on campus, students may wish to exchange child care hours or participate in playgroups that allow students to study while their children play together. Students may find this cooperative association lends well to a variety of needs; such as, time, socialization for both student and offspring, and reduced childcare expenses.

Counseling

Students may need to avail themselves of counseling services during their educational process. Counselors are a valuable resource in terms of helping students with personal exploration and decision making that relate to the ultimate goal of becoming a nurse. Typically, services offered by counselors include individual counseling for personal concerns. Schools may also establish a liaison in counseling who works primarily with nursing students. For schools that do not have someone in a counseling position, faculty may consider filling these needs if their background and expertise has prepared them for this role.

Personal difficulties. Individual counseling may involve management of personal problems to allow better focus on educational pursuits. In some instances, students may need referral to a community or private agency. Consider the following scenario. A student in the process of a divorce has several concerns. The counselor reviews options for the student and provides the student with a list of resources to assist the student to procure legal council, temporary housing, and work-study. The student's unease relative to divorce proceedings, where to live, and necessary financial means are addressed by the counselor's assessment of the student's concerns and appropriate referrals. The counselor schedules a follow-up appointment with the student to ascertain if the student requires further assistance. Of course, a divorce is a major crisis for most people. The best approach may be for the student to request a "stop-out" for a year to manage this personal issue.

Students who suffer from test anxiety may also benefit from sessions with counselors knowledgeable about measures to enhance testing abilities and decrease test anxiety.

Liaison for nursing students. Establishing a liaison with counselors who work primarily with nursing students and understand the rigors and demands of the nursing program is especially beneficial. Faculty who enjoy close associations with liaisons are able readily to refer students to someone who understands what it means to be a nursing student. Counselors who have a solid grasp of what the nursing program entails are in the best position to provide guidance and extend helpful resources to the students. When confronted with concerns, the student wants a solution. A liaison familiar with the nursing program can clarify information and will not need to spend time gathering details relative to the program itself. This is more time saving and less stressful for the student than if the counselor had to gather background information relative to how the program functions to understand the nature of the problem.

Students should meet the counseling liaison at the beginning of the nursing program and learn what services are offered. Services provided may be outlined and given to students in the form of pamphlets or other written materials. Personally meeting the counselor lends a special touch and provides a familiar face for the student should the need arise to take advantage of services offered.

It is important for faculty to have a working relationship with counseling services. Faculty may find it helpful to establish sessions with counseling to facilitate their understanding of factors that trigger stress for students. Such opportunities to discuss student needs with counselors facilitate faculty referrals.

Chapter 6: A Student Success Program for Currently Enrolled Students

Cultural Considerations

A national goal is to increase the ethnic and racial diversity within the healthcare professions to provide culturally competent care (Department Health and Human Services, 2005). We are an increasingly diverse nation, for whom multicultural nursing is imperative. Multicultural nursing, while essential, is difficult to achieve due to the high attrition rates of nursing students who comprise under-represented groups. This is especially true of those nursing students for whom English is a second language (Klisch, 2000).

English as a Second Language (ESL)

Klisch's literature review of the 1990s examined twenty articles that addressed the issue of retention strategies for culturally diverse students in general and students with ESL in particular. Nursing schools have responded to this need to decrease attrition for nursing students with ESL via:
- enhanced faculty knowledge of transcultural nursing theory
- course development to reflect cultural awareness, knowledge, and skills

Malu and Figlear (1998) offered an analysis of the problem of language development that both nurse educators and nursing students with ESL face. Data from admission files of all first-year immigrant nursing students with ESL were analyzed and periodic, open-ended interviews were conducted. Data analysis revealed four problems: language development, differing expectations of nursing education, a fear of failure, and unfamiliarity with a participatory learning model.

Malu and Figlear (1998) posited that satisfactory command of cognitive academic language proficiency takes five to seven years of intensive academic language study for a person who begins to study English as a teenager to compete successfully with native English speakers. "Language learning goes well beyond words" (p. 44). Faculty need to be aware that language involves the sociocultural, cognitive, and affective domains of learning.

Sims-Giddens (2000) points out that the student with ESL has to develop strategies to "learn, remember, and use new vocabulary appropriately" (p. 25). These students can initiate and monitor generative reading strategies (peer teaching, crucial term identification, personal word lists, relating words to ideas, and imagery) to build vocabulary and become independent in their learning.

Based on the above cited difficulties, following are suggestions for helping nursing students with ESL (Malu & Figlear, 1998; Sims-Giddens, 2000).
- students with ESL should maintain a vocabulary notebook wherein the student writes a word in English, its synonyms, and any personal connections, to help develop language.
- beginning nursing students with ESL should be allowed to access a bilingual dictionary and have additional time to complete exams.
- faculty should provide synonyms for everyday words on exams that students with ESL do not understand. However, a "nursing content word, such as 'asepsis,' should not be clarified because all students are expected to understand that word" (Malu and Figlear, 1998, p. 45).
- faculty should use computer-assisted instruction (CAI) for students with ESL.

CAI provides further exposure to new vocabulary in multiple contexts and immediate feedback to the student.

Faculty-student collaboration and familiarity with the school's facilities and resources are encouraged along with active involvement in school functions and study groups (Malu & Figlear, 1998).

Conversation Circles

In an effort to gain insight into the particular learning needs of the nursing student with ESL, the authors designed what was termed Conversation Circles. Recognizing their inexperience in regard to students with ESL, the authors turned to a colleague whose expertise in the field, and interest in promoting positive student outcomes, provided an ideal compliment to the authors' needs and interests.

Conversation Circles were held a total of three times during the term. The objectives were:
1. Establish a channel (Conversation Circles) for students with ESL to share their thoughts and concerns about being a student nurse.
2. Explore the shared experiences of first and second level nursing students as they relate to impediment to, or enhancement of, their success in the nursing program.
3. Identify learning needs of students with ESL and share them with nursing faculty.

Chapter 6: A Student Success Program for Currently Enrolled Students

4. Determine faculty development requirements relative to the cultural and educational needs of the students with ESL such as knowledge pertaining to advising, educational assessment, and necessary interventions.

While the authors met only three times with the seven students who participated in this study, certain insights were garnered that faculty may consider in their design of instruction (Caputi, Engelmann, & Stasinopoulos, 2006). See Table 6.5 for an overview of these insights. See the CD-ROM accompanying this book for an in-depth discussion of this topic.

Establishing a Culturally Diverse Program

"Cultural diversity is the state of affairs that exists when the values and beliefs of different cultures are acknowledged and when these values and beliefs are given equal consideration when decisions are made" (Leonard, 2001, p.16). Establishing a culturally diverse nursing program involves creating an awareness of cultural differences and honoring the special attributes each person has to offer. This translates to sensitivity toward cultural differences in relationships among all individuals the student will encounter while obtaining a degree in nursing and extends to the institutions in which the learning takes place. A culturally diverse nursing program refers to a diverse faculty educating a diverse student population to care for an increasingly diverse client population. Valuing diversity is at the heart of establishing a culturally diverse program.

Create awareness. Covington (2004) highlights the need to establish clinical experiences that provide students with an opportunity to work with culturally diverse client populations. Faculty may foster cultural appreciation by describing cultural and societal dimensions of groups and involving students in the discussion of culturally specific considerations for nursing care (Cook & Cullen, 2000). Discussion of stereotypical portrayals and dimensions of cultural values in given situations are two examples of behaviors to meet the objective of enhanced cultural awareness (Cook & Cullen, 2000).

Foster a diverse learning environment. To address the needs of a multicultural society, nursing education must foster a diverse learning climate, rich with many perspectives which add to the profession of nursing as a whole. Although some believe that minority students are best served by minority faculty,

Table 6.5 – Faculty Insights from the Conversation Circle Experience

1. Use real situations taken from nursing practice, so pieces of the puzzle fall into place.

2. Prior to beginning a new lecture session, conduct a review, so students have an opportunity to clarify information prior to the start of a new topic.

3. Consider if there is ample time for review of class material or test results.

4. Be as organized as possible when teaching. Students with ESL have difficulty framing a lecture that is out of sequence, or jumps from one topic to another without making smooth transitions.

5. Students with ESL struggle with context and grammar. Speak slowly and provide information in writing. Explain abbreviations and provide a list to accompany the explanation.

6. Many students have problems with testing, and students with ESL are no exception. Teach them how to prepare for and take tests.

7. Allow additional testing time. Gradually reduce this testing time as students progress through the program.

8. Create learning situations that enable students to speak, or present to others, during class or clinical postconference, so their English language skills may be refined.

9. Implement Conversation Circles upon admission to the nursing program, during the very first nursing course. The bond the Conversation Circles created was greatly appreciated by the students. Students also appreciated the fact that faculty took the time to discover their learning needs.

10. Learn about the resources within your institution. Establish a liaison for reading and writing assistance.

11. Include cultural aspects of caring for patients in this country. Students with ESL commented that they need help to prepare for dealings with difficult patients. Role playing might offer one avenue to model nurse-patient interactions.

(All text in the above table is drawn from a survey and is presented verbatim.)

Campbell and Campbell, as cited by Griffiths & Tagliareni (1999) concluded that the most important match between mentor-protégé should be that their personality and compatibility of outlook compliment one another. Overall, "students should be supported in their attempts to use and express their cultural attributes in the classroom without feeling uncomfortable" (Campinha-Barcote, 1998, p. 3). In other words, all are respected and feel safe to be a part of the culture.

How well faculty embrace diversity sets the climate for the student's learning and appreciation of diversity. Stacciarini (2002), a native of Brazil, reflects on her personal experience becoming a nurse educator in the United States. She advocates face-to-face communication and more personal interactions with other faculty, such as having a chat over coffee, avoiding e-mail or voice-mail interchanges as sole modes of communication, and avoiding the use of jargon. Because many aspects of her position were bewildering, she felt having a faculty mentor would have been helpful. All these factors impacted to some extent the ease with which she acclimated to the culture of nursing education in the United States. These insights are offered from a personal perspective and consider the feelings of a faculty member in nursing education. There is much universal application in these simple suggestions to enhance interpersonal interactions. Nurse educators and students everywhere must value differences that impact their own teaching and learning.

Emphasize culturally sensitive teaching and learning. Addressing cultural sensitivity in the classroom and in clinical learning environments to create a culturally sensitive milieu is essential. This is important for both the student and the student's clients. If faculty are unable to model culturally sensitive care, students will experience difficulty in valuing such care. For example, in the provision of individualized client care, a care plan would reflect interventions that are respectful and mindful of the diversity of the client (Cook & Cullen, 2000).

Appreciation and respect for one another is a basic tenet of caring. Students who participated in the Conversation Circles specifically stated that faculty who were respectful of their differences made them feel welcome and free to learn. Cultural sensitivity communicated through acceptance affected their comfort level when seeking help with matters relating to the class (Caputi, Engelmann, & Stasinopoulos, 2006).

Heighten appreciation of cultural differences. Specific opportunities should be planned to foster socialization and an appreciation of one another. One very simple, yet effective, way to foster appreciation among students and faculty is to plan a gathering where everyone shares food native to their own culture. This informal gathering offers a non-stressful avenue to exchange information about cultures and provides a foundation for future interactions.

Stokes (2003) discussed the benefit of gatherings as a retention strategy for minority students in relationship to the social climate of a nursing program. This empowerment initiative, which was described as an opportunity for minority and international students to interact and share concerns, involved 76 students over a five year period. While the impact the gatherings had on academic success is not known, 65 of the 76 students completed the nursing program. The gatherings provided opportunities for fellow students to share their success strategies for program completion.

Implementation

Implementing a Student Success Program is aimed at achieving the outcomes of retention, on-time graduation rates, and NCLEX pass rates. Following are steps necessary to implement the Student Success Program.

Plan the Components of Your Student Success Program

Based on the data collected in the admissions process and the self-assessment, determine which components discussed in this chapter to include in your Student Success Program. Plan a program that addresses both class and individual needs.

Meet with the Retention Specialist to design and implement a specific approach for all student needs. Plan to address needs in common for the class with necessary interventions.

Examples of planned interventions designed for the entire class include seminars in study skills, test-taking strategies, and time management. If assessment data point to curricular choke points, plan strategies to improve these elements in instruction. Interventions for student success should be implemented as soon as feasible. The sooner a problem is identified, the sooner the intervention should occur.

Meet with individual students considered at-risk for failure and plan an individualized approach for success. Plan referrals to the Retention Specialist. Work with the Retention Specialist to pinpoint exact student needs and interventions best suited to that individual. For example, a student experiencing difficulty grasping a particular concept may benefit from peer tutoring.

Notify Students About the Student Success Program

Announce the Student Success Program and how it will be used to help students succeed. Convey the Student Success Program in a positive light, so students perceive it as integral to success, not a punishment or only indicated for weak students. Inform students that faculty work closely with students and the Retention Specialist to design interventions for the class as a whole and for individual students. Provide students with details concerning the Student Success Program, so students know when and where to meet with faculty or the Retention Specialist.

Carry Out the Program

Meet with the Retention Specialist to implement the Student Success Program for the entire class. Discuss the components of the program with the students to ensure they understand the purpose of each intervention and the outcomes expected. Establish short- and long-term goals and a timeline for these goals to be realized.

The results of class testing may reveal learning needs for the entire class. For example, testing reveals a curricular choke point when students miss two-thirds of the items about nursing care for the client with safety needs. A review is planned to discuss this content during the last 15 minutes of the next class. Items will be added to the next test, to retest students' knowledge of this content. Faculty also plan to use classroom assessment techniques to ensure students have an understanding of the material being discussed.

Individual student needs are also addressed through discussions between faculty and the Retention Specialist. Following are examples of individual learning needs and the interventions planned by faculty and the Retention Specialist.

Example # 1: Student learning need – classroom

A student is experiencing difficulty mastering content related to the client with congestive heart failure. The short-term goal is the student will re-test on this content and achieve a minimum of 75%. The long-term goal is the student will pass the entire course. The interventions stipulate the student is to meet with the peer tutor one hour a day, three days a week, for the next two weeks. By the end of week two, the student is to submit to the peer tutor a concept map that illustrates the student's understanding of the client with congestive heart failure. In week three, the student will re-test on content related to congestive heart failure.

Identifying any student who, on the first examination for the course, receives a failing score is important. Interventions are immediately planned and might include computer programs to remediate the topic of concern, or use of critical thinking tools that apply information from theory to clinical practice. The point of contact occurs as soon as possible after the poor test score is obtained, so an intervention can be implemented prior to the student taking the second test. Refer to the exam analysis tools in Figures 6.2 through 6.7 discussed earlier in this chapter, which may be used to provide objective analysis of a student's test results.

Example # 2: Student learning need – clinical

If the learning need is clinical in nature, faculty should meet with the student as soon as possible after the precipitating event and communicate which aspects of clinical performance need improvement. For example, when the student has just completed an injection with less than optimal technique, the time to discuss the student's performance is right after the occurrence, not six weeks later in a final evaluation conference. Any part of the performance that was performed well should also be highlighted.

The faculty will establish a time for a follow-up meeting with the student. It may be helpful to set weekly goals. Progress should be documented. A clinical contract between teacher and student may be helpful to delineate the exact nature of the problem, the necessary steps to resolve it, and expected outcomes. If possible, the student is afforded time to remediate the skill and perform it again, to provide an opportunity to successfully master the skill.

Chapter 6: A Student Success Program for Currently Enrolled Students

Ongoing communication among the faculty and support personnel is essential to ensure the plan is functioning as anticipated.

Evaluation

Faculty evaluate the efficacy of the overall Student Success Program on an ongoing and timely basis, according to the type of intervention that is employed and a reasonable time frame for a response to occur. Evaluation is specific to the indicators of success established for the nursing program.
Steps used to evaluate the Student Success Program include:
- use established indicators for success to measure outcomes as discussed in Chapter 4. Indicators of success might include:
    o students earn a minimum of a C in all nursing courses
    o program achieves an 85% retention rate
    o program achieves a 15% graduation rate with one stop-out
    o students earn 75% on all exams
- establish set points when evaluation data will be collected, trended, and analyzed. Compare outcomes with indicators of success. Note any variances from the established indicators of success and determine personal, academic, or cultural variables that might have impacted the outcome.
    o document students' grades at the end of each course and identify content areas that were problematic for the students
    o calculate attrition rate at the end of each nursing course and determine variables that contributed to a student's reason for leaving the program
    o calculate the percentage of graduates who have one stop-out and track reasons for student exit and subsequent performance upon returning to the program
    o calculate the percentage of correct test items and if less than 75% is achieved in any one content area, a curriculum choke point is identified

Evaluation might also entail review of specific interventions designed to meet a student's needs enacted as part of an individual's success plan. The following examples demonstrate how an individual student's interventions might be evaluated.

Example # 1: Evaluation of Tutoring Program

Faculty design a tutoring program for a student who achieved less than passing on the first two course examinations. Together, faculty and student identify specific areas in which the student needs help: not enough time for studying, test-taking skills deficiencies, inability to understand the textbook used in the course, and lack of clinical application of the material studied in class. To evaluate the tutoring process, faculty plan to meet with the student once weekly for three weeks to assess any further needs and determine how the tutoring process is working. The student's status will be re-evaluated after each subsequent test. This evaluation process is both formative and summative. The faculty of the Student Success Committee will track this process to determine if tutoring is a worthwhile intervention to continue.

Example # 2: Interventions to Address Personal Concerns

A student shares with faculty a major concern about going through a divorce and states it is very difficult to cope. The student is distraught and admits to being depressed. The student states no family members live in the state, nor are there close friends to talk with about concerns. The faculty phones the counseling liaison for nursing and makes a referral for the student. In this case, the intervention was immediate and the student will require ongoing support and monitoring for emotional stability and functional ability in the clinical setting. No immediate resolution for this problem is possible; however, it is expected that the student will gain the necessary ongoing support to continue in the program and meet personal needs. The Student Success Committee will track how this particular student progresses, making a note in the student's file. With the student's permission, this data may be accessed to provide additional information about this particular student's success, which impacts program indicators of success for graduation and retention rates.

Chapter 6: A Student Success Program for Currently Enrolled Students

Student Perspectives on Success

Viewing the educational process through the eyes of the students is also important. Students can shed light on factors they feel impact their ability to succeed and provide insights faculty can use to adjust teaching and plan interventions for optimal student performance. Using student perception appraisal questionnaires, both at the beginning and end of a clinical course, Jeffreys (2002) examined students' perceptions of variables that influence retention. The study included students who participated in an enrichment program's study groups led by peer mentors or tutors. The enrichment program was included as one of the select variables on the pre-test instrument. The Likert-type scale used to measure student evaluations follows:

1. Does not apply
2. Severely restricts
3. Moderately restricts
4. Does not restrict or support
5. Moderately supports
6. Greatly supports

Findings suggested the highest ranked variables viewed as "severely restricts," on both the pre-tests and post-tests, were environmental variables of finances and family. In addition, "moderately restricts" variables were also environmental (finances, family, and employment). Faculty advising and tutoring service were viewed as "greatly supports" by more students on the post-test measurement than on the pre-test (Jeffreys, 2002). Students perceived the enrichment program, tutoring, and faculty advisement as supportive for retention, which highlights the value of such support measures in programs of nursing.

Plan to gather input from both individual students and from the entire class. Determine the purpose of gathering feedback and plan the best time to collect it. When this information is collected will determine the ability to respond at a point when it can positively impact students. Some aspects of teaching and learning lend well to immediate feedback, such as a special event, which could be surveyed at the end of the event. Test review conducted immediately after the exam provides an opportunity to gain insights that faculty can use to perform test analysis or to write a better test the next time the test is administered. It may be better to evaluate other aspects of the course at the end of the term, with use of a course evaluation tool. Ask questions on the evaluation tool that pinpoint interventions employed to determine if they were successful in the students' eyes. Be specific. Ask for ways to improve course delivery. A sample course evaluation tool is presented in Figure 6.9.

Figure 6.9– Example Course Evaluation Tool

DIRECTIONS: Using the scale of 0-5, circle the number that reflects your degree of satisfaction with each element of this course and the course overall. Please add additional comments that can help guide future revisions of the course. Thank you.						
0 = Not at all satisfied 5= Very satisfied						
1. The course syllabus.	0	1	2	3	4	5
Comments:						
2. The course orientation.	0	1	2	3	4	5
Comments:						
3. The textbooks.	0	1	2	3	4	5
Comments:						
4. The study guides.	0	1	2	3	4	5
Comments:						
5. Extent to which preparation for the pediatric presentations helped me to understand the dimensions of wellness in relation to the pediatric client.	0	1	2	3	4	5
Comments:						
6. The pediatric paper.	0	1	2	3	4	5
Comments:						
7. The laboratory components:						
a. Tracheostomy care and suctioning	0	1	2	3	4	5
b. Medication administration via G-tube	0	1	2	3	4	5
c. IV content	0	1	2	3	4	5
d. Case study presentations	0	1	2	3	4	5
Comments:						

Chapter 6: A Student Success Program for Currently Enrolled Students

8.	The PhysWhiz programs.	0	1	2	3	4	5
	Comments:						
9.	The Critical Thinking Case Studies.	0	1	2	3	4	5
	Comments:						
10.	The clinical orientation.	0	1	2	3	4	5
	Comments:						
11.	The extent to which the clinical facility met my learning needs.	0	1	2	3	4	5
	Comments:						
12.	The extent to which clinical staff were helpful.	0	1	2	3	4	5
	Comments:						
13.	The pediatric clinical.	0	1	2	3	4	5
	Comments:						
14.	The rotations to the critical care units.	0	1	2	3	4	5
	Comments:						
15.	The option for additional review.	0	1	2	3	4	5
	Comments:						
16.	The option for use of the index card during testing.	0	1	2	3	4	5
	Comments:						
17.	The extent to which group testing helped increase my understanding of the material.	0	1	2	3	4	5
	Comments:						
18.	The extent to which faculty demonstrated care and concern for you.	0	1	2	3	4	5
	Comments:						
19.	What behaviors by faculty were helpful for your learning?	0	1	2	3	4	5
	Comments:						

20. What is your expected grade?	A　　B　　C　　D　　F
Comments:	
21. Strengths of this course:	
Comments:	
22. Suggestions for improvement:	
Comments:	
23. Overall, how would you rate this course?	0　　1　　2　　3　　4　　5
Comments:	
24. Please include any additional comments you would like to share about any aspect of this course.	
Comments:	

 The Example Course Evaluation Tool may be accessed on the CD-ROM accompanying this book.

Once feedback is collected, seek clarification if needed. Let students know how faculty responded to their suggestions. Students appreciate knowing their feedback is valued. For example, when beginning a new term explain how feedback from previous evaluations informed the rationale for changes or implementation of a new instructional design. Or, if changes were not made, discuss with students the reasons why the course is structured as it is and the goals faculty hope to achieve by using the current design.

Faculty Behaviors

The impact faculty behaviors have on student success, as noted by the caring curriculum portion of the Student Success Model in Figure 1.1, cannot be overemphasized. Perceived faculty support on the part of students, a caring environment, and faculty assistance are frequently noted as key factors contributing to persistence in nursing education (Shelton, 2003).

Chapter 6: A Student Success Program for Currently Enrolled Students

The actualization of a caring curriculum is only as good as it is perceived to be by those who should benefit – the students. Perhaps the least attended consideration in our hurried, knowledge to impart, additive curriculum approach, is the validation that we create an environment that is in fact perceived as nurturing and conducive to learning in our students' eyes. Evaluation of the extent to which the curriculum was a caring environment would be important to include on the course evaluation tool and would offer students a chance to comment on their perception of the learning climate. Questions might include:
- were faculty respectful in their attitude toward you?
- do you believe faculty demonstrated care and concern for you?
- what behaviors by faculty were helpful for your learning?

Revision

Evaluation data provide the basis for revision of the Student Success Program, both for individual students and the program as a whole. Revisions that address the overall Student Success Program focus on meeting goals based on indicators of success, such as student retention and program aspects that students or faculty identify as needing improvement. The following steps comprise the revision process:
- review data and compare results with indicators of success and program outcomes.
- consider salient features of the evaluation and whether revision is indicated. The need for revision is determined by processing the following factors:
  o data to support conclusions presented in the evaluation phase
  o degree to which previously enacted interventions have been successful
  o outliers which represent any factor that skewed results, either positively or negatively
  o adequate time for interventions to be realized

Based on the following indicators of success, examples of revisions might include:
- *Indicator of Success:* Students earn a minimum of a C in all nursing courses. Ninety-three percent of students in their first nursing class earned

Cs on their final course grade. This is an improvement of 4% from the previous year. Evaluation data for the students who were not successful are reviewed. Based on their findings, faculty retain the current outcome criterion of students must earn a minimum of a C in all nursing courses. Efforts are concentrated to meet individual student needs and identify curriculum choke points.

- *Indicator of Success:* Program achieves an 85% retention rate. The present retention rate is 80%. Faculty determine their current strategies seem to be working because the retention rate in the previous year was 75%. Faculty decide they are making some progress; however, not enough. Plans are made for the Retention Specialist to meet with students to discern any student needs that might be addressed to improve student retention. Faculty will consider input from the Retention Specialist before making any changes.
- *Indicator of Success:* Program achieves a 15% graduation rate with one stop-out. The current graduate rate with one stop-out is 17%. Since enacting this indicator of success three years ago, faculty have noted significant progress. They decide to wait another year before revising this goal or making changes to their plan. Faculty will continue to monitor the graduation rate with the number of stop-outs.
- *Indicator of Success:* Students answer all test items with a 75% success rate in each content area: This goal was not met for all content areas in nursing courses. Students in two courses answered less than 75% of the test items correctly in three subject areas. Faculty in the two courses where choke points occurred plan to meet and discuss alternative teaching strategies to enhance student learning in the coming year. Students in the current year will be retested after remediation on identified content. Faculty also plan to evaluate each test that contains content identified as choke points to ensure the tests are reliable and valid. Level of difficulty and item discrimination will be reviewed. Faculty will use their test blueprint to identify any test items that do not match course objectives and content, are not appropriately weighted, and do not reflect NCLEX-style items, with the majority of items written at the application level or above. The indicator of success is not altered at this point. Faculty will evaluate student command of the identified content areas once again the next academic year. Further additions or revisions will be determined at that point.

Chapter 6: A Student Success Program for Currently Enrolled Students

Any changes to the Student Success Program for an individual student are based on the evaluation of how well the interventions are working for that student. To illustrate, consider the student who was prescribed individualized tutoring sessions. If the tutoring fails to help the student achieve higher test scores, faculty will need to determine if a different intervention is necessary. Perhaps tutoring was not an effective strategy for that particular student or it may be the student did not follow the prescribed interventions the tutor offered. Faculty will need to determine why the tutoring was not successful. Interventions will be designed after the data are collected. Interventions may require a referral to counseling, if a learning disability is suspected, or a referral to academic learning skills center if reading or math skills are deficient. The important point is that evaluation of the intervention takes place in a timely manner and, if the plan is not working, a new plan is devised. It may be necessary to employ a number of interventions simultaneously to establish the most effective solution to the identified needs or concerns.

A Hypothetical Nursing School Example

Hypothetical Nursing School (HNS) faculty designed their Student Success Program for their current students. They planned their Student Success Program as indicated by assessment of the at-risk student and the class at-large to meet student needs in three realms: academic support, non-academic support, and cultural considerations. Each student's progress was tracked throughout the program and measured against indictors of success.

Academic Support

Academic support began with the first point of contact with the student, when the climate for learning was established, and concluded when the student graduated.

A welcome open house was scheduled prior to the start of the year. Students were given the opportunity to meet fellow students and the faculty who would teach their courses. The first hour was spent mingling and refreshments were served. Next, an overview of the year was presented, with agenda specific to each class. Scheduling, grading, advising, and academic assistance were discussed. For freshman and newly transferred students, orientation included a synopsis of the entire program, with a special emphasis on the first year of the program. Continuing students received information specific to the next year. The Retention Specialist presented an overview of the assistance provided by this position.

At the conclusion of orientation, each student was given an opportunity to ask questions, then completed an evaluation of the day's activities. The evaluations were reviewed and any areas needing further attention were noted and addressed by a follow-up letter from nursing faculty to the students.

Creative Class Scheduling

Faculty determined they would like to be more flexible in their class scheduling. This year they offered two different lecture times. The first option was to schedule all lecture hours in one day. This made for a long day, but required only one trip to campus. The second option was to schedule lecture hours over two days, with time allotted for class divided between the two days, necessitating two trips to campus. Faculty presented these scheduling options to students well in advance of orientation, which allowed students to select the class time which best met their needs and provided ample time for planning purposes. The Retention Specialist was asked to share any concerns students expressed about class scheduling, and adjustments were made if indicated. Faculty planned to evaluate student feedback about these two scheduling options.

Retention Specialist

HNS faculty worked closely with their Retention Specialist, who functioned as a consultant, counselor, liaison, and advocate for the students. Faculty planned for the Retention Specialist to address factors that impact academic performance and persistence such as:
- organizational strategies
- suggestions for better note-taking
- ways to use the student's learning style to the student's advantage
- direction and focus for study
- ways to effectively plan and manage time

Chapter 6: A Student Success Program for Currently Enrolled Students

The Retention Specialist was viewed as an integral part of the Student Success Program. HNS faculty designed several interventions to foster student success in their program.

Grading Options

The grading policy was explained to all classes. A sample assignment sheet with associated point distribution for each assignment was reviewed. Students were provided a tracking sheet to help them keep a record of their progress in the course. The sheet listed all assignments, the point value for each assignment, and the point total for the course. Students were asked to bring their tracking sheet to any meetings they had with faculty or the Retention Specialist. Assignments with their associated grading rubrics were explained, so students understood how their work would be evaluated.

Academic Advising

Faculty believed a new policy would help meet their goal to increase retention by 10%. Sometimes students are not aware they need to take action to improve their course standing until it is too late. A new policy was written that stated: students are appraised that if at any point they achieve less than 75% on an exam, they are to make an appointment with the Retention Specialist. Together, the student and Retention Specialist will design a plan delineating the timeline, focus, and method of study to meet student learning needs. The Retention Specialist will share the interventions that have been planned to meet student needs with the faculty in the course. The Retention Specialist and faculty will plan periodic meetings to review student progress.

The faculty identified skill performance in the clinical as a factor that contributes to attrition. Faculty designed a contract to use when a student demonstrates difficulty meeting clinical objectives. This contract is designed to address the difficulty in clinical practice, detail the nature and scope of the problem, and offer a means to address the concern. Students received a nursing skills remediation slip if faculty identified any skill deficiencies. This intervention allowed the student an opportunity to practice the skill first, then return demonstrate the skill with laboratory staff. Students were then given another opportunity to perform the skill in clinical, thus building confidence and expertise in skill performance.

Faculty Office Hours

Faculty explained to students they hold office hours, and are also available via e-mail and voice-mail, to address any concerns. General announcements were also posted in a common area easily accessed by students. Open lines of communication were established and students were made to feel welcomed. Students received a copy of faculty office hours, phone numbers, and e-mail addresses. The best time and method to reach faculty was noted for each faculty member.

Academic Assistance

HNS faculty provided each student with a listing of academic assistance resources they might use in the school of nursing and the college in general. A written overview of particular offerings, such as assistance with math, reading, and writing was provided, along with information about accessing these support services. Information about accessing computer programs and websites was also included.

Test-taking Analysis and Strategies

If a student achieved less than 75% on an exam, the faculty and students completed the LLUSN-LAP Exam Analysis Program (see Figures 6.2 through 6.7). The students then met with the Retention Specialist who focused on test-taking skills with the students. All students who experienced test-taking difficulty were mandated to take the study skills course. If any of these students had obtained a C in their anatomy and physiology course, or if more than three years had passed since completing anatomy and physiology, an optional review of these courses was highly recommended. Students retested on the topics in which they achieved a low test score after their work with faculty and the Retention Specialist. If students achieved an 80% or above on the retest, an additional five points were added to their cumulative points earned in the course. If they retested and scored below 75% a second time, students met with faculty once again to go over problem areas as identified by the LLUSN – LAP tool, then scheduled another appointment with the Retention Specialist to probe further to identify the problem.

Chapter 6: A Student Success Program for Currently Enrolled Students

If, after the second appointment with the Retention Specialist, the student did not achieve 75% or above on the subsequent test, the student must complete modules based on the content the student needed to learn. The student was required to meet with the Retention Specialist every two weeks until the student was consistently achieving 75% or above on course tests.

Reinforcing Course Content – Tutors

Faculty determined they would like to have two tutoring options available to provide academic assistance, peer tutors and faculty tutors. They provided two peer tutors for each class who were available to students for six hours each week. Administrators agreed to hire two faculty tutors from the part time faculty who would be on campus three days each week, for four hours each day. There was no charge to students for tutoring. The tutors met with the students to review course content that students found difficult to master and provide suggestions for more effective study.

Reinforcing Course Content – Critical Thinking Skills

Of particular interest to HNS faculty was the development and application of critical thinking skills by their students. To address this objective, faculty asked students to write one critical thinking test item at the completion of each class, and explain the reason why each option was either correct or incorrect. Students were also asked to develop a critical thinking case study, which they presented on a client they cared for during their clinical experience. Both activities were selected to help students apply information.

Exit Interviews

HNS faculty had scattered data about why or when a student leaves the nursing program. They decided to track this information, to see what they might learn. They established that whenever a student exited the program, the nursing department administrator would meet with the student to discuss reasons for leaving. These exits were tracked by the HNS Retention Committee to determine any problems faculty might need to address.

HNS faculty also realized they had little information about what they were doing well, what students liked about the program, and what they should continue to do. They asked the Evaluation Committee to develop a survey that would gather this information as students exited each course. The HNS faculty adapted the tool in Figure 6.9 to evaluate each nursing course.

Non-Academic Support

HNS faculty identified several areas in which they could provide support of a non-academic nature. Based on areas the majority of students indicated as concerns on the *Start Right in Nursing School* self-assessment tool, faculty addressed financial aid, job opportunities, child care options on campus, and counseling services.

Financial Aid

HNS faculty researched available financial aid for their students and were able to recommend several resources. These included scholarship funds and student loans. The liaison from counseling attended orientation and provided students with contact names and written information about these options.

Part-time Employment on Campus

Students were informed that job opportunities on campus are posted and faculty use grant money to hire students as aides for their courses. Students were told how they could interview for those positions and job applications were distributed during orientation and the first class session.

Child Care

During an advising session prior to admission to the program, several students indicated they would like to explore child care arrangements at the school. The HNS campus offers child care services to employees and students. An open house was scheduled for the 11 students potentially interested in using this facility. A brochure was provided which detailed the hours of operation and cost to the students.

Some students wished to explore the option of establishing exchange of child care hours with fellow students. A room and time were set aside for students who had used such an approach in the past to discuss how they formed their group and established rules for a cooperative effort. Several students attended this session and determined they would form a cooperative association among their class and make plans for their first meeting.

Counseling

The counseling liaison who works with nursing students was present for orientation to introduce services and allow students to place a name with a face. Availability and types of help offered were explained at this time. Students were provided an opportunity to ask questions and explore options available to them.

Cultural Considerations

To foster socialization and a greater cultural appreciation, HNS faculty planned an open house to welcome all students on the first day of school. All students were encouraged to attend. Certain cultural items were placed on display and faculty encouraged an appreciation of each other's cultures and customs.

As a result of curriculum review, faculty assigned a cultural assessment tool to enhance culturally sensitive nursing care in the first nursing clinical rotation. Students in advanced clinical courses were assigned a reflection tool to discuss their incorporation of culturally competent care for a client not of their culture.

Both strategies, an appreciation day and development of a cultural assessment for a particular client, met the objective of creating an awareness of cultural differences.

HNS faculty recognized they needed to thread culturally competent care throughout their nursing program and charged the Curriculum Committee with the task of presenting course objectives which highlight cultural considerations so they could address any gaps in the curriculum. Faculty also agreed to bring one article to share about designing instructional strategies that place an emphasis on multicultural nursing.

Two faculty decided they would like to attend a conference on multicultural nursing practices and creating a caring curriculum. They submitted their request to administration to enhance their knowledge of multicultural nursing in educational practice.

Implementation

The HNS faculty established a Student Success Committee to evaluate trends and make recommendations to full faculty regarding student needs and potential interventions, particularly for those at-risk for failure. Faculty reviewed student progress every two weeks and met with the Retention Specialist to identify any student concerns.

Faculty analyzed this data and identified student needs. Interventions were implemented to enhance HNS student success and will be evaluated and revised according to established indicators of success.

Indicator # 1: Attain an 85% retention rate.
- each student was assigned to a faculty advisor who tracked the student's progress throughout the program. The Checklist of Positive and Negative Factors (refer to Table 2.6) was completed with the student. Using this checklist, all students in the program were assessed for any problems or concerns.
- full faculty met and reviewed the findings. All findings were summarized and filed for counseling purposes during the student's time in the nursing program.
- faculty determined that seven students felt quite stressed. A small group session was arranged with the liaison from counseling to help address each student's needs. The counselor offered suggestions for ways to reduce stress.
- faculty met to review academic progress at two points during the term, after the first test and after midterm. Ten students in the program were found to be in academic difficulty, receiving less than a C on their first two nursing exams. Faculty met with these students to complete the LLUSN-LAP tools and mandated the students meet with the Retention Specialist.
- faculty conducted exit interviews with students who left the HNS program prior to graduation. Exit interview data were submitted to the Evaluation Committee for analysis.

Indicator # 2: Improve grades by 10% on the retest of content identified as curriculum choke points for those students who failed to achieve 75% on the first test. Content of the retest included the pediatric client with alterations in cardiac function and the client with neuromuscular dysfunction.

- faculty reviewed test items that addressed the two content areas of concern. Test items were revised to NCLEX-style items.
- students were provided with study guides to focus their learning.
- faculty planned learning activities that included case study and student presentations to address the two content areas of concern.
- students retested on identified content with an outcome of a 10% improvement of their previous test score.

Indicator # 3: Attain 5% or greater improvement on exams for those students who complete the optional review of anatomy and physiology, receive tutoring, or complete the study skills course.
- faculty mandated students experiencing test-taking difficulty take the study skills course. If any of these same students obtained a C in their anatomy and physiology course, or completed the course more than three years ago, the optional review of anatomy and physiology was highly recommended. Mandatory tutoring was implemented for those students who completed the mandatory study skills course and continued to experience test-taking difficulty.
- faculty tracked student performance of those who took the mandatory study skills course, completed the optional review of anatomy and physiology, and participated in mandatory tutoring, noting subsequent student exam performance.

Indicator # 4: Attain student satisfaction average of 3.75 or higher on all course evaluation items.
- faculty conducted course evaluations at the completion of each course.
- faculty reviewed course evaluations for the courses they taught. Faculty made any changes they deemed necessary and shared the rationale for their decisions with the students. In this way, open lines of communication were maintained regarding student concerns.
- faculty invited a student representative to discuss student concerns during a faculty meeting. Faculty allowed 15 minutes for discussion of student concerns and possible solutions to identified problems. Resolution to any concern identified was noted in faculty minutes and shared with the student representative.

Indicator # 5: Increase NCLEX pass rate by 5%.

- faculty attended workshops to enhance their ability to write NCLEX-style test items.
- faculty planned an exit exam to help identify students who need further study.
- faculty implemented an NCLEX review course.

Evaluation

Members of the Evaluation Committee met to determine whether established program indicators of success were realized. The results for each outcome were addressed with HNS faculty.

Indicator # 1: Attain an 85% retention rate.

Result: Outcome not met, retention rate is 83%.

- five of the seven students who reported difficulty with time management stated they felt much better and their grades were improving. Two were still struggling and thinking about leaving the program. These two students were referred to outside agencies for help with elder care and psychiatric counseling for depression. The student who needed help for elder care received community resource recommendations and was able to obtain the services needed to continue with the program. The other student decided to leave the program and seek treatment for the diagnosed depression. All other students in the HNS program developed a personal success plan to capitalize on positive factors.
- despite compliance with faculty recommendations, three students failed their first nursing course.
- faculty conducted exit interviews with students who left the HNS program prior to graduation. Most students left the HNS program due to personal reasons (90%).

Indicator # 2: Improve grades by 10% on the retest of content identified as curriculum choke points for those students who failed to achieve 75% on the first test. Content of the retest includes the pediatric client with alterations in cardiac function and the client with neuromuscular dysfunction.

Result: Outcome met, all students tested at least 10% higher on retest of content identified as curriculum choke points.

Indicator # 3: Attain 5% or greater improvement on exams for those students who complete the optional review of anatomy and physiology, receive tutoring, or complete the study skills course.

Result: Outcome met for those students who completed the mandatory study skills course and received tutoring. All students in this group who had obtained a C in anatomy and physiology, or had completed it more than three years ago, participated in the optional review.

Indicator # 4: Attain student satisfaction average of 3.75 or higher on all course evaluation items.

Result: Outcome met with the exception of one course, which indicated a student satisfaction average of 3.25. Faculty from the course met and determined which course elements were rated low in satisfaction by students. Based on student feedback from the course evaluation tool, HNS faculty in the course made adjustments to two assignments, which will be evaluated the next time the course is taught.

Indicator # 5: Increase NCLEX pass rate by 5%.

Result: Outcome met and exceeded. NCLEX pass rate increased from 84% to 92%.

Generally HNS faculty are pleased with the outcomes they effected by careful planning and implementation of designed interventions. Based on the results of this evaluation, faculty have the information to make necessary revisions to their Student Success Program. The next section discusses the revisions faculty planned, to further improve their program.

Revision

Faculty made revisions to their Student Success Program based on data analysis and recommendations from the Student Success and Evaluation Committees. These two committees worked together to evaluate data at the end of each term and made recommendations for future planning. Faculty from these committees invited their Retention Specialist to participate in the evaluation process to determine what recommendations and revisions might be of help. In addition, HNS faculty planned to use the data analysis to support their request to administration for more resources to implement identified revisions to their current Student Success Program.

Faculty met to consider revisions that addressed each indicator of success. The following recommendations were offered:

Indicator # 1: Attain an 85% retention rate.

Recommendation: No revision, continue current plan. HNS faculty believe student factors beyond their control contributed to the 83% retention rate. While the goal of an 85% retention rate was not attained, considerable gains were evidenced from the previous three years, when retention rates barely approached 80%. Faculty will continue with the current plan for one more year before making any revisions.

Indicator # 2: Improve grades by 10% on the retest of content identified as curriculum choke points for those students who failed to achieve 75% on the test covering this content.

Recommendation: No revision, continue current plan. This outcome was met and interventions suggested positive results. It was recommended that faculty consider additional active learning and critical thinking strategies, and continue to assess curriculum choke points.

Indicator # 3: Attain 5% or greater improvement on exams for those students who complete the optional review of anatomy and physiology, receive tutoring, or complete the study skills course.

Recommendation: Continue to offer all planned interventions to current and future students and track results.

Indicator # 4: Attain student satisfaction average of 3.75 or higher on all course evaluation items.

Recommendation: Continue course evaluations and faculty meetings with student representative in attendance. In addition, offer students the opportunity to send a student representative to standing faculty committee meetings, to provide further insights about interventions that might benefit students. Re-evaluate the extent to which students are satisfied after implementing the two revisions to the course that received a 3.25 satisfaction rating.

Indicator # 5: Increase NCLEX pass rate by 5%.

Recommendation: Continue current plan. Investigate obtaining and administering specialty exams, offered by Health Education Systems, Incorporated (HESI). Specialty exams are customized based on course syllabi to cover content throughout the curriculum, which provide a comparison of individual students taking the exam with all students who have previously answered the test items. Consider writing a mandate that students receive tutoring to address student content and knowledge needs identified by these exams.

Faculty Development

As a result of implementing the Student Success Program, HNS faculty recognized the need to expand their teaching skills to include visual learning cues and at least one learning strategy for the kinesthetic learner. To address this need, faculty were invited to attend a presentation by a guest speaker who offered teaching strategies that addressed a variety of learning styles. This presentation was offered at no expense to faculty.

Faculty set aside 30 minutes in their faculty meeting and shared the new learning strategy they plan to implement in the classroom. HNS faculty also determined similar faculty development opportunities should be made available to all new faculty. Current faculty were encouraged to continue their exploration of teaching strategies that address a variety of learning styles.

Closing Thoughts

A Student Success Program is crafted with care and knowledge of students' needs. Establishing a Student Success Program necessitates commitment from each member of the team: faculty, students, support staff, Retention Specialist, and administration. Faculty design interventions and evaluate their impact through a dynamic process that includes critical analysis of results and new or revised methods to meet established indicators of success.

All students require follow-up to implementation of interventions. Follow-up ensures that action was taken and the outcome measured. If the outcome was less than desired, the plan or intervention is modified.

No matter what the intervention, or how long it is employed, it is couched in such a way that students know that faculty truly care about their well-being and accomplishments. The merging of the art and science of nursing education is nestled within a caring curriculum. Faculty expect students to demonstrate caring in their clinical practice with clients. Students should be afforded similar care by the faculty who teach them.

Faculty need to make concerted efforts to understand the student experience and be compassionate. Nathan (2005), anthropologist and professor, describes her undercover experience living as a college freshman:

> I also had my own trials and tribulations as a student, and though I did "A" work in a couple of courses, in another I was easily the worst student in the class. As I found myself dropping further and further behind, it became a struggle for me to go to class. I came to understand what it means to be on the fence between giving up and making more of an effort. If there is one lesson that I have found most supported by my freshman experience, it is the lesson of compassion (p. 134-135).

Learning Activities

1. Identify needs and implement planned interventions for students. At the end of the term, compare your attrition rate in your current nursing class with attrition rates of previous years. What was the impact of your interventions?
2. Develop an evaluation tool that focuses on aspects of caring. Include faculty behaviors that students perceive as reflective of caring, such as comfort level in approaching faculty, extent to which students perceive faculty entertain student concerns and respond in a positive manner. Administer this tool to your students. Do students perceive faculty care about their ability to succeed in your program?
3. As a result of identifying interventions to meet student needs, what faculty development needs have you personally identified? Discuss with faculty colleagues the ways in which these needs might be met.

References

Blowers, S., Ramsey, P., Merriman, C., & Grooms, J. (2003). Patterns of peer tutoring in nursing. *Journal of Nursing Education, 42*(5), 204-211.

Campinha-Barcote, J. (1998). Cultural diversity in nursing education: Issues and concerns. *Journal of Nursing Education, 37*(1), 3-4.

Caputi, L. (2004). Operationalizing critical thinking. In L. Caputi & L. Engelmann (Eds.), *Teaching nursing: The art and science, Vol 1 & 2,* Glen Ellyn, IL: College of DuPage Press.

Caputi, L., & Blach, D. (2007, in press). *Integrating concept maps into a nursing curriculum.* Glen Ellyn, IL: College of DuPage Press.

Caputi, L., Engelmann, L., & Stasinopoulos, J. (2006). An interdisciplinary approach to the needs of non-native speaking nursing students: Conversation circles. *Nurse Educator, 31*(3), 107-111.

Condon, V. M., & Drew, D. E. (1995). Improving examination performance using exam analysis. *Journal of Nursing Education, 34*(6), 254-261.

Cook, P., & Cullen, J. (2000). Diversity as a value in undergraduate nursing education. *Nursing and Health Care Perspectives, 21*(4), 178-183.

Covington, L. (2004). Cultural diversity: Teaching students to provide culturally competent nursing care. In, L. Caputi, & L. Engelmann (Eds.), *Teaching nursing: The art and science, Vol 1 & 2,* Glen Ellyn, IL: College of DuPage Press.

Dictionary.com. (2006). Retrieved May 25, 2006, from http://dictionary.reference.com/search?q=tutor

Engelmann, L., & Caputi, L. (2005). Ideas to develop critical thinking in the classroom and clinical. In, L. Caputi (Ed.), *Teaching nursing: The art and science, Vol 3,* Glen Ellyn, IL: College of DuPage Press.

Gaines, C. (1996). Concept mapping and synthesizers: Instructional strategies for encoding and recalling. *Journal of New York State Nurses Association, 27*(1), 14-18.

Gaines, C. (1999). Clearing up the "concept fog." *ABNF Journal, 10*(2), 52-53.

Griffiths, M. J., & Tagliareni, M. E. (1999). Challenging traditional assumptions about minority students in nursing education: Outcomes from Project IMPART…Improving minority professionals' access to research tracks. *Nursing and Health Care Perspectives, 20*(6), 290-295.

Hickey, B. L. (2006). Lessons learned from collaborative testing. *Nurse Educator, 32*(2), 88-91.

Higgins, B. (2004). Relationship between retention and peer tutoring for at-risk students. *Journal of Nursing Education, 43*(7), 319-321.

Hsu, L. (2004). Developing concept maps from problem-based learning scenario discussions. *Journal of Advanced Nursing, 48*(5), 510-518.

Ironside, P. (1999). Thinking in nursing education. Part I: A student's experience in learning to think. Part II: A teacher's experience. *Nursing and Health Care Perspectives, 20*(5), 238-247.

Jeffreys, M. R. (2002). Students' perceptions of variables influencing retention: A pretest and post-test approach. *Nurse Educator, 27*(1), 16-19.

Jeffreys, M.R. (2004). *Nursing student retention: Understanding the process and making a difference.* New York: Springer.

Klisch, M. (2000). Retention strategies for ESL nursing students: Review of literature 1900-99 and strategies and outcomes in small private school of nursing with limited funding. *Journal of Multicultural Nursing & Health, 6*(2), 18-25.

Leonard, T. (2001). Exploring cultural, ethnic, and racial diversity in baccalaureate nursing education programs. (Doctoral Dissertation, Georgia State University).

Ligeikis-Clayton, C. (1996). Shared test taking. *Journal of the New York State Nurses Association, 27*(4), 4-6.

Lusk, M., & Conklin, L. (2003). Collaborative testing to promote learning. *Journal of Nursing Education, 42*(3), 121-124.

Malu, K., & Figlear, M. (1998). Enhancing the language development of immigrant ESL nursing students: A case study with recommendations for action. *Nurse Educator, 23*(2), 43-46.

Mitchell, N., & Melton, S. (2003). Collaborative testing: An innovative approach to test taking. *Nurse Educator, 28*(2), 95-97.

Nathan, R. (2005). *My freshman year: What a professor learned by becoming a student.* Ithaca, NY: Cornell University Press.

Owens, L. D., & Walden, D. J. (2001). Peer instruction in the learning laboratory: A strategy to decrease student anxiety. *Journal of Nursing Education, 40*(8), 375-378.

Ramsey, P., Blowers, S., Merriman, C., Glenn, L. L. & Terry, L. (2000). The NURSE Center: a peer mentor-tutor project for disadvantaged nursing students in Appalachia. *Nurse Educator, 25*(6), 277-281.

Rossignol, M. A. (2004). Dyad testing: Promoting skills used in the workplace. *Nurse Educator, 29*(2), 80-83.

Scheffer, B., & Rubenfield, G. (2000). A consensus statement on critical thinking in nursing. *Journal of Nursing Education, 39*(8), 352-359.

Shelton, E. N. (2003). Faculty support and student retention. *Journal of Nursing Education, 42*(2), 68-76.

Sims-Giddens, S. S. (2000). Graduation and national council licensure examination pass rate of Mexican-American undergraduate nursing students. (Doctorial dissertation, Northern Arizona University 2000), 89.

Speziale, H. J. & Jacobson, L. (2005). Trends in registered nurse education programs 1998-2008. *Nursing education perspectives, 26*(4), 230-5.

Stacciarini, J. (2002). Experiencing cultural differences: Reflections on cultural diversity. *Journal of Professional Nursing, 18*(6), 346-349.

Stokes, L. G. (2003). Gatherings as a retention strategy. *The ABNF Journal,* 80-82.

Tracey, G. (2003). A national study of support programs (efforts) in baccalaureate and associate degree nursing programs to enhance retention and success of students. (Doctoral dissertation, University of Central Florida, 1003). *Dissertation Abstracts International, 64* (2598).

Valencia-Go, G. (2005). Growth and access increase for nursing students: A retention and progression project. *Journal of Cultural Diversity, 12*(1), 18-25.

Vinten, S. A., & Ellett, M. L. (2000). Are two heads better than one? Students and educators explore dyad testing. *Excellence in Nursing Education, 2*(4), 1-2.

Wink, D. M. (2004). Effects of double testing on course grades in an undergraduate nursing course. *Journal of Nursing Education, 43*(3), 138-143.

Chapter 7:
A Case Study:
Creating A Success Program for Nursing Students

Imagine this event: your school's NCLEX® pass rate drops below 60%. What would you do to remedy the problem? Where would you begin? This chapter is about one nursing program's effort to implement interventions specifically tailored to deal with high attrition and low NCLEX pass rates, and how those interventions came to define a success program for nursing students. The second phase of the research first introduced in Chapter 4: *How Faculty Assess and Make Use of Learning Styles* is also presented in this chapter. Lessons learned went well beyond improving NCLEX outcomes. As you read this chapter, consider how the interventions implemented within this nursing program might benefit faculty and students in your program of nursing.

Overview: Case Study Methodology

Case study methodology is not governed by a single scientific approach, which is different from quantitative methodologies, where specific measurable concepts are identified and the researcher controls and interprets the data. Instead, one entity is examined in depth then studied and analyzed for patterns (Langford, 2001). Unlike traditional empirical research, case study is not built upon a foundation of an elaborate theoretical framework.

The goal of case study methodology is to provide the most complete description of the case as possible (Zucker, 2001). With case study research, data is collected about particular instances of a phenomenon, and understanding is sought for each instance relative to its own terms and context.

According to Gall, Gall, & Borg (2003) case study may serve one of three purposes:
1. Detail descriptions of a phenomenon
2. Develop possible explanations for the phenomenon
3. Evaluate the phenomenon

In this study, the authors selected case study for the first purpose, describing a phenomenon. The phenomenon is the evolution of a success program for one nursing program administered on four college sites. Gall, Gall, and Borg (2003) refer to a good depiction as one that will provide a thick description of the phenomenon. The authors recreated as much of the context of the evolution of this success program as possible. Constructs were inferred from interviews with case study participants and their descriptions of this phenomenon that occurred within their nursing program.

Case study methodology provided the means for a humanistic and interactive dynamic (Creswell, 2003). For the purposes of this research, the case study approach is particularly useful as a research method to appreciate the subjective richness of an account by nursing faculty as they discuss their experiences with, and responses to, low NCLEX-RN pass rates in 1998. A high attrition rate was also a concern during this year. A descriptive narration is used to present the findings and salient features in this case study.

All participants involved in this case study consented to share their comments personally, recognizing the tone and intent of this descriptive study was to provide insights and meaning about their experiences. With their permission, comments from participants are shared throughout the chapter to highlight key insights and reflections. Quotations from the participants as well as the authors' interpretation of the interviews are used in this qualitative narrative (Creswell, 2003).

Purpose

One purpose of this case study was to describe the development of a success program for nursing within Illinois Eastern Community Colleges (IECC) that may have contributed to increased retention and NCLEX-RN pass rates from 2000 through 2005. Four colleges comprise the IECC District: Olney Central College, Frontier Community College, Lincoln Trail College, and Wabash Valley College. The nursing program is administered through Olney Central College and is offered at all four colleges. Research questions one and two address this goal:
1. What events led to the development of your success program?
2. What elements comprise your success program?

A second purpose of this case study was to explore how faculty within the nursing program used knowledge of students' learning styles when teaching nursing. This particular program tailored teaching to student learning styles and strengths as one aspect of their success program. Therefore, the program was selected to illuminate the ways in which knowledge of students' learning styles impacts teaching and learning and enhances student program completion and NCLEX-RN pass rates. Research questions three and four address this goal:

3. Why is knowledge of student learning styles helpful for faculty as they develop teaching-learning strategies?
4. What variables are important to consider when developing instruction relative to student learning styles?

Chapter 4 presented the first phase of a research study the authors designed to address assessment and use of learning styles. This chapter presents the second phase of the research designed to address learning styles within the context of what the authors will refer to as IECC's success program for nursing.

Research Method and Technique

Interviewing was the primary research technique used in this study. Meetings were planned for this qualitative research on two occasions. First, the authors met with the Associate Dean of Nursing and Allied Health, faculty from the nursing program, and the Learning Skills Center director to discuss the roles the skills center staff play in skills assessment, and the recommendations they offer on behalf of students. Following the first meeting with faculty and staff from the colleges the authors met and discussed the information they had gathered during the meeting. The authors compared their data for similarities and differences. Specific questions to redirect or collect further information from the first meeting were prepared and incorporated into questions posed during the second meeting.

The second meeting was held on campus at one of the colleges the subsequent day. Faculty and personnel present included:
- Director of the Title III grant
- Associate Dean of Nursing and Allied Health
- Faculty from one of the campuses
- Department heads of nursing from three campuses

Chapter 7: A Case Study: Creating A Success Program for Nursing Students

The second meeting was taped and the authors transcribed all notes and compared them for accuracy and completeness. The transcripts from the interviews were examined closely to derive elements that comprise the success program, including why faculty tailor their teaching to student learning styles and strengths.

Research Questions

The following four research questions were explored in this case study specific to the success program, and assessment and use of student's learning styles:
1. What events led to the development of your success program?
2. What elements comprise your success program?
3. Why is knowledge of student learning styles helpful for faculty as they develop teaching-learning strategies?
4. What variables are important to consider when developing instruction relative to student learning styles?

Purposeful Selection

The Colleges of IECC were of interest to the authors because faculty had implemented strategies that brought the desired results of improved NCLEX-RN pass rates and decreased attrition. The authors came to know about these findings through a conference presentation by two IECC faculty when they described their use of learning styles as one component of a success program for nursing students.

Data Analysis and Interpretation

The authors followed the process outlined below adapted from Creswell (2003) to analyze and interpret the data from this case study, which included:
- organizing and preparing the data for analysis
- transcribing and reading through the data, to gain a general sense and impression of the information collected

- interpreting the data based on responses to questions posed to the participants
- validating that the interpretation of data was correct by asking the Associate Dean of Nursing and Allied Health to review the initial transcription and final summary of the case

All data were organized, categorized, and summarized from two interview sessions and written documents the four college site members supplied to the authors. Interview data were recorded and transcribed. Both authors compared transcripts to provide a description of the case.

Validation of Data

The authors took notes during both meetings and the second meeting was taped. Permission from all parties involved was obtained prior to the beginning of each session. Transcriptions and written notes were reviewed for accuracy by the Associate Dean of Nursing and Allied Health. Data were regrouped to present a thematic, yet chronological presentation of the case.

Researcher Actions

The authors construed, synthesized, and clarified information to produce a case history. This process involved recording, constructing, and presenting a chronicle of events that reflect the development of the success program within the nursing program of IECC.

Entry and Disclosure

The authors sought entry to this setting by communicating with two nursing faculty and the Learning Skills Center director to discuss the possibility of conducting a case study to learn about their success program and their use of learning styles. These three individuals agreed to meet with the authors and suggested other faculty who were interested in sharing their insights about their experiences in designing and implementing instruction based on student learning styles. Issues of confidentiality were addressed and each person consented in writing to participate in the study. The second meeting was recorded and transcribed then reviewed for accuracy by the Associate Dean of Nursing and Allied Health.

The remainder of this chapter presents the salient features of the discussion that ensued among the authors and all participants in the case study. Data were synthesized into meaningful categories. Concepts were illustrated with excerpts from discussions that occurred during the two interview sessions. Where appropriate, select dialogue is quoted to explicate meaning and substantiate conclusions. Although the authors developed interview questions to guide discussion prior to their visit, in some instances the questions were not posed, as the natural progression of the discussion allowed for discovery of information sought. A copy of the interview tool is on the CD-ROM accompanying this book.

Brief Description of the Nursing Program

The four colleges of IECC District #529 admitted 187 nursing students for the 2004-2005 academic year. There were 16 full-time and 3 part-time faculty within the district during this time. There has been a 75% turnover in faculty since 2000. Four of the five faculty who were present during the year of the low NLCEX pass rate remain with the district. Currently, there are 18 full-time and 2 part-time faculty who teach within the district. A full-time load for faculty is 15 credit hours per term. Faculty generally teach an average of 2.7 hours of overload. With the help of preceptors, the clinical ratio is twelve students to one faculty, with a maximum of 10 students in the clinical setting and two students under the supervision of preceptors in the college laboratory. Faculty are assigned to one college site but may teach a clinical session for another college site. Such faculty sharing is based on enrollment. In the past seven years, faculty have taught theory between college sites only when they were hired for that position (twice). In some cases faculty travel many miles to clinical sites in order to provide learning experiences in larger facilities.

The colleges use a ladder curriculum with an exit for a certified nursing assistant, exit for a practical nurse, and entrance for practical nurses to articulate into the associate degree nursing program. The first year resembles a licensed practical nurse (LPN) program. Content is expanded in the second year with a wellness to illness progression.

Curriculum is structured so students may exit after the first semester as a certified nursing assistant. Students may also exit after the first year prepared for the licensure exam for practical nurses after completion of an optional summer course which is presented between the first and second year. This option allows students to work as practical nurses prior to graduation. Most students who take the optional summer course do not exit the program. Many students believe work experience as a practical nurse positions them for future employment as an RN. If students opt to work as practical nurses, they are advised to balance work and school. Students are counseled to take care of themselves physically to avoid returning to the program exhausted.

Students who continue in the program exit with an associate's degree and are prepared to take the NCLEX-RN. The total number of semester credit hours for the two year program is 72. The nursing laboratory courses are two clock hours to one credit hour; the clinical portion is two clock hours to one credit hour. The student has 10 clinical hours per semester.

Technical support for instructional purposes is readily at hand for use of faculty, and the Learning Skills Center's director is closely involved with evaluation of students' learning problems and personal needs. This involvement is addressed throughout the case study. On interview, faculty describe a "real team approach." Everyone is involved.

How the Success Program Started

This section discusses the events that put the success program in motion. Research question one is addressed:
· what events led to the development of your success program?

In 1998 the NCLEX pass rate dropped to 51%. Formulating a response to the drop in NCLEX pass rates required faculty to conduct a critical data review. As faculty began to investigate their low NCLEX pass rate, they discovered eight of the 103 graduates did not test in the first or second testing period after graduation; therefore, of the 95 students who did write the NCLEX during that time period, 49 passed. They also found that 65 of their 103 graduates did not take the free review course offered on campus the first week after graduation.

Of the 65 who did not take the review course, 46 did not pass NCLEX. The course was not mandatory and many of the students who failed were not "at-risk" students.

When faculty asked students why they did not take the review course, the students responded they did not think they needed the review. Students said they always did well in the program and they had heard the program's NCLEX scores were pretty good, so there was no need to take the review. Several students indicated that they knew they could repeat the test if they failed on the first attempt.

Faculty offered all graduates who failed NCLEX the opportunity to return to the program with an option to repeat the last semester or take a specially prepared review course free of charge. Very few graduates accepted either of these offers of help.

Possible Reasons for Low Scores

Faculty needed to gain a sense of why the low NCLEX score occurred. The following sections describe facts faculty discovered as they explored this issue.

Student Preparedness

Faculty were observing changes in their student population which led them to believe students were unprepared for college. For example, students did not always complete assigned readings or homework (bibliography cards, care plans, teaching plans). With respect to homework completion, students made comments such as, "I know what to do so why should I have to write it down?" Students were satisfied with their grades as long as they did not receive unsatisfactory or failing grades.

The Associate Dean of Nursing and Allied Health recalled a student who failed one of the nursing courses. Upon discussing the situation with the student, it was determined this student had experienced a light senior year of high school, with a study hall, a microbiology class, and one other course. The student's GPA from high school was a 4.0. Both the student and the student's parents were quite upset when the student failed a course in the nursing program as the student "had never failed anything." At the exit interview with the student and her parents, the Associate Dean of Nursing and Allied Health shared the student's journal entry with the student's permission, "I read for this test and it helped." The

Associate Dean of Nursing and Allied health who had worked with this student to enhance test-taking skills commented she never thought to ask the student if she was completing the assigned readings. As educational preparation and study habits came to light, faculty decided student lack of preparation needed to be addressed.

Diverse Population

Students who entered any of the four colleges came from different areas. The colleges range widely in geographic location. Some students were from the local high schools; however, there were also older students who entered the program. In addition, IECC draws students from neighboring states. There were several LPNs who entered to pursue an associate degree in nursing. All these students varied greatly in their background and educational foundation. Faculty determined they needed a mechanism to evaluate applicant needs and identify necessary interventions to meet those diverse needs.

Preliminary Interventions that Helped Students

Two preliminary interventions sparked the beginning of the success program. One of these interventions included development of a success course titled, Strategies for Success. Prior to assuming her present role, the Associate Dean of Nursing and Allied Health worked with students teaching math and study skills. Upon assuming her present role, the Associate Dean instituted the Strategies for Success course students take in the summer prior to beginning nursing coursework their freshman year. The Strategies for Success course includes sections on learning styles, study skills (preparation for class, note taking, reading for understanding), time management, stress management, self-care, and test-taking skills. Students complete the Learning Style Inventory (LSI) during this course and the College Student Inventory ™.

A second intervention included development of a math skills course offering general math review and drug calculation skills. While the math course was not mandatory, the course was offered on all four campus sites and students were strongly encouraged to take it. Students are counseled into the math skills course either concurrent with or before the first nursing course, when pharmacology content is introduced. Because pharmacology content is integrated into each nursing course, one faculty developed an online component for each nursing course, which includes general review, many practice questions, and quizzes related to pharmacology.

Several other strategies were implemented early in the development of the success program and included a mandatory review course, exit exams, educational computer programs, and critical thinking activities to facilitate student learning.

Mandatory Review Course for NCLEX

One of the first interventions that became part of the success program was the inclusion of a mandatory NCLEX review course. Each college donated money to hire tutors and IECC allocated funds to pay for a mandatory review course for students to take upon completion of the nursing program. These donations reflected a substantial investment to promote student success.

The mandatory review course was added as two credit hours. This course is part of the 72 credit hours required for the associate degree.

The mandatory review course was contracted with National Education Consultants (NEC) in 1999. NEC tailors its review based on the student composite results from the Health Education Systems, Inc. (HESI) exit exam.

Faculty use an NCLEX-RN review program online and require students to complete a certain number of test questions as part of the mandatory review course. Faculty have not required a specific passing score.

Faculty Development

To facilitate professional growth and ensure faculty were prepared to write critical thinking test items and promote critical thinking in their classrooms, NEC conducted a workshop with faculty. Test item construction focused on methods faculty could use to upgrade the cognitive level of questions from knowledge/comprehension to application/analysis. Strategies were offered to stimulate critical thinking in the classroom and included integration of case studies and discussion of actual clinical situations based on instructor and student clinical experiences.

Exit Exams

Two exams are administered to evaluate student learning needs as students approach the end of the program. These two exams are administered as a component of the mandatory review course. The HESI exam is administered in March. Faculty counsel students about areas of concern the HESI exam identifies. Students who score less than 850 on the HESI are required to take additional NCLEX-style tests before the review course is completed. Students can not graduate without completing all requirements of the review course.

The ARNETT exam is administered in April to compare with the outcomes from the HESI exam. The ARNETT is a computer-adaptive exam designed like the NCLEX. The more questions the student answers correctly, the higher the degree of difficulty. With the ARNETT exam, the computer shuts off when the student has achieved the passing score.

Technology

A major change for faculty has been more extensive use of technology as part of instructional strategies to meet learning needs. This use of technology was made possible in large part due to Title III grant money, first awarded in September, 2001. Title III grant money has provided instructional training for use of technology, enabled upgrades in technology in the classroom, and provided a data management system to track student outcomes.

The ways in which faculty and students learn have been enhanced with use of technology. Faculty believe that they learn when they are willing to make changes. Faculty avow the changes they have made to incorporate technology in their teaching have made a difference for both students and faculty.

One faculty commented that the Title III grant helped get faculty started with technology. The Colleges of IECC have implemented Entrata, a program that provides students with e-mail access and a method for students and faculty to communicate. Faculty enter grades, post assignments, and provide outlines in advance of class so students know what to expect and can prepare before attending class. One faculty poses a question online before and/or after students attend class to help determine students' understanding of the material.

Computer Programs

Students have been required to complete computer programs and keep instructional logs since 1997. This requirement was implemented because students were taking tests via the computer and faculty wanted to be sure students were comfortable with the process. Faculty decided to explore learning activities students could complete at home via the computer. This allowed faculty to make online assignments and evaluate any problems students experienced using computer-assisted instruction. The faculty use a tracking program to determine if students complete assignments. Funding for these online resources is provided by administration.

Critical Thinking Activities

Critical thinking activities were also cited as instrumental to student success. Faculty instituted use of *Strategies, Techniques, and Approaches to Thinking – Critical thinking Cases in Nursing,* by de Castillo (2003), which moves through different levels of critical thinking. Students are also encouraged to engage in group discussions. Much more interaction takes place in current classes than prior to implementing this strategy. Several group activities involve the use of case studies. More activities that encourage critical thinking are discussed in later sections of this chapter.

Putting It All Together: Success Program Elements

The authors were interested in delving further to explicate those elements that reflect aspects of the nursing program's success with raising NCLEX pass rates. Main topical areas and responses of those who participated in the two interview sessions are discussed in this section and address research question number two:
- what elements comprise your success program?

Admission Testing

Students take the COMPASS® placement assessment test at any of the colleges within IECC for academic advisement into appropriate courses. The nursing program uses the college standard of the 34th percentile, which is necessary to be admitted to a degree seeking program, as one part of their admission criteria. A student's score determines if the student can be admitted to the program and identifies remediation needs.

One concern identified with COMPASS testing was that this test did not reveal time since last exposure to content, such as algebra and chemistry. Another concern was that while other tests offer tutorials, the COMPASS does not. Faculty thought, "Why have a student take the test cold and mandate remediation? Why not enable the student to succeed in the first place?" A tutorial would allow the student to arrive prepared for the COMPASS exam and provides a better picture of the student's abilities than if the student takes the exam without knowing what to expect.

Faculty discussed these concerns with the director of the Title III grant, who wrote an online tutorial that students use to refresh their knowledge prior to taking the COMPASS exam. The tutorial presents the types of problems students will encounter on the COMPASS and affords students practice opportunities prior to testing. Learning needs are augmented with websites. A favorite is mathhomework.com. Faculty and personnel in the Learning Skills Center also help refresh students' knowledge of math and science. All these opportunities to prepare help build student confidence and position them to score well on the COMPASS exam.

In this situation, faculty and the director of the Title III grant took steps to address the issue that the COMPASS exam may not accurately reflect student abilities without students' receiving adequate review. College policy mandates students who do not score in the 34th percentile to take a four credit hour math class. Students may complete this course on their own or with a tutor. This is a time-consuming process. Use of the tutorial enabled better assessment of student learning needs and the development of tailored review and/or remediation for those students who needed it.

Ranking System for Admission

Faculty use a computer program to rank students for admission using a predetermined rubric. See Figure 7.1 for the rubric used to rank students for admission. Students must earn a minimum score of 6 to be eligible for admission.

Figure 7.1 – Rubric for Ranking Applicants to the Associate Degree Nursing Program

---

Rubric for Ranking Applicants to the Associate Degree Nursing Program

Applicants to the Associate Degree Nursing Program are ranked according to the following criteria:

COMPASS/ASSET Test Scores: Student must meet minimum entry-level scores at or above the 34th national percentile. Nursing applicant may take the COMPASS or ASSET test twice during an application process.

Grade Point Average (GPA): Grades earned in the <u>nursing support courses</u> are used to calculate the GPA. The same formula is used as for the cumulative.*

High school students' GPAs are calculated on the courses they have taken that will prepare them specifically for nursing – math, English, science, psychology and sociology.

Composite Science Score: If the student has one or all of the science courses (Human Anatomy & Physiology I & II and Microbiology) completed and has been successful in the first enrollment in the course, the student will earn extra points as follows:

$$A = 1.0$$
$$B = 0.75$$
$$C = 0.5$$

If a student has repeated a science course(s), a -1 point will be computed for each repeat. A student who has a lapse of five years or more between repeating a course will not have a deduction in points.

The minimum entry level composite score is 6.0, which is derived from the COMPASS or ASSET test, GPA, and science courses. All students are ranked according to this score with in-district residents given preference.

A cumulative GPA of 2.5 is required to make application to the nursing program.

---

* The college criteria for converting letter grades to a numerical score is used: A = 4 points, B = 3 points, C = 2 points, and D = 1 point.

The COMPASS score, grades in prerequisite science classes, and overall GPA earned in nursing support courses are used to determine the admission score. The COMPASS test is required. For students with special needs, the ASSET test is provided because there is no print version of the COMPASS test. There is a correlation table for the COMPASS and ASSET scores. There is a point system for each of these criterion.

Faculty implemented new measures to address the retention rate. NCLEX scores had improved but attrition rates had also increased. The GPA of 2.5 for admission is a new 2007 criterion. Previously, the GPA admission requirement was 2.0. Also, the deduction of a point for students who repeat science courses is a 2007 addition. In collaborating with science instructors, faculty perceived that persons who repeated science courses were less likely to be successful in completing the program. Faculty looked at data on 120 students admitted to the nursing program who had repeated a science course. Of those, 66 failed to complete the nursing courses.

A lighter academic load is the incentive for students to complete science courses prior to entering the program. While students might be able to manage their nursing coursework while maintaining a 17- or 18-hour course load, it is very difficult. In addition, completion of science courses prior to entering the program provides students with a knowledge base that facilitates understanding of pathology and the rationale for many nursing actions. Faculty believe students who complete their science courses prior to beginning the nursing program are much more successful. In essence, a two year program is spread over three years.

Tutoring

The Learning Skills Center provided tutors for biology and other classes; however, there were no tutors designated for nursing. Each of the four colleges contributed $1100 a year to hire alumni tutors. One of the current nursing faculty tutored students while she was a student in a baccalaureate program and found it a worthwhile effort. The Associate Dean of Nursing and Allied Health commented alumni have provided tutoring services which have provided the "best tutoring for the program." Alumni know the curriculum as no other peer tutor can. This is a major advantage in the use of alumni tutors over peer tutors. Some second level students have tutored other nursing students; however, this

Chapter 7: A Case Study: Creating A Success Program for Nursing Students

was a heavy load for them and less than ideal. Most tutoring needs have been met through use of alumni tutors.

Identifying Learning Needs

Staff in the Learning Skills Center work with students to identify needs and plan interventions to promote learning. These identified needs are useful for classes as a whole, but also provide information about individuals. Individual student reports are typically completed in October, allowing faculty to intervene or refer early in the student's course of study.

Conditions such as attention deficit hyperactivity disorder (ADHD) are not diagnosed by staff in the Learning Skills Center. A condition of this nature would need to be documented by a licensed psychologist or healthcare provider. Learning Skills Center staff assess learning needs and make recommendations to students. For example, staff in the Learning Skills Center suggested a student experiencing difficulty seek a healthcare provider for further evaluation. The student was a middle-aged adult diagnosed with ADHD. The student received treatment, returned to the program, and graduated. The student likened the difference to "walking into the sunlight – the clarity it made."

E-mail and phone communications between staff in the Learning Skills Center and the Associate Dean of Nursing and Allied Health serve as reminders and follow-up about student status. For example, staff in the Learning Skills Center might report they tested a student the first term of the nursing program and what their testing revealed.

Faculty always know when students visit the Learning Skills Center. Both students and the Associate Dean of Nursing and Allied Health receive a report which is kept in the student's file.

Student Examples

The Associate Dean of Nursing and Allied Health commented that a high number of students are successful because they do make necessary adaptations. However, she also postulated that paying attention to the student is what really matters. For example, a student preparing to take a test forgot to bring a purple transparent overlay. Blue or light purple transparent overlays are helpful in the reduction of glare from the test paper and serve to reduce vision stress. The student was shaking when requesting colored paper for the test. When the student was informed faculty would obtain the colored paper, the student was greatly relieved. The Associate Dean of Nursing and Allied Health commented, "I would say a lot of students are definitely impacted by what we do. Taking time for students really matters."

Accommodations for testing for another student stipulated she be allowed to test alone with unlimited time and walk around and talk out loud during the test. To accommodate this student's needs, the student was provided a private room and allowed to walk around as needed during testing. The room was equipped with a camera. The student passed NCLEX without need for the additional time granted by the testing site.

Another tool used to assist this same student was a magnifying bar to delineate lines of text for easier reading. Use of this tool enabled the student to read the medication administration record in the clinical setting.

Faculty counseled this student throughout the program. One faculty commented, based on the student's needs, "We knew right away this student was going to need to be selective about the type of nursing chosen for practice. We followed the student closely and documented everything."

Interestingly, the Associate Dean of Nursing and Allied Health received a call from a hiring specialist in a human resources department who stated they hired this graduate to work on a cardiac step down unit. The hiring specialist had a few questions about the graduate's performance. With the graduate's permission, the Associate Dean of Nursing and Allied Health addressed the questions, then entered into a discussion about how the faculty had worked with the graduate. The hiring specialist shared she had the same problem herself (ADHD), and they could work it out. The six month employer survey indicated the graduate remained at that hospital. The Associate Dean of Nursing and Allied Health remarked, "This employee was noted fair in three areas and average in others. The graduate was able to adapt."

This student example illustrates the challenges faculty face when determining a student's success or failure. Faculty determined this student was safe in practice and met all learning objectives. Faculty concluded that the interventions implemented for this student during her time in the program were worthwhile, and they would continue to provide similar interventions for other students.

Personal Contact

The authors asked how faculty viewed caring and personal interactions in relation to student success. Faculty responded they employ considerable thought developing strategies for students to be successful. On their final survey of students prior to graduation, they asked the students what one factor made a difference. The students' response was individual contact with the faculty. The Associate Dean of Nursing and Allied Health explained it is the real feeling the students have that faculty want students to be successful, not just graduate. It is also about knowing students on an individual basis. All faculty teach in the classroom and in the nursing skills laboratory. This teaching arrangement provides an opportunity for faculty to interact with students on a one-to-one basis. These interactions build trust and knowledge of the student as an individual.

Faculty Development

Faculty recognized the need for enhanced teaching strategies and understanding of the technology available to them. These two needs were met via faculty development courses offered through Performance Learning Systems, Inc. and through training courses offered at each college site provided by the Title III funding.

Faculty learned to develop a discussion board to use with students. Faculty use the discussion board to pose reflection questions and require students to respond weekly. Faculty are also using the discussion board to address clinical questions and concerns.

New learning strategies were also a part of the faculty development courses. One strategy was "think, pair, share," which involves dividing the students into small groups and posing a question. To use this activity with students, ask students to think first individually about the answer to a question. Next group each student with a partner to discuss the answer. The third step is to ask the student pairs to share with the class the answer they derived as a pair.

Faculty also participated in discussions where they sit toe-to-toe or knee-to-knee for the purpose of brain-storming. Faculty have since used this technique to enhance communication skills in their students.

Faculty development also included creation of WebCT courses and use of electronic whiteboards, online grade books, and internet links to PowerPoint®. Faculty development was also supported by mini-grants, one of which enabled a faculty member to become familiar with PowerPoint. As new technologies were mastered, faculty used their skills to create presentations for state and national conferences.

Instructional Strategies

Faculty identified several select instructional strategies as instrumental in the formation of the success program. These strategies are discussed in this section. Associated faculty development needs are also discussed for their impact on faculty ability to enact new teaching strategies. Strategies included:
- development of a test bank
- implementation of a math review
- teaching alternatives to straight lecture
    o active discussion
    o small group work
    o advance assignments
    o visual aids
    o skits
    o commercials
    o videotaping
    o concept mapping

Test Bank

With the assistance of the administrative assistants and what is described as a monumental effort to input test items into a data base, faculty compiled a large test bank all faculty use to construct their exams.

There are no identifiers indicating who wrote the test items. A test blueprint is maintained and test items are periodically revised to ensure they are high level items. As students learn more complex content, faculty ask questions that reflect a higher level of difficulty. Higher level items may be selected from the test bank when faculty construct tests.

Math Review

The department head of one of the college sites created a math review for students. This review included medication administration, not simply math calculations. The review is available to all four college sites online via Web CT and is leveled for each course. Students are required to pass the math drug calculation test with an 85% each semester.

Teaching Alternatives to Straight Lecture

The faculty described how their teaching has shifted from straight lecture to a variety of interactive techniques. These teaching alternatives to lecture are described in this section.

Active discussion. One of the strategies faculty implemented involves student discussion of journal articles. The students are instructed to read an article, answer questions, and engage in discussion. Subsequent to this classroom activity, faculty provide students an opportunity to apply this knowledge to client care scenarios.

Small group work. Another technique faculty employ is to assign students to small groups. One group might work on a computer program, while another group works with an instructor doing some activity. The groups switch, so students complete all activities.

Advance assignments. One faculty shared she was struck by the need to change her teaching approach when one of the students asked her why nursing faculty expect students to write everything down, when in medical school there are transcriptionists who supply the lecture notes, enabling students to listen and participate during class. The faculty thought, "Why don't I give the students an outline of what I am going to talk about in advance of class?" Now this faculty provides a case study or class outline prior to class and students use their book to answer questions. Students are actively engaged in learning, asking questions, and arriving at class prepared.

Visual aids. One faculty described how she used visual aids to help students learn about the endocrine system. She had several visual aids: a light bulb for a uterus, hard boiled eggs for ovaries, golf balls for testes, milk bones for bones, and a bra for the mammary glands. As the class talked about the target organs, the faculty would pin the organ on the student. Students found the experience both fun and educational.

Skits. Faculty assigned students to develop and perform skits. In one class, students were assigned a particular endocrine gland function to present. The directions were to create a skit to convey the function of the endocrine gland assigned. The faculty conducting the class brought visual aids (described above) to help students design their skits. For one of the skits in this class, a student brought a phone and he was the connection between the blood sugar and the pancreas. Students would come as food to raise blood glucose, then use the phone to call the pancreas and tell the pancreas about the need for insulin. In this skit, students demonstrated knowledge of how the pancreas functions.

In another class about electrolytes, students set up campaigns for their electrolyte since that content is usually taught around election time. Students wrote slogans and developed their political action committee and who supported them in the house (cell) and outside the house (extracellular). They identified major contribution groups (foods) and why their electrolyte was most important and should get the vote.

Faculty believed students were actively engaged in learning when performing and viewing these skits as evidenced by the types of questions the students asked. One faculty prepared review questions to help facilitate student discussion and process information.

Commercials. Another approach faculty used was to assign students to write commercials. Students responded in creative ways. Some students wrote commercials during which they had an assigned number of minutes to sell their disease. Faculty commented this type of learning is fun for students and teachers. While students are not awarded points for this activity, they freely participate.

Videotaping. Faculty have designed camera evaluations for skills, interactions, and teaching plans. Students work in pairs and tape one another's performance in the nursing laboratory. Students self-evaluate their own performance and submit the videotape to faculty when they have completed necessary revisions. Faculty review the tape and provide recommendations for improvement. Students may be required to submit a second tape. Due to a class size of 80 students and limitations in video-recording equipment, faculty alternate taped assignments. Some of the students use their own cameras.

Faculty use a skills checklist from the textbook for evaluation purposes. For select skills, students may earn a total of 15 points. The scoring is:
- 3 points if perfect first time

Chapter 7: A Case Study: Creating A Success Program for Nursing Students

- 2 points if first resubmit and satisfactory
- 1 point if second resubmit and satisfactory
- 0 points if four or more resubmits but must be completed and must be satisfactory

Types of videotaping. Students videotape interaction recordings, teaching plans, and assessments. Students role-play an interaction recording, which usually addresses some type of psychiatric condition. Evaluation sheets for interaction recordings are provided in the syllabus.

Faculty also design scenarios about client teaching plans that students role-play. One scenario faculty devised involves students providing information on sexual activity after a birth. Evaluation sheets for teaching plans are also provided in the syllabus.

For an assessment class, students are asked to perform an assessment, such as head-to-toe, neurological, and psychosocial assessments. The requirements are that the student perform the proper assessment and know what types of questions to ask.

Students submit a videotape of their assessment to faculty for evaluation. Students turn in a self-evaluation with the tape, which prevents students from turning in their assignment with an expectation faculty find the errors and places responsibility with the students to evaluate their submissions. The process of self-evaluation enables students to literally see what they are doing and identify changes they need to make to their submission. As one faculty noted, "Taping is a good way for students to look at how they interact, how they respond to a situation. I have required students to review the tape with me. I can point things out and ask the student why a particular action was implemented."

Concept mapping. Both faculty and students have been excited about concept map development. Faculty believe use of concept maps allows students to think in a different way. Faculty comment students have pride in what they accomplish and their work is often very good. One student used a picture of a little dog for a client with a dog bite who was very sick and had tubes in every orifice. The student designed a concept map using the picture of the dog. The student used bags that were yellow to represent the urinary drainage device, brown for the bowel collection device, and red for the IV solution.

Faculty introduce the concept maps in stages, moving from simple to complex, to apply what is covered in each course. Students complete some beginning components of the concept map the first semester. The second semester students create an entire concept map, when they have knowledge of a complete client assessment. The creation of concept maps in stages compliments student development.

Faculty commented these students expressed a great deal of excitement in the learning experienced from making concept maps. The process enabled students to see how everything relates.

Associated Faculty Development Needs

The faculty discussed how these instructional strategies could be realized, considering development needs for all faculty and the lack of preparation or teaching experience common to many faculty new to nursing education. Teaching skills and faculty development are impacted by a large learning curve. It is difficult for new faculty to learn the curriculum and learn to teach it, especially simultaneously.

An orientation is provided to help guide new faculty in their teaching. Examples of written work, such as student care plans, are provided to illustrate expectations for each level of the program. In addition, certain faculty are assigned to work with new faculty. Many times, relationships develop among faculty that enhance faculty development for both new and experienced faculty.

There are also incentives for faculty development from the school district. If faculty complete courses and workshops, their salary is increased. This incentive led faculty to several Performance Learning Systems courses, one of which was the *Teaching the Skills of the 21st Century*. This course was described as "wonderful networking where real learning occurs." Techniques learned in this course that faculty now use with their students include:

- discussion: think-pair-share, toe-to-toe meetings, or five minutes to discuss a topic.
- sayings: you can charge for your electrolytes.
- questions: are you in or out of the cells (referring to electrolyte location).
- group work: groups are established, roles and tasks are assigned, and participation of group members is encouraged.

Faculty also took advantage of a variety of conferences and workshops about teaching and nursing education.

Chapter 7: A Case Study: Creating A Success Program for Nursing Students

Enthusiasm for Teaching

Faculty are excited about the opportunity to bring life to their classrooms. They believe this excitement translates the idea to students that faculty want to teach and enjoy being with students. Faculty meet a variety of learning needs using different instructional strategies. They use the internet to augment presentations and the active learning strategies previously described. Faculty stated, "We can't stand up there and lecture because it doesn't get across ...it doesn't develop critical thinking. Students can't just take notes."

One faculty encountered the student view that the teacher is supposed to present the material and the student is supposed to come, take notes, and successfully pass the test. This faculty believes students might not fully appreciate these active learning components, but believes students will use the teaching and communication skills they have developed as a result of completing assignments that require active participation. For example, students who are required to present their concept maps to faculty and other students gain experience formulating and presenting their knowledge. This experience prepares them to discuss aspects of care with their clients and other healthcare professionals.

An important aspect of these experiences is that faculty hold students accountable for their learning and expect them to engage in the learning process. The teaching tools faculty use to promote this engagement have served them well.

Faculty Assignments

Faculty assignments have also changed. IECC uses "creative calendar planning" which provides a mechanism for faculty to teach on both levels of the nursing program. For example, faculty might teach mobility on first level and orthopedic nursing on second level. This structure allows faculty to teach to their area of expertise. An additional advantage is faculty know both levels of learners and the content students have learned in their early courses. This structure provides continuity in instruction and an ability to build on previously taught content.

One faculty commented about this system, "Once you get it – it works. So far this semester was my best semester. I had my content down and it really moved for me."

Faculty described several advantages to teaching on both levels. A major advantage of this structure is that faculty can hone and know particular content completely. With knowledge of specific content on both levels, faculty have the ability to address learning needs for students who might be returning or newly transferred to the program. Faculty plan instruction for content not yet covered for these students based on knowledge of where that instruction is placed within their program. In this way, individual student learning needs are met without having students repeat or omit material. It is also possible to develop a two-year content plan because faculty know precisely which topics need to be addressed in a given portion of the course. When full faculty come together to determine curriculum, they have collective knowledge of content and can plan revisions accordingly. Faculty believe this structure for class instruction is a time saver and has led to better faculty relationships. The change to more creative calendar planning was morale building.

Faculty were asked if they saw a difference since implementing creative calendar planning in terms of student attitude or student characteristics. Major changes cited include:
- students state they feel very comfortable seeking any faculty for help.
- students are exposed to a variety of teaching styles, which is helpful: no one faculty will appeal to every student's learning needs.

Relationships among faculty have also changed with this structure for class delivery. Faculty commented, "We know other people do things differently and that's what's so nice about it. I think we try to play our strengths."

Faculty recognize the importance of an environment that supports communication and understanding among students and provide an atmosphere where students feel nurtured. Because faculty move between levels in the program, students feel comfortable faculty will know their learning needs. In addition, students are exposed to a variety of faculty skills that enable fresh and exciting learning.

Tracking of the Success Program

The ability to access data is essential to IECC's assessment plan. For example, IECC might evaluate attrition and completion using variables of age and gender to determine if these variables are affecting student success. Data may be accessed

Chapter 7: A Case Study: Creating A Success Program for Nursing Students

for the entire district or for individual college sites. This capability to access data enables better planning – if a pattern is found on one site, the intervention would be different than if the pattern is the same on all sites.

One of the major initiatives of the Title III grant was to examine issues related to student retention. Faculty were tabulating data by hand and identified they needed a better means to access information about program outcomes. IECC does not have an institutional research department, so faculty sought a way of organizing and retrieving information for their purposes. A district committee composed of the Associate Dean of Nursing and Allied Health, the director of the Title III grant, staff from information technology (IT), faculty, and administration concluded they would purchase software that allowed them to manipulate data rather than develop their own program. The purpose of obtaining software was to bring the ability to access data to all stakeholders: faculty, administration, and personnel in student services.

Working together, the district committee designed data sets based on existing reports and information outlined by the management information systems manual published by the state's community college board. This information encompassed state and federal data such as: enrollment, course resource data, completion rates, and student data (age, gender, ethnicity, student intent, disability, limited English, previous degree, high school rank, ACT scores, remedial courses, and enrollment type) (http://www.iccb.org/HTML/pdf/manuals/mismanualfy02.pdf, 2002).

The software purchased did not work well for the IECC faculty, staff, and IT. They then developed an internal system that is flexible in data retrieval. This internal system provides IECC with longitudinal data that can be manipulated for forecasting and trend analysis.

The director of the Title III grant relayed, "We have redesigned existing information. It was a high learning curve, especially for me, because that is just not my area of expertise. I worked with our IT department for district data and I collaborated with them to structure the collections."

The advantage for the nursing program was whatever information they wanted to view could be obtained district-wide or by college site. For example, first semester attrition was examined relative to campus environment and faculty at each site, to determine differences or similarities among schools. No differences were found in attrition rates among the four schools.

251

Factors Key to Success

This section provides an overview of factors faculty identified as key for their successful implementation of a student success program: fiscal support, the role of the Learning Skills Center staff, and use of the learning style inventory. These factors comprise the elements integral to development of the success program.

Fiscal Support

After a rigorous application process, the district was awarded a competitive Title III grant. This grant provides assistance to eligible institutions of higher education to become self-sufficient by providing funds to improve and strengthen their academic quality, institutional management, and fiscal stability. One-year planning grants and five-year development grants are awarded. Funds may be used for faculty development, administrative management, development and improvement of academic programs, joint use of facilities, and student services (U. S. Department of Education, 2006).

The district was awarded a five-year development grant with three components: developmental education, student information systems and retention, and faculty and staff development. As a way to encourage faculty to explore and utilize technology, Title III staff developed a mini-grant process. Faculty applied for and received mini-grants each year of the Title III grant, which ended September 30, 2006. Mini-grant projects were shared district-wide and used as a catalyst to inspire other faculty to consider the use of technology in teaching. Nursing faculty were the single largest program group to utilize Title III grants and have used these grants to enhance their use of technology in the classroom. The nursing program also piloted the College Student Inventory as part of the retention initiatives component of the Title III grant.

Learning Skills Center Staff

While each college site has a Learning Skills Center that serves students at that site, the Learning Skills Center located at Olney Central College offers developmental support for nursing students. Students from the nursing programs are referred to the Olney Learning Skills Center site for help with a variety of concerns. When a student is referred to the Olney Learning Skills Center, the

Chapter 7: A Case Study: Creating A Success Program for Nursing Students

director assesses the student to identify needs and potential interventions. The following are addressed:

- dietary intake – is the student eating a well-balanced diet with adequate nutrients? Alternative dietary patterns are suggested, such as reduction of sugar and increased protein.
- study skills – how adept is the student in terms of study skills? What suggestions are indicated?
- time management – does the student use time wisely and efficiently? What improvements could be made?
- stress reduction
    - personal stress – what help might the student need to be less stressed? Are there financial or personal concerns that referrals might help address?
    - vision stress – is the student experiencing visual difficulties? Vision stress is described as a reader experiencing spatial distortions while viewing or reading text. Readers may report the text appears to dance on the page or the letters appear jumbled. The solution is to place a sheet of blue or light purple transparent vinyl over each page. The overlay of transparency helps to reduce glare and text distortion. Tests may be printed on paper of these colors to help reduce vision stress.
- tutoring needs – does the student need a tutor? If so, nursing has money budgeted to provide an alumni tutor. IECC graduates employed as registered nurses are hired. If additional hours are needed for tutoring, the Learning Skills Center provides funding for tutoring.
- multitasking skills – how well does the student manage to complete multiple tasks simultaneously? How might the student improve in the ability to multitask?
- testing time – Is extra time needed for testing? Faculty implement additional time for students to test based on recommendation from the director of the Learning Skills Center.
- referrals (not diagnoses) for student with a possible learning disability – students are referred to a licensed therapist or primary care provider for further evaluation.

Information is communicated to the college site Nursing Department Head and to the Associate Dean of Nursing and Allied Health regarding each student referred to the Learning Skills Center. The Nursing Department Head shares the information with the college site faculty. A report is filed on each student the Learning Skills Center director evaluates.

The Learning Skills Center is integral to the success nursing students experience as they matriculate through the nursing program. The Learning Skills Center director and associates maintain a close relationship with nursing faculty. Skills center staff communicate with faculty about the needs of the students and the progress students make. One example of the assessments Learning Skills Center staff perform is discussed in the next section, learning style inventory.

Learning Style Inventory

The district uses the Center for Innovative Teaching Experiences (C.I.T.E.) LSI to obtain a baseline assessment on all students who enter the nursing program. This inventory tool was selected based on knowledge of other tools available and the information this tool measures. Students meet with skills center personnel and review the results of their LSI.

Faculty receive feedback about ways students learn based on their learning style. Research question four incorporates faculty knowledge of student learning styles and poses the question:

- what variables are important to consider when developing instruction relative to student learning styles?

To address this question, consider the following report about a student's learning style in three categories: visual numeric, tactile concrete, and oral expressiveness. Faculty must consider these learning styles when they design instruction.

- visual numeric – when learning math, the student prefers seeing the process. The implication for faculty is to provide a visual representation of the math concepts being taught. For example, when teaching intravenous infusion rates, faculty might provide an intravenous bag with all the necessary tubing, the infusion pump, and the doctor's order for the infusion rate so the student can visualize how to set the hourly rate and total volume to be infused.
- tactile concrete – the student prefers hands-on activities when learning. To address this learning style, faculty would design class to include an activity such as concept mapping.

Chapter 7: A Case Study: Creating A Success Program for Nursing Students

- oral expressiveness – the student prefers to discuss learning material with another student rather than alone. Designing group activities or projects would foster this student's learning need.

Suggestions to Address Identified Concerns

The report from skills center personnel identifies specific student needs. For example, a report might read: the student makes careless and sloppy errors in math, has difficulty seeing decimal points, has problems with fractions and other math concepts, experiences extreme frustration when working higher level math problems, and has difficulty working word problems. When reading, the student skips words or lines, often rereads lines and loses line placement, is easily distracted, finds it harder to read the longer the time period, blinks and squints, finds words swirl on a page, and omits word and word units.

When particular concerns are identified, skills center personnel meet with the student to offer suggestions. Suggestions to the student to address the concerns about math and reading noted in the above report include:
- extend time for testing
- test in a quiet area
- undergo vision and hearing screening
- tape record classes
- have a list of math rules when studying for math tests
- avoid fluorescent lighting; read under lamp light; sit near a window
- use a place keeper when reading
- practice visualization exercises
- use blue or purple transparent vinyl overlay when reading
- use peach colored paper for tests and handouts
- practice mnemonic devices for memory
- take frequent breaks

Using Learning Style Data to Develop Teaching-Learning Strategies

One aim of this study was to address faculty assessment and use of learning styles. Prior to implementation of teaching and learning strategies, faculty were provided a four-hour workshop on strategies to enhancing learning. During this workshop, faculty assessed their own learning styles and explored how to address learners with different learning styles.

The following section offers insight to research question three related to this aim:
- why is knowledge of student learning styles helpful for faculty as they develop teaching-learning strategies?

During meetings, faculty discuss the learning styles of the students who will be in class, based on the LSI data. Faculty use knowledge of learning styles to design instruction to accommodate a variety of learners. For example, if faculty find their class is largely comprised of visual learners, they will include a variety of visual cues in their classroom instruction and nursing skills laboratory sessions. Faculty have also completed the LSI, to learn about their own learning styles. Faculty have found knowledge of their own learning styles helpful to their teaching.

The information provided by the learning center staff about the results of the LSI is also used to counsel students based on their strengths. Faculty offer suggestions based on the LSI profile. For example, if the inventory points to recording lecture, faculty will use that information to work with and encourage students to implement that strategy for learning. Having the information from the LSI has enabled faculty to understand that for some students, recording lecture is a useful and necessary intervention.

Program Outcomes

IECC began their success program in the fall of 2000. Data was recorded and assembled for analysis. Table 7.1 presents an overview of data compiled since 1998.

Faculty established a program completion rate with an expected level of achievement that 50% of students on the midterm roster in fall semester of the first year would complete the associate degree nursing program within three years. Between 1998 and 1999, for example, NLCEX pass rate improved by 34%; however, the completion rate for those completing in 2 years dropped by 17.5%. Completion rates for the two-year time frame are not available for comparison during this time period. Comparing three-year completion rates between 2001 and 2002, the NCLEX pass rate improved by 8% and the completion rate improved by 1%. There appears to be some leveling of NCLEX pass rates and three-year completion rates for 2003, 2004, and 2005. To date,

Table 7.1 – Program Outcomes

Variables	Year								
	1998	1999	2000	2001	2002	2003	2004	2005	2006
Student enrollment (LEVEL I) Fall	128	104	83	103	138	155	188	178	179
Student enrollment (Level II) Fall	115	98	110	98	94	113	137	133	140
Graduates per year (students complete the program just once a year, in the Spring)	103	68	56	78	72	82	96	100	119
Completion rates*:									
Completed in three years	Not Available	37.1%	32%	45%	46%	53%	54.4%	50.5%	43.4%
Completed in two years	51%	33.5%	Not Available	Not Available	43%	50%	50.5%	42.5%	44.1%
NCLEX Pass Rate	51%	85%	87%	85%	93%	85%	84%	83%	90%**
Student Satisfaction with program	Not Available	Not Available	87%	89%	100%	100%	94.1%	92.8%	Not available
Employer satisfaction (Rated students good to excellent)	Not Available	Not Available	94%	91%	98%	100%	100%	100%	Not available

*Completion rates are calculated noting the students who are on the mid-term roster in the first semester of Level I and are on the graduation roster two years or three years later. For example, the completion rate for 1999 considered the midterm roster of Level I fall of 1997 (2 year completion rate) and 1996 (3 year completion rate). There are a total of four nursing courses. Level I fall is NUR 1201 and spring is NUR 1202. Level II fall is NUR 2201 and spring is NUR 2202. Students' names on midterm rosters are noted in NUR 1201 and upon graduation/completion in NUR 2202.

** In 2006, IECC had a 91% pass rate for those who had taken NCLEX. At the time of this report, seven graduates had not taken NCLEX, and of these, six had not made application to take the exam. There is one graduate from 2005 who has not applied to take NCLEX. Reasons cited for students not applying over the last two years include personal (having a baby, family illness, death in the family) and financial issues (not having money for application, college debt).

data from 2006 reflect an improved NCLEX pass rate with a decreased three-year completion rate, but an increased two-year completion rate when compared with 2005. To assist with completion rates, faculty have adopted the criterion, beginning fall 2007, that students must be certified nursing assistants or have equivalent credentials/experience before admission. Students may apply and be ranked without this criterion, but must meet it before classes begin in August.

The *2005 Report to Constituents* (National League for Nursing Accrediting Commission, 2006) establishes graduation rate as the number of students who complete the program within 150% of the time of the stated program length. A mean graduation rate of 69.2% for diploma, 73.2% for associate, and 80.85% for baccalaureate programs are posted for the 2003-2004 academic year.

In their review of NCLEX outcomes, faculty assess every graduate's past program performance, including testing abilities in coursework and on standardized exams, and nursing skills laboratory abilities. In addition, faculty personally contact graduates who fail NCLEX. In 2006, two students reported test anxiety and failed after taking the minimum number of questions. Both students retook and passed; one student earned Bs and was a good practitioner in school. Both graduates stated they were too stressed to think – and knew it at the time of testing. Another student who experienced test anxiety all through the program failed NCLEX and stated anxiety as the reason. Faculty had found this student to be an excellent practitioner.

Other reasons cited that lent to NCLEX failure included taking vacations, delivering a baby, moving, and experiencing the death of a family member. In 2005, six students from one site failed NCLEX. One of these six students left the review early. Several students were observed to sleep during the review. Faculty expressed concern about attitude on the part of these six students as a deterrent to NCLEX success.

For the years 2004 and 2005, the program seems to have reached a plateau in both completion rates and NCELX pass rates. The Associate Dean of Nursing and Allied Health has been looking at possible reasons for this occurrence, as well as the pattern for 2006. One potential variable includes significant faculty changes. There were two faculty hired in 2006, four faculty hired in 2005, three faculty hired in 2004, four faculty hired in 2003, and two faculty hired in 2002. These newly hired faculty replaced faculty who retired or took other positions. In some cases, faculty were hired due to new positions created by increased student enrollments. Of the total faculty, four were experienced teachers (have greater than five years with the district). The Associate Dean of Nursing and

Chapter 7: A Case Study: Creating A Success Program for Nursing Students

Allied Health commented, "My feeling is that with a lot of change in faculty due to retirements (five), job changes (four), a faculty death in 2005, and new hires, the student and program outcomes have been fairly constant."

Measures have been in place since 1999 to address faculty development needs regarding test item construction. In March 1999, NEC staff reviewed test items faculty were using on tests and conducted a workshop that provided faculty an opportunity to work within groups to upgrade questions to application and analysis cognitive levels. ARNETT Development Corporation conducted a workshop in September 1999 to talk about NCLEX structure, format and changes, and how to prepare students.

In November 1999, an interactive workshop on relating curriculum objectives and test questions in terms of Bloom's taxonomy was presented. Using concepts from the curriculum, faculty established unit objective, activities, and questions that increased in difficulty as the student progressed. These workshops were provided in response to a need identified by faculty and students for changes in the approach to teaching and testing.

IECC continues to address faculty development needs. Faculty have attended several faculty development workshops between 1999 and 2006. Many of these workshops have been offered on site. In February 2006, NEC staff talked with faculty and student representatives about testing and practice for NCLEX. Also discussed was how to stimulate critical thinking/analysis in classroom discussions and activities via integration of case studies and actual clinical situations from instructor experience and student clinical experience. A workshop for faculty on clinical evaluation and communication with students was planned for September, 2006. The focus of the September workshop was also on test items and methods to upgrade the cognitive level of questions from knowledge and comprehension to application and analysis.

Faculty and administration continue to attempt to target factors that may be impacting student success. Faculty report watching outcomes closely and will continue to monitor student characteristics. Faculty conduct student surveys prior to students completing the nursing program and have noted the major reasons students leave before completion are personal/family concerns and economics (need to work), rather than program problems. Increasing numbers of student responses to the surveys indicated they had not developed adequate study habits and that the courses were too difficult and time- consuming. Faculty plan to explore the issues of study habits and course difficulty in relation to the number of students who also indicate work is too time-consuming.

The percentage of exiting students who indicated they did not plan to return to the program increased from 17% in 2004, to 20% in 2005, and to 26% in 2006. Faculty will explore why these students do not plan to return to the program.

Faculty have also looked at data that reflect student commitment to nursing as a career choice. Survey data reflected an increase in responses (from 5% in 2003 to 11% in 2005 and 2006) indicating students changed their major, were not interested in nursing, and had no clear goal.

To address these issues partially, the nursing program adopted the admission criterion of 2.5 GPA to apply – an increase from the previously established 2.0 GPA, and the requirement of certified nursing assistant, so students will better understand aspects of the profession before they begin nursing school. In addition, incoming freshman students take the success course, which has a study skills component. Until the 2006 - 2007 academic year, the success course was taught by non-nursing faculty except for one component which was directly related to nursing. In 2006, nursing faculty taught/facilitated the entire success course at each college site, with faculty incorporating more emphasis on critical thinking, with examples of sequencing, prioritizing, and analyzing situations. Additionally, faculty emphasized the commitment involved in the educational process and the rewards of the profession.

Implications for Nursing Faculty

The National League for Nursing Accrediting Commission (NLNAC) suggests an 80% benchmark for program completion (Personal communication with Carol Gilbert, October, 2006). Forrest (2004) provides the following example of a program goal and completion rate: the goal is to promote an awareness of the roles of the professional nurse. Outcomes suggested for this goal include: 90% of students will complete each nursing course successfully and 90% of students that are admitted to the program will graduate.

Nursing faculty should establish program completion rates in keeping with the mission and philosophy of their school with consideration of a national standard as reported by NLNAC. Student characteristics that place students at-risk for program completion are one component to consider when establishing the expected level of achievement. For example, if faculty decide to target underprivileged students to help these students become nurses, and the school has a low retention rate, many would view this as more acceptable than admitting students with high entrance scores on whatever measurement is used, and still having a high attrition rate. When examining factors related to completion rate and NCLEX pass rates, faculty should consider their population as well as variables that either positively or negatively impact a student's ability to complete the nursing program within the timeframe established as a program goal. What variables are operating? Would a success program allow more students to complete the nursing program? Programs that establish stringent admission guidelines may dramatically improve their retention rates; however, at what expense to students who may have successfully completed their nursing program and passed NCLEX? Programs should carefully evaluate their admission criteria to ensure it provides for admission of qualified applicants while not excluding applicants who would have succeeded.

Limitations of the Study

This study was an attempt to report what constitutes a success program and how faculty assess and use learning styles. The main limitation of this study is generalizing this case to other programs of nursing. Case study findings could have been augmented if multiple case studies were undertaken and reported by the authors.

The events described in this study are specific to IECC and probably not replicable. However, readers may view descriptions presented in this study for their similarity to their own nursing programs.

Recommendations for Future Research

The following recommendations are offered in relation to the findings of this case study.
1. Future research should examine other programs known to develop a success program, to identify similar or different interventions to promote student success.
2. Students should be tracked from admission to exit from a nursing program to identify strategies that promote program completion and student success on NCLEX.
3. Faculty should explore the best methods to address student learning styles when planning instructional strategies.

4. Faculty should examine teaching methods and instructional design to discover the best ways to meet student learning needs.
5. Faculty should examine their personal learning needs and engage in self-development to promote effective teaching.

Closing Thoughts

The case study presented in this chapter represents a process of self-evaluation, enactment of student success strategies, and growth in faculty development that crystallized the success program within a four college site nursing program. Nursing programs everywhere need to perform their own evaluations to best determine ways to establish programs of success. While each situation will differ, the meanings implicit in this case may be used by faculty as they consider approaches to curriculum design and instruction in their programs of nursing. Lessons learned included an overall student success program that:

- identified student needs, both prior to and after admission to the nursing program
- obtained necessary resources to meet identified students needs
- met faculty development needs to employ teaching strategies specific to student needs, promote critical thinking, and enhance test-taking skills
- promoted program retention
- promoted success on NCLEX

The authors are grateful to all who participated in this study and would like to extend a special thank you to Donna Henry, Associate Dean, and the following individuals: Jervaise McGlone, Director, Title III grant, Donita Kaare, Director of Learning Skills Center, Charlotte Bruce, Director of Library, Theresa Marcotte, Instructor, Kathleen Nelson, Department Head, Nancy Buttry, Department Head, and Freda Neal, Department Head.

References

Creswell, J. W. (2003). *Research design: Qualitative, quantitative, and mixed methods approaches*. Thousand Oaks, CA: Sage Publications.

Gall, M.D., Gall, J.P., & Borg, W.R. (2003). *Educational research: An introduction* (7th ed.). Boston: Pearson Education, Inc.

Illinois Community College Board. (2002). Management Information Systems Manual, Retrieved, June 26, 2006 from: http://www.iccb.org/HTML/pdf/manuals/mismanualfy02.pdf

Langford, R.W. (2001). *Navigating the maze of nursing research: An interactive learning adventure.* St. Louis: Mosby.

Martinez de Costello, S.L. (2003). *Strategies, techniques, and approaches to thinking: Critical thinking cases in nursing.* Saunders (3rd ed.). St. Louis: Elsevier.

National Center for Education Statistics. (2006). Retrieved, October 4, 2006 from: http://nces.ed.gov/programs/digest/d05/tables/dt05_310.asp

US Department of Education. Retrieved, June 12, 2006 from: http://www.ed.gov/programs/iduesannh/legislation.html

SunGard. Retrieved, June 18 from: http://www.sungardhe.com/

Zucker, D.M. (2001). Using case study methodology in nursing research. *The Qualitative Report, 6(2),* 1-12. Retrieved, June 15, 2006 from: http://www.nova.edu/ssss/QR/QR6-2/zucker.html

Chapter 8: Passing, Failing, and Readmitting

Readmission policies are necessary because retention rates of 100% are rare. Students cannot continue to an on-time graduation for a myriad reasons. As these students request readmission, a school must be prepared to meet their needs through written policies and procedures that are fair, considerate, and consistently applied.

This chapter looks at the issue of readmission. The discussion addresses the many factors that influence readmission policies. The chapter concludes with a model for developing a readmission policy and applies this model to the development of a readmission policy for the Hypothetical Nursing School.

Differentiating Terms

Students leave a nursing program for many reasons, and there are a variety of terms used to describe these reasons. Because no universal nomenclature of reasons exists, these terms are used differently from school to school. Having an agreed upon definition of these terms facilitates communication among faculty. The following are commonly used terms and definitions.

- **attempt**
  The word attempt is a positive term that indicates a withdrawal for any reason, regardless if the student was passing or failing when exiting the program.
- **drop-out**
  Drop-out refers to the act of leaving a nursing program with no intention of returning.
- **inactive Status**
  Inactive status indicates a period of time during which a student in a nursing program is not enrolled in a nursing course. Same as leave of absence.

- **leave of absence**
  Leave of absence indicates a period of time during which a student in a nursing program is not enrolled in a nursing course. Same as inactive status.
- **readmission**
  Readmission refers to a return to a program after leaving for any reason, such as a previous failure or leaving for personal reasons.
- **reinstatement**
  The term reinstatement is sometimes used to refer to the situation when a student reenters a nursing program after leaving due to an academic failure.
- **stop-out**
  Stop-out refers to the act of leaving a nursing program with the intention of re-enrolling in the program.
- **withdrawal-passing and withdrawal-failing**
  Depending on the reason for withdrawing from a nursing program, the student can leave as withdrawal-passing (WP) or withdrawal-failing (WF). Many faculty find it helpful to make this distinction as a criterion for readmission. The student who withdraws passing is more likely to be considered positively by the faculty when faced with a decision regarding that student's readmission than the student who leaves the nursing program with the status of withdrawal-failing.

Abbreviations

Some nursing programs use abbreviations to classify student status. These abbreviations are presented in Table 8.1.

A student may have more than one classification; such as, NC-P and WF meaning the student did not continue for personal reasons and was failing at the time of withdrawal. Classifying students to indicate the reason for not continuing in a nursing program is helpful when considering a request for readmission and plan for success. For example, if a student withdrew for financial reasons, targeting financial assistance might be a helpful intervention upon readmission.

Table 8.1 – Abbreviations Related to Failing and Withdrawing from a Nursing Program

Abbreviation	Definition
F	Failed; the student completed the course (did not withdraw) but earned a D or F.
I	Incomplete; the course is over but the student has outstanding work to complete The student must complete all deficiencies prior to continuing to the next course. If not completed by the time the next course begins, the grade is changed to an F.
NC	Not continuing because of a failing grade in a support course.
NC-Fi	Not continuing for financial reasons.
NC-P	Not continuing for personal reasons.
R	Returning to the nursing program after meeting the re-admission criteria.
WF	Withdrew from the course before completing the course while earning a failing grade.
WP	Withdrew from the course before completing the course while earning a passing grade.

Program Policies

All policies written for the nursing program should be in compliance with the institution's mission, policies, and procedures. These policies should be reviewed and approved by the institution's lawyer to ensure they are legally sound. This intensive review of policies also ensures the wording of the policies accomplishes what nursing faculty are trying to effect.

Communication to students about nursing program withdrawal and readmission policies cannot be overemphasized. Students need this knowledge to make an informed decision. Nursing faculty are acutely aware of this responsibility and require students to provide evidence they have read the program policies. These policies are best contained in the nursing student handbook. Students may be required to sign and submit a statement verifying they have read the policies.

Even when the students' awareness of withdrawal and readmission policies is ensured, it is best for faculty to guide each student in the decision to leave a nursing program. Leaving a nursing program can be a stressful experience for the student; as the stress level rises, cognition often becomes impaired. Every student in this situation deserves a supportive, caring faculty response.

Faculty often have difficulty in issuing a failing grade, or counseling about withdrawal, and may experience some degree of distress. However, the faculty is the professional who must maintain emotional control, and support the student through the process. Faculty may need support during this process. For new faculty, having a mentor to talk with about a problem and support from administration are ideal. It is always helpful to alert administration to the situation.

Early Identification and Intervention

The best approach is for faculty immediately to implement interventions when a student is identified as having difficulties rather than waiting until there is no hope for passing. At the very least, faculty should identify at mid-term any student not passing or in jeopardy of failing either academically or clinically. These students should be counseled and a plan of action developed that guides the student in the remainder of the course for successful completion. Examples of instruments that can be used include a tool to direct students who are failing theory examinations (Figure 8.1), a tool for identifying clinical skills deficiencies (Figure 8.2), and a learning contract (Figure 8.3). Electronic versions of these tools are on the CD-ROM accompanying this book. The faculty should be careful to document all these interventions.

Faculty's Role

The tools in Figures 8.1 through 8.3 are helpful to frame the problem and identify factors that can help or hinder students' efforts to reach their goal of successful completion of the nursing program. These tools also provide an objective means of discussing student needs and ensure due process. Completed tools may be included in the student's file and used as a point of reference for determining progress in meeting identified goals or the need for further intervention. Remember that faculty behaviors can have powerful influence on students' success. As you help students complete these tools, consider your role in the following:

1. Assist the student to make the decision to stop out, drop out, or persist.
2. Help the student to attain the goals identified on these tools.
3. Consider aspects of the nursing school's Student Success Program that can be beneficial for the student, then make the appropriate referrals.

Figure 8.1 – Theory Examination Advisement Tool

Theory Examination Advisement Worksheet/Theory Contract

Your performance on the most recent test was below 78%. Please carry out the interventions indicated in the below checked items. Include dates for completion of each activity.

☐ Attend all classroom sessions and stay for the entire class time.

☐ Consult with the teacher writing the test and review each question to determine why the item was missed.

☐ With the teacher, review your class notes and talk about how to study for the next test.

☐ Complete the chapters in the Student Study Guide that accompanies your textbook for the units covered on last test and for the remainder of the assignments for this term.

☐ Establish times to meet with your teacher to clarify any material.

☐ Complete pertinent *TLC Medical Center* integration plans.

☐ Other interventions as agreed upon by you and your teacher.

_____

_____

_____

Student's Signature   Faculty's Signature

_____
Date

Figure 8.2 - Skill Performance Deficiency Tool

Nursing Skill Review Sheet

The below skill must be practiced then demonstrated to the nursing skills laboratory faculty prior to performing the skill in the clinical setting. Please follow the below procedure.

Procedure:
1. Review the assigned readings, audiovisuals, and computer programs listed below.
2. Make an appointment with the manager of the nursing skills laboratory to return demonstrate the skill.
3. Practice the skill prior to the appointment time.
4. Upon completion of the skill return, the nursing skills laboratory faculty will provide written feedback on your performance.
5. Return the signed, completed form to your clinical teacher.

Student: _____

Clinical Teacher: _____

Skill(s) to be Practiced/Demonstrated: _____

Deadline Date: _____

Readings, audiovisuals, and computer programs to complete prior to your return demonstration:
_____
_____

Date skill practiced: _____

Date of return demonstration: _____

Nursing Skills Laboratory Faculty's Comments/Signature:
_____
_____
_____
_____

Student's Signature _____

Clinical Faculty's Signature _____

Date _____

Figure 8.3 - Learning Contract

Learning Contract and Plan of Study

Student's Name _____
Date _____

Areas in need of improvement:

Plan for improving the above and demonstrating satisfactory performance, by <date>:

Please address the following:
1. Obstacles that may interfere with completion of this plan of study
2. Benefits and costs related to continuing in the nursing program
3. Benefits and costs related to not continuing in the nursing program
4. What financial factors may be influencing your performance?
5. What emotional factors may be influencing your performance?

_____   _____
Student's Signature   Faculty's Signature

Grading Policies

Although many factors can result in withdrawal from a nursing program, those factors often manifest as poor grades, thus necessitating a withdrawal because of substandard academic performance. Faculty often debate what percent should be the minimum for passing. This is frequently a topic discussed among faculty colleagues as they gather at nursing education conferences and workshops. The goal is to set the percentage high enough to ensure students have the necessary knowledge base and cognitive abilities to pass NCLEX and practice safe nursing, yet not so high that large numbers of students fail.

In an effort to determine current practice in undergraduate, pre-licensure registered nursing programs, we visited 50 websites of schools of nursing from all parts of the United States to determine if this information was available. Approximately 50% of the schools included on their websites the minimum percentages required for earning a passing grade in a nursing course. The remaining 50% of the websites either stated that a C grade is required but did not state the percentage; or, they noted that the grading scale would be presented during orientation to each nursing course. Table 8.2 presents the data from this review of websites.

In this very small sample the percentage most commonly cited was 75%. Slightly less than half of the schools used 75% as the minimum passing percent. The range was 73% to 78%.

Table 8.2 – Percentage Required to Pass a Nursing Course

Type of Program	73%	74%	75%	76%	77%	78%	Total
ADN	0	0	6	0	1	2	9
BSN	2	5	5	2	2	0	16
Total	2	5	11	2	3	2	25

A Few Thoughts on Grading

None of the 50 websites visited indicated how the percent was calculated. That is, was a 75% required on all tests or was the 75% earned by averaging the scores of all objective tests and subjective assignments. Following are a few considerations about grading.

Test Construction and Scoring

Faculty must understand that a percentage earned on a test is only valuable if the test is well written. That is, a poorly constructed test that results in students earning less than 75% is not a reliable indicator of the student's ability. Or, perhaps the faculty decides the test was too difficult because a large number of students failed the exam, so the teacher decides to give credit for more than one option for many of the items on the test, boosting scores to the passing level. The contrived scores on this poorly constructed test do not provide any measure of confidence of the students' knowledge level.

Equally important is the cognitive level at which the test items are written. If a test contains primarily knowledge and comprehension items, the test is only a measure of the students' knowledge of facts and concepts, not a measure of the student's ability to think at a higher level. When the student does not receive a test that is written at the application level and above, the student is ill prepared for the transition to the next level and may not test well. Non-existent or poorly conceived test plans that do not include the cognitive level of the test items hinder student growth in testing. The test plan design should allow gradual increases in difficulty to compliment student knowledge acquisition.

The use of reliable and valid tests is an important educational tenant. Faculty must institute testing policies that ensure the implementation of this tenant. With these thoughts in mind, each nursing program should establish a testing policy that includes:

1. Using a test blueprint relating test items to course objectives, cognitive level, and the NCLEX test plan
2. Adhering to a consistent format when writing items
3. Writing critical thinking, NCLEX-style test items
4. Analyzing items after administering the test and making a determination about scoring
5. Rewriting flawed items based on item analysis and student feedback

A highly valid and reliable test is often a difficult goal to achieve with teacher-made tests. Students often question the validity of teacher-made tests. Remarks such as, "I have no idea where those test questions came from!" or "Nothing that was discussed in class was on the test!" are commonly heard from nursing students. These types of student responses to teacher-made tests must be eliminated through the thoughtful construction of all nursing tests.

The bottom line is that the percent selected as the minimum for a passing grade in a nursing course is only useful if valid and reliable tests are administered. If necessary, faculty should take course work, attend workshops, and read current literature on construction of nursing exams. Faculty must maintain high standards and continuously update their knowledge on how to compile a valid and reliable test. Students should pass a nursing course because they know the material and can apply it to nursing practice, and they should fail because they do not know the material or cannot apply it to nursing practice. Students should not pass or fail on the basis of poorly constructed tests.

All Measurement Contains Error

Think about this quote: "…all measurements contain error" (McDonald, 2002, p. 187). What does this mean relative to determining if a student passes or fails? What if your student is a few points (not percentage points) from passing? For example, if the student needs 500 points to pass and has earned 498, does the student fail? If "all measurements contain error" might this student be failing because of an error in your test measurement?

This is an intriguing dilemma to consider. How might faculty recompense for this error in measurement? One mechanism may be to offer students "surprise" bonus points. As the end of the term nears, provide students with an optional extra-credit assignment. The assignment should focus on course objectives and preferably course objectives specific to each student's needs. That is, the assignment should require the student to focus on areas of course content that represent the lowest scores for the student. The student could construct a care plan or concept map addressing these weak areas. The points allowed for this extra-credit assignment would vary depending on the statistical analyses of the objective tests administered throughout the term. If the teacher believes the tests were extremely valid and reliable, only a few bonus points might be offered. If the test analyses demonstrated the tests were marginal, more bonus points are offered. This provides a mechanism for addressing the notion that all measurement contains error while providing remediation for individual students in their demonstrated areas of weakness. Bonus points that are a surprise, or announced near the end of the course, have a particular impact on student performance. If students are not aware that bonus points will be available as they go through the course, students do not intentionally avoid doing the work of the term, banking on the fact that they may make up low score with bonus points. In this case, the surprise bonus points not only enhance students' knowledge, but the students' sense of empowerment that they can take a positive action to remediate their areas of weakness.

What Constitutes a Failure?

Nursing is a very complex discipline. Although there is a knowledge base specific to nursing, that knowledge base is derived from both the natural and social sciences. Information from these sciences is interwoven with the science of nursing practice, making nursing a very eclectic discipline. Nursing also involves the cognitive, psychomotor, and affective domains of learning. All these influences make nursing an exciting and diverse field of study. However, all these influences can render nursing difficult to learn and difficult for faculty to evaluate if learning has occurred.

Test grades are only one dimension that contributes to a grade in nursing. Nursing education is complex and other factors influence grading; therefore, the question becomes, "What constitutes a failure in nursing?" The answer to that question may be a combination of events. Following are aspects of nursing education that contribute to a failing status.

Classroom Aspects of a Nursing Program

1. Final grade in a nursing course below the minimum percentage established
2. Final grade in a support course below the minimum grade established
3. Need to repeat more than two non-nursing courses that apply to the nursing degree

Clinical Aspects of a Nursing Program

1. Failure to meet attendance requirements. Some schools allow alternate assignments for missed clinical days. However, some states require a minimum number of hours in the clinical setting and only a portion of those hours can be "observational" or non-client care experiences.
2. Behavior not consistent with established standards such as those prescribed by the nursing department or the American Nurses' Association Code for Nurses
3. Unsafe clinical performance; dismissal may be immediate without prior warning.

Nursing Skills Laboratory Aspects of a Nursing Program

1. Not successfully demonstrating competency in performing nursing skills
2. Not passing a dosage calculation exam by an established date

General Nursing Program Policies

1. Failure to comply with nursing program regulations and policies
2. Failure to meet objectives of a learning contract by a specified date
3. Cheating or plagiarism

The fact that so many variables impact a student's grade demonstrates that evaluating nursing students is a very complex process. Time and experience are necessary to master the skill of evaluating students resulting in a fair grade assignment. New faculty need support in learning this process.

Issues Related to a Readmission Policy

As is apparent from the above listings, evaluating learning in nursing for the purpose of issuing a pass or fail grade is not as simple as averaging scores on objective tests. The following issues are often considered when developing grading guidelines for a readmission policy.

1. Do the guidelines eliminate some students from readmission to the nursing program who would have otherwise succeeded?
2. What is the number of times a student can repeat a nursing course?

3. Is the nursing program restricted by state rules and regulations that do not allow students in public schools to repeat a course more than twice?
4. Does repeating a course affect financial aid that may be perceived wasted if the student does not complete the nursing program?

Limits on Readmission

Students should be aware that the standard for passing nursing courses may be higher than in other courses. Nursing requires higher standards to protect the safety and well-being of clients. This higher standard increases the attrition rate and, therefore, the number of students seeking readmission. Additionally, limited clinical space restricts the number of students accepted into a nursing program. This impacts the availability of space for reentering students. Faculty must contemplate who will be most successful and what resources are available to support students who have previously demonstrated difficulty with the nursing program courses.

A major question facing nursing faculty is how many times a student should be allowed to return to the same nursing program. To obtain a perspective on what is occurring in schools of nursing, we visited 100 nursing school websites. Only 42 of the 100 schools provided information about their program readmission policy on their websites. Although the number of schools is small, the data provide an indication of the trend in schools of nursing related to the number of readmissions allowed. Table 8.3 contains this data.

Nearly 79% of these schools allowed only one readmission after a failure. No schools were found to allow more than three readmissions. Some schools had variations on the strictly one readmission rule. For example, one school stated that if the student fails during the first year, one readmission is allowed. If no failure in the first year, the student is allowed two readmissions during the second year. If readmitted once in the first year, the student is allowed one readmission during the second year.

Some schools may also base readmission on the reason the student left the nursing program. If a stop-out is due to a failing grade, the student may be readmitted just once. If a stop-out is for personal reasons, the student can be readmitted more than once.

A final consideration is the length of the break in coursework. Schools may consider a long time away from nursing courses a risk to successful completion.

Table 8.3 – Number of Readmissions

Number of Readmissions Allowed	Number of Schools
1	33
2	7
3	2

A policy may be written to handle this consideration. For example, the readmission policy may state that a student is readmitted only if the last nursing course was successfully completed within three years of the stop-out. If more than three years, the student must enter at a point earlier in the program. Some schools require the student to reenter at the beginning of the program if too much time has lapsed.

Whatever number of readmissions are allowed, faculty need to track progress of readmitted students. Future decisions about numbers of readmissions should be based on data collected and trended over time. While many of the programs surveyed had similar numbers of readmissions allowed, it is not known if these policies functioned to promote student success upon readmission. The number of readmissions is not as important as the mechanisms for success that are in place for the readmitted student.

Requirements for Readmission

Once it is established that a student may reenter the nursing program, the next question facing faculty is, "What are the requirements for readmission?" Typically the first step involves some process whereby the student petitions for readmission. This process may be simple, with the student required to submit a written request for readmission. Or, it may be more involved, with the student completing a form stating the student's intent and strategies that would be implemented to ensure success. Figure 8.4 is an example of the type of form that may be required. An electronic version of this form is on the CD-ROM accompanying this book.

Figure 8.4 – Readmission Request Form

Request for Readmission in the Hypothetical Nursing School

Name _____

Date _____

Requesting to enroll in nursing (course #)
_____

Reason for previous stop-out
_____

Success Plan: Your plan for successfully completing the nursing program on your return.
_____
_____
_____

Student Signature
_____

Faculty to Complete:
After reviewing the student's success plan, comment on the student's potential for success and any further interventions you believe will be helpful to the student.
_____
_____
_____

Faculty Signature
_____

Readmission Committee Recommendation
_____ Approved   _____ Not approved

Reason for denial:
_____
_____

Readmission Committee Members' Signatures
_____
_____
_____

Leave of Absence

Some nursing schools have specific provisions in place for a leave of absence. An approved leave of absence with subsequent continuation of courses is not considered a readmission if the student left prior to completing the course and was passing when taking the leave, or the student left the nursing program at the end of a course and earned a passing grade in the course. A leave of absence typically involves an unwanted or unplanned absence due to extenuating circumstances such as military service, pregnancy, illness, family crises, or financial difficulties. Students requesting a leave of absence must do so in writing. Figure 8.5 is a sample leave of absence request form. An electronic version of this form is on the CD-ROM accompanying this book.

Additional Requirements for Readmission

Petitioning for readmission and preparing a plan for success are basic elements of a readmission policy for a school of nursing. With these two basic elements, additional requirements may be included in the policy in an effort to ensure the student is successful upon returning to nursing school. Examples of additional requirements include the following:

1. Show competency for selected nursing skills from previous terms. The student is provided two opportunities to pass these skills.
2. Complete additional course work as directed by the readmission committee to facilitate success in required nursing courses.
3. Undergo special counseling activities to improve study skills or time management skills.
4. Retake the last clinical course completed prior to leaving.
5. Complete a remediation plan which includes testing at the course level at the time of the stop-out.
6. Pass a competency exam for all previous courses completed and return demonstrate all previously learned nursing skills. If a minimum grade on a course test is not earned, the student will stop taking tests and reenter the program at that level.
7. The student may be required to work as a CNA or in some other health care related position prior to reentry.
8. If readmission occurs more than a specified number of years after leaving

Figure 8.5 – Leave of Absence Request Form

Leave of Absence Request Form for Hypothetical Nursing School

Name _____
Date _____

After completing this form, submit to the Dean of the Hypothetical Nursing School.

Reason for requesting a Leave of Absence:
_____
_____
_____
_____

Semester you expect to return:
_____

Plan for review of nursing content prior to your return:
_____
_____
_____
_____

Leave of Absence Committee Recommendation

_____ Approved   _____ Not approved

Reason for denial:
_____
_____

Leave of Absence Committee Members' Signatures
_____
_____
_____

the nursing program, the student must retake all nursing courses.

Other Qualifiers Placed on Readmission

Some schools of nursing place additional qualifiers that students must consider prior to requesting readmission. While these qualifiers have merit, careful consideration is necessary prior to their adoption. Faculty should have sound rationales and reasons for including these qualifiers. Following are examples of qualifiers that may be included in a readmission policy.
1. If the set number of readmissions has been met, the student can return only with faculty approval.
2. If failing the beginning fundamentals course, the student must reapply to the nursing program, after meeting the current admission criteria.
3. Readmission must occur within two calendar years from the time the last nursing course was successfully completed.
4. If all return options have been exhausted, the student may complete the LPN program after the eligibility requirements are met (for schools that have both an LPN and RN program). Once completing the LPN program, the student can be readmitted one more time to the RN program.

Faculty may consider counseling students in academic difficulty to withdraw rather than fail because failing will negatively impact the student's GPA. This lower GPA may prevent the student from meeting the admission criteria to reenter the nursing program or fail to meet the GPA needed for graduation.

Ranking Students for Readmission

The faculty must consider how students will be ranked for readmission. Some schools use a "first-come, first-served" philosophy and readmit students in the order in which their request for readmission was received. Other schools rank students by other means. Following is an example prioritizing system indicating the order in which students are considered for readmission to a nursing program.
1. Students on an approved leave of absence
2. Students who withdrew with a passing grade

3. Students transferring from another nursing program
4. Students who withdrew with an unsatisfactory grade or completed the course with an unsatisfactory grade
5. Students who have been out more than one year

As always, when an ordering system is used to determine which students are admitted first, the faculty must have sound rationale to support the process. Special consideration should be given to students who are seeking readmission into the first nursing course of the program. Faculty must keep in mind that whatever policy they adopt, readmission into the first term impacts students applying for first admission. For example, students placed on a waiting list who were not admitted into the program from the previous year and have already met admission requirements, are also viable candidates for admission to the program. Who has priority into the first nursing course when space is limited? The policy enacted should consider all potential ramifications for admission scenarios.

Transfer Students

Transfer students may be of special concern for a school of nursing. What occasionally occurs is the student exhausts all options for readmission into a nursing program then applies for admission to a neighboring school. Faculty of schools of nursing have looked upon this situation in a variety of ways. Some schools admit the student with advanced placement without regard to the number of times the student has enrolled in another school. Other schools consider this student at risk for failing based on the student's history.

The reason for a restrictive policy for transfer students is because the faculty of a nursing program is reluctant to admit a student considered not likely to succeed. Although this policy may seem reasonable, the policy may not be fair to the student. For example, consider Nursing School A with a policy that students must earn a 78% to pass a nursing course and only one readmission will be granted. A student earns a 76% in a nursing course, retakes the course, earns a 78%, and then proceeds to the next nursing course. In the next course the student earns a 77% so is not allowed to retake the second nursing course. Nursing School B is close to this student's home. Nursing School B has a policy that will not allow this student to enter because the student is ineligible for readmission at Nursing School A. However, the minimum passing grade in Nursing School

B is 75%. This student has earned a higher percent when attending Nursing School A than is required for passing in Nursing School B, yet the student is not allowed to enroll in Nursing School B.

There are a number of ways a school can handle requests for admission from transfer students. Following are some points to consider.

1. If the readmission policy at your school is the same as that of the student's previous school, the student will not be allowed to enroll. In other words, if the student is ineligible to return to the original program, the student would not be allowed to enter your nursing program.
2. If the student is eligible for readmission in the former nursing school, the student will be considered to have no withdrawals at the time of admission to your nursing program.
3. If the student is ineligible for readmission in the former nursing school, the student will be admitted and considered to be entering the new program with one withdrawal. Therefore, if the current nursing program only allows one readmission, this transfer student will be ineligible for readmission upon failing a nursing course.
4. The student's grades in percentage from the former school will be compared to the standards in your school to determine if admission is granted.

Exit Interviews

An exit interview is an important activity that can provide valuable information regarding the needs of students. An exit interview addresses the issues that contributed to the student's exit from the program and provides insights about the student's exit that faculty may otherwise not discern. Input from the student, faculty, and preceptor, if applicable, is included. The exit interview can reveal reasons for failure that were not previously considered by faculty. Exit interviews provide faculty with an idea of why their students are exiting prior to graduation. This information can be used to make changes in various components of the program to prevent losing students in the future. This information can also help faculty when evaluating admission criteria and requirements related to passing and failing a course.

However, exit interviews can sometimes yield unreliable data for several reasons (Jeffreys, 2004).

1. The student may give a reason for leaving the nursing program, but may be unaware of the actual reasons that contributed to that decision. For example, poor grades may be cited as the reason for leaving, but the student may be unaware what factors contributed to the failing grade.
2. The student may rationalize the decision to withdraw to provide a socially acceptable reason. For example, the student may be experiencing abuse by a spouse and is unable to concentrate. To hide the abuse, the student may give what is believed to be a more socially acceptable reason for withdrawing.

Even with these limiting influences, exit interviews should be conducted with each student. Valuable data is collected during these sessions that can be used to determine the effectiveness of your Student Success Program. Students who withdraw for personal reasons such as surgery or to care for a family member should not be included when determining the rate of attrition and retention to determine the effectiveness of your student success program (Jeffreys, 2004). These are factors that influence student success that are outside the scope of a student success program.

Steps in Developing Your Readmission Policy

Readmission policies of schools across the country or across program type are not standardized. To write a readmission policy the same as another school simply because it is what everyone else is doing is not supportive of the needs of your students. The components of a readmission policy should be considerate of the school's population of students. Use evidence to support the components of the readmission policy and why specific components are best for the students. As you work through the following six steps in developing a readmission policy, consider what works best for **your** students in **your** school.

1. Identify any institutional restrictions.

Prior to developing your readmission policy, you must consider any institutional or governmental constraints. For example, some institutions only allow a student to retake a course two times.

2. Develop the purpose for your readmission policy.

Consider the purpose of your readmission policy. The purpose may be simply to ensure fair and equal access to the nursing program for all returning students. Another purpose may be to establish a mechanism whereby students returning to the program are likely to be successful on a second attempt.

3. Collect, analyze, aggregate, and trend student data.

The purpose of this step is to ensure an understanding of the characteristics of returning students so your policy meets their needs. A good starting point is to collect data from primary sources that provide information about the major reasons students leave your nursing program. If exit interviews have been conducted, extract relevant information from those interviews. Also, readmission requests from students may contain pertinent information.

A secondary source of information is student records from the previous five years. Student records can reveal grades earned prior to leaving the nursing program. Earned grades can be helpful in some ways; however, having a grade without the students' explanation about why that grade was earned, yields limited information. Having difficulty understanding nursing content can lead to a failing grade; but, working too many hours in a job limiting hours for study, can also lead to a failing grade. Clarification of why the grade was earned is an important piece of information.

Interview your current students. Ask students who drop out what factors most influenced their decision to drop out. Ask students who stop out what factors most influenced their decision to stop out.

Survey the students who persist. Ask them what factors most influenced their decision to stay in the nursing program. Asking students about why they persist may reveal information that can be used to justify offering certain services and discontinuing others.

You may begin by using open-ended questions, followed with a Likert-type scale with factors listed to assist students who find it difficult to identify the actual reasons for leaving the nursing program or reasons for persisting. Answers to these questions can help guide revisions to your success plan which will influence student retention and aspects of your readmission policy.

Once the data have been gathered, aggregate and arrange the data into a meaningful format that can be used as a reference and rationale for your readmission policy.

4. Identify available resources.

Assess your resources. What resources are available to address the needs of students who are leaving your program? Do you have resources that can address these needs when they first occur so strategies can be implemented that result in successful completion rather than dropping out?

Resources also include personnel to carry out the various aspects of your readmission policy. Specific aspects of a readmission policy may include testing competency in performing nursing skills, testing prerequisite knowledge, or completing additional course work. Are faculty available for these tasks if they become part of your readmission policy?

5. Develop a readmission policy.

Using all the information acquired in steps 1 through 4, write your readmission policy. Consider the number of readmissions allowed, the requirements for readmission, and, if space is limited, your system for prioritizing students to determine who will be admitted first.

5a. Consider the Number of Readmissions Allowed

Consider how many times a student will be allowed to return to your nursing program. Also influencing the number of readmissions may be the level of the student upon leaving and the reason for leaving.

Another consideration is the timing when the student withdraws or fails a nursing course. If the student fails the first nursing course of the program and the policy is that students are readmitted on a "space available basis" and all available seats are filled each year, there will never be a "space available" for this student. Will this student need to reapply to the nursing program and start the process over again? If the student failed and GPA is a factor considered for admission, this student will have a lower GPA because of that failing nursing course grade. This GPA may prevent the student from joining the pool of viable applicants. Is this fair to a student who has met some, but not all, of the course objectives and may be reentering the course knowing more than the other students who have yet to take the course? Perhaps this student is more likely to succeed on readmission because the student is keenly aware of what is required for passing and better prepared to meet those requirements than the student who is new to the nursing program.

Now consider the student who has failed one nursing course in the first level then successfully passed on readmission and advanced to the second level. This student has invested time, money, and energy progressing far into the program. This student fails a second level course, perhaps even the last course of the program. With a policy stating just one readmission, this student is no longer able to return to the program. Both the student and the school have no return on their investments. Can this type of policy be justified? Perhaps with remediation and the opportunity to repeat that final nursing course, the student will complete the nursing program. Perhaps a better option is to invest one more term in this student and produce a graduate nurse rather than take a chance on a completely new student who may or may not progress to program completion.

5b. Identify Requirements for Readmission

Requirements for readmission are based on the aggregate data collected on students who have left the program as well as data about individuals seeking readmission. Refer to earlier sections of this chapter for examples of specific requirements to include in a readmission policy.

5c. Prioritize Students for Readmission

Establishing a fair and impartial system with rationale for the system used to prioritize students for readmission is important. Perhaps past experience indicates that students who withdraw passing are more successful on readmission than students who withdraw failing. This would be a strong indicator for assigning available space first to students who were passing at the time of withdrawal. Other aspects to consider may be length of time students have been out of the program and if issues that interfered with their success have been addressed.

6. *Evaluate your readmission policy.*

Your readmission policy should undergo yearly evaluation to determine if the policy is meeting its stated purpose. Take a close look at your readmission policy and consider if it truly reflects the needs of your student body. Consider the following questions.
- does the policy help or hinder admission for students seeking reentry?
- does the policy help or hinder students' success when readmitted to the nursing program?
- does the policy correlate with success in completing the program?
- if the readmission policy states that a student can only be readmitted one time, is there evidence that students who are readmitted two times are unsuccessful?
- is there data that shows that students who return three or four times are draining the system, failing to complete the program, or not passing NCLEX?
- is the readmission policy evidence-based?

Admission and readmission policies are not independent entities but are parts of a system and, as such, each part affects the other parts. Therefore, use the data collected about attrition and readmission when considering revisions of admission criteria.

Finally, assemble a nursing appeals committee to evaluate special circumstances and determine if students should be readmitted beyond that allowed by your readmission policy. This would require guidelines for overriding the readmission policy. This committee should be available for all students seeking readmission.

Figure 8.6 presents a model of the steps for developing a readmission policy.

Unsafe Performance

Schools may consider adopting a policy stating that if a student is deemed unsafe while caring for clients, that student is dismissed from the nursing program and not allowed to return, even if this is the student's first dismissal. Unsafe practice is dangerous. Because of the seriousness of the consequences of unsafe clinical behavior, it is important that unsafe behavior be clearly described.

The nursing teacher supervising the student considered to be unsafe is unable

Figure 8.6 – A Model for Developing a Readmission Policy

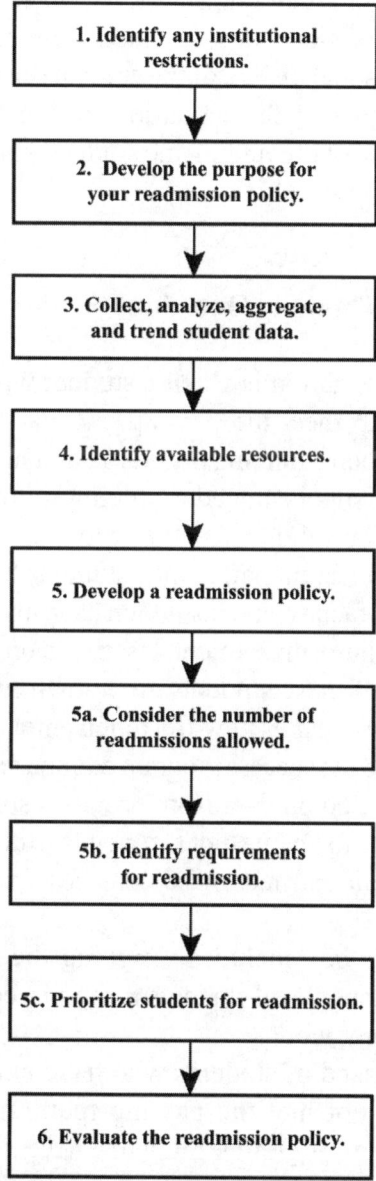

to accompany that student on a one-on-one basis throughout the clinical day. The teacher may be responsible for eight to nine other students in the clinical group. Because close supervision to ensure client safety is not possible, it may be best to not have the student in the clinical.

The faculty deeming a student unsafe must be ensured of administrative support of the "unsafe" decision. Also, that faculty member must be certain that personal opinion or a personal dislike of the student does not cloud the faculty's judgment resulting in an unsafe evaluation, rather than an unsatisfactory evaluation, for the purpose of preventing the student from reentering the nursing program at a later time.

Thinking Outside of the Box

A most unfortunate situation is when a student withdraws from a nursing program and is unable to meet the passing criteria for readmission. This is especially unfortunate when a nursing program has a high attrition rate in upper level courses. Some students just need a little more time. With the traditional educational system, students must meet the criteria in a set time frame with no opportunity to follow a different path. Once students have reached upper level course work, the students, faculty, and institution have invested much time, money, and energy. Perhaps this huge investment deserves a unique approach. After all, the specific difficulties of these students are known factors, factors a success program can target. Every year as new freshmen enter a nursing program, they are virtually unknown, and the success program administered to these new students provides a plan that is based on data from previous students; faculty can only hope the plan will address the new students' needs. But, for a returning student, previous difficulties are identified and the success program can target those difficulties.

Thinking outside the box includes weighing the possibility of a second readmission with these upper level students forming a cohort group. Let's take a look at how this idea might work.

The cohort is comprised of students who have entered the final year of a nursing program, have not met the passing requirements, and are granted readmission. The nursing program's Student Success Committee studies the characteristics of this cohort group and meets individually with each student. The Student Success Committee develops a specific success plan precisely targeting the needs of this group. If a Student Success Program is already in place, the components of that program that can directly help this group of students are used. The faculty teaching this group are in close communication with the Student Success Committee to be sure all aspects of the success plan are implemented in their courses.

This may appear to be an expensive plan; however, consider the investment that will be lost if these students are not readmitted, or are readmitted and fail. Faculty are encouraged to consider such a plan and seek grants and other special funding such as establishing a partnership with local healthcare providers to fund such a cohort program.

Hypothetical Nursing School Example

The faculty at the Hypothetical Nursing School (HNS) developed a new readmission policy with the goal of developing a policy that correlates with student success. The faculty then followed the steps listed in the model in Figure 8.6 to develop their readmission policy.

1. Identify Any Institutional Restrictions

The Hypothetical Nursing School is a program in a public institution. The number of times a student may retake a course is not restricted. The school's financial base is tax dollars, grants, and personal and corporate donations. The faculty believe it is important to be fiscally diligent as the readmission policy is developed.

2. Develop the Purpose for Your Readmission Policy

The faculty of HNS developed the purpose statement for their readmission policy. The statement reads, "The purpose of the readmission policy at the Hypothetical Nursing School is to identify students who will most benefit from readmission into the nursing program and to assist those students to accomplish their goal of successfully completing their course of study."

3. Collect, Analyze, Aggregate, and Trend Student Data

The faculty collected data from student records and interviewed persisting students. Student records indicated that 75% of students leaving the program earned a D or F or had a D or F at the time of withdrawal. Twenty-five percent of students had a passing grade when withdrawing. The faculty determined the difficulties identified with passing the nursing courses involved the following:
- students working in a job and not having enough time to study
- students for whom English is not their first language
- students with outside family responsibilities that imposed restrictions on study time
- students who believe their studying did not produce the test scores they had hoped to achieve

4. Identify Available Resources

The faculty at Hypothetical Nursing School had previously established a success program with many resources available for students. The success program included advice on financial aid, organizing time, and study skills. However, no specific assistance is available for students who were non-native English speakers. The faculty will investigate ways to help these students.

5. Develop a Readmission Policy

After much discussion and consideration of all the student data, the faculty at Hypothetical Nursing School developed a readmission policy. Components of the policy include the following:
- all readmissions will be on a space available basis.
- students will be allowed one readmission into first level courses.
- students will be allowed two readmissions into second level courses.
- any student deemed unsafe when providing client care will not be allowed readmission.
- when a student leaves Hypothetical Nursing School for any reason, if the student intends to seek readmission, the student must write a letter of intent within 60 days of the last day of attendance. The student must meet with a faculty adviser to develop a success plan incorporating the reason for leaving. If the reason for leaving impacted the student's school performance, the student must discuss how that issue has been resolved.

- prior to returning to the nursing program, the student will meet with a faculty advisor and register for a one-hour course based on the nursing school's Student Success Program.
- if the student's break in enrollment is longer than one year, the student must pass a written test demonstrating knowledge of nursing content for all the courses passed to date. The student must also return demonstrate all the critical nursing skills identified in each nursing course.
- if more than one student is seeking readmission to the nursing program for the same course, the order in which students will be granted readmission is as follows:
    o students leaving with a passing grade.
    o students leaving with a D or F will be ranked according to the percentage they earned in the course.
    o transfer students.

6. Evaluate the Readmission Policy

As part of the Hypothetical Nursing School's evaluation efforts, the readmission policy will be evaluated every year. The students who are readmitted will be tracked and their success in completing all nursing courses with an on-time graduation will be recorded. Students who are readmitted will be assigned a faculty advisor who will meet with the student throughout the student's remaining course work and determine if the success plan is effective, if the plan needs to be revised, and what additional resources will be needed. The faculty will meet at the end of each school year to review this data and determine if revisions in the readmission policy are warranted.

Closing Thoughts

After establishing a readmission policy, faculty must engage in ongoing critical evaluation of the entire process. The policy is evaluated to determine if it is fulfilling its stated purpose. Retrospective studies are conducted to determine if the policy is meeting the students' needs and program goals or outcomes. The policy must encourage success on readmission rather than merely readmitting a student without appropriate interventions. Readmission without a success plan most likely will result in the student failing once again. Readmission without a success plan is clearly irresponsible behavior that impacts both students and financial stakeholders.

Learning Activities

1. Talk with faculty from three different schools of nursing about their readmission policy. Compare and contrast the three policies.
2. Search the websites of schools of nursing. Find ten websites that address a readmission policy. Consider the philosophy of each school to determine if the school's philosophy is reflected in its readmission policy.
3. Interview five students who are currently readmitted to a nursing program. Compare and contrast the reasons why the students left the nursing program and their plans for successfully completing the nursing program with this readmission.

References

Jeffreys, M. R. (2004). *Nursing student retention: Understanding the process and making a difference.* New York: Springer.

McDonald, M. E. (2002). *Systematic assessment of learning outcomes: Developing multiple-choice exams.* Sudbury, MA: Jones and Bartlett.

Chapter 9:
A Model for NCLEX® Success

Because successfully passing the NCLEX is mandatory for entry into nursing practice, pre-licensure nursing programs must always consider the importance of preparing students for passing that examination. A student success program must include a planned approach to assist students to be successful on the NCLEX.

This chapter provides an overview of the elements that impact NCLEX success including nursing knowledge, student characteristics, and thinking skills. Faculty influence these elements through teaching strategies and evaluation methodologies.

Overview of NCLEX

The NCLEX serves to safeguard the public from unsafe practitioners and assist state boards of nursing in determining candidates' capabilities for performing at entry-level practice. Licensure is compulsory in all states and U.S. territories (National Council of State Boards of Nursing, 2004).

NCLEX-RN and NCLEX-PN are computer adaptive tests. Registered nurse (RN) candidates take a minimum of 75 and a maximum of 265 items during a six-hour maximum period for completion. Licensed practical/vocational nurse (LPN/LVN) candidates take a minimum of 85 items and a maximum of 205 items during a five-hour maximum period for completion. A tutorial, sample questions, and all breaks are included in the time allotment (National Council of State Boards of Nursing, 2005, 2006a). The length of a candidate's examination is based on the performance of the candidate. Each question posed is based on the candidate's response to the previous item. Testing concludes when the candidate reaches competency, once the minimum number of items has been answered. If competency is not met, the candidate continues to answer questions until competency is established. If competency has not been met after taking the maximum number of items, or if the time expires before competency is determined, the candidate fails (National Council of State Boards of Nursing, 2006a). The percent of each school's candidates passing the examination is reported each quarter – January through March, April through June, July through September, and October through December – and as a yearly total (National Council of State Boards of Nursing, 2006b).

The Importance of NCLEX Success

Success on NCLEX is the gateway to professional practice. Although a common goal for all nursing programs is a 100% pass rate on NCLEX (Williams & Bryant, 2001), at a minimum, each school must meet their state-mandated required pass rate. When a program does not meet the state-mandated required pass rate, that program must address this issue with the state board of nursing. In addition, first-time NCLEX pass rates are used as a benchmark by accrediting commissions for program accountability (Siktberg & Dillard, 2001).

NCLEX failure affects several stakeholders. Among these are the graduates who failed, the employers who seek additional staff, the community members who require healthcare services, and the programs that teach nursing.

Students may be devastated by failure on NCLEX and suffer loss of self-esteem (Beeman & Waterhouse, 2003). Emotional and financial hardships related to decrease in salary, demotion, or loss of job may be incurred (Poorman & Webb, 2000).

As a consequence of low NCLEX pass rates, programs may be under scrutiny by their administration and executive boards, prospective students who seek entry, agencies who hire the school's graduates, and current and prospective faculty who seek continued or new employment. Schools whose pass rates fall below acceptable standards may lose accreditation or state approval and be unable to attract qualified students to their program (Beeson & Kissling, 2001).

Delaying NCLEX

The longer a candidate delays taking the exam, the more likely a decrease in pass rate. Spector and Alexander (2006) reported for the graduates testing in 1998 to 2000 who took the NCLEX-RN zero to 26 days after graduation, the first time pass rate was 89.2%. For graduates who tested 27 to 39 days after graduation, the first-time pass rate was 86.1%. If graduates delayed taking the exam 40 to 62 days after graduation, the first-time pass rate was 81.1%. The pass rates of graduates who delayed 63 to 1,568 days after graduation dropped to 51%.

In addition, problems arise for graduates in accessing help in addressing deficits after NCLEX failure. Schools of nursing may not have mechanisms in place for graduates to receive help on subsequent attempts to pass NCLEX. Therefore, graduates should be in the best position possible for success on NCLEX on the first attempt.

Variables Used to Predict NCLEX Success

Use of NCLEX pass rates as an indicator of program quality has sparked nursing faculty to find measures to predict students' chances of passing NCLEX (Tanner, 2006). Over the past two decades, many studies have reported academic and non-academic variables for their ability to predict NCLEX success. Prediction of success on the NCLEX is often reported as a multifaceted phenomenon (Barkley, Rhodes, & DuFour, 1998). The Caputi Model for NCLEX Success (Figure 9.1) groups these multiple factors into three categories or components. These components are nursing knowledge, student characteristics, and thinking skills. All three components must be present and in a relationship with each other, with each impacting the other for NCLEX success.

The three central components – nursing knowledge, student characteristics, and thinking skills – are influenced by two encompassing components, teaching strategies and testing/evaluation techniques. These two additional components represent ways faculty influence student success on NCLEX. This model shows that considerations for raising NCLEX scores require a multifaceted approach with active involvement of both students and faculty (Personal communication with Linda Caputi, July, 2006).

Application of the Caputi Model for NCLEX Success

The Caputi Model is used as the framework for the rest of this chapter. The model attempts to explain how student characteristics, thinking skills, and nursing knowledge as impacted by teaching strategies and testing/evaluation techniques,

Figure 9.1 – The Caputi Model for NCLEX Success – A Multifaceted Model

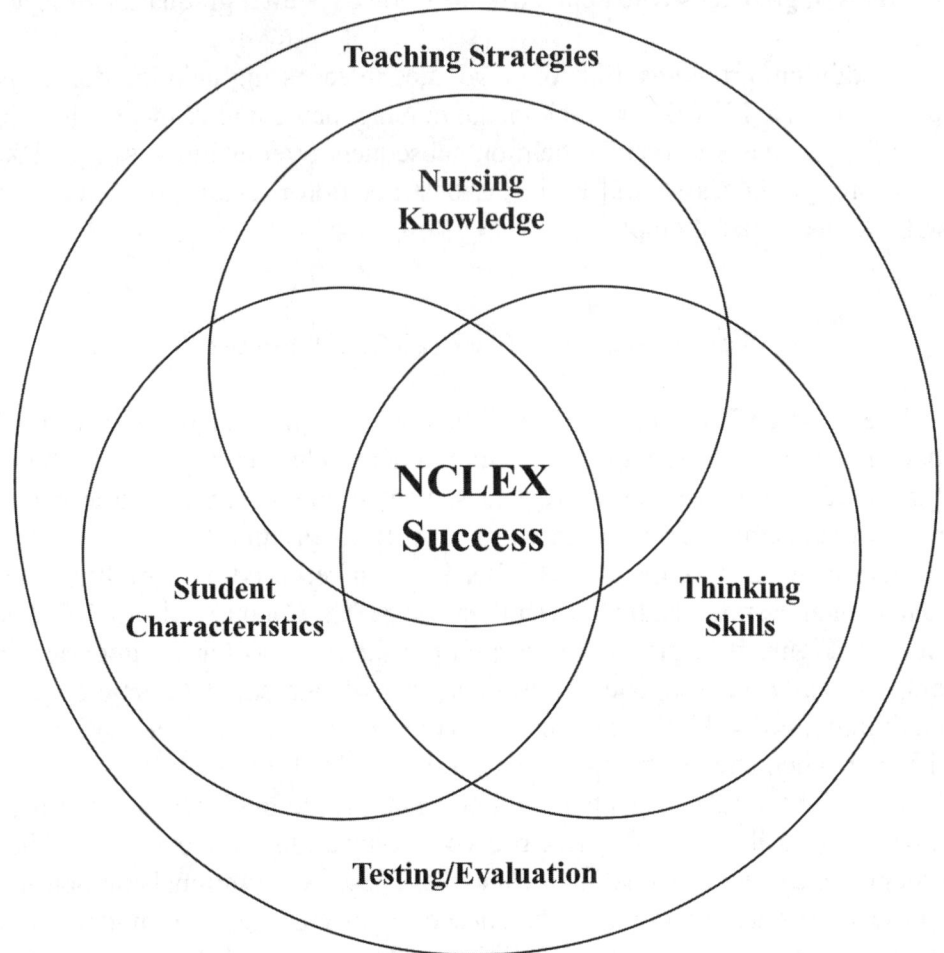

©2006, Linda Caputi, Inc. Used with permission.

create a dynamic environment as the basis for the NCLEX success component of the Student Success Program.

Student Characteristics

Faculty must be aware there are a number of characteristics that each individual student brings to the educational environment. These include characteristics such as English as a second language (ESL), family responsibilities, number of hours of work per week, and age, gender, and ethnicity, each having the potential to impact performance on NCLEX (Arathuzik & Aber, 1998; Beeman & Waterhouse, 2001; Beeson & Kissling, 2001; California Board of Registered Nursing, 2000; Daley, Kirkpatrick, Frazier, Chung, & Moser, 2003; Endres, 1997; Gallagher, Bomba, and Crane, 2001; Higgins, 2005; Yin & Burger, 2003). Many of these variables indirectly affect NCLEX success; that is, they interfere with the student's ability to study adequately (too many work hours; family responsibilities competing for time). Others may interfere with the student's ability to process information or communicate that information, as may be the case with students for whom English is not their primary language. Other factors are non-modifiable ones such as age, gender, and ethnicity. However, none of these factors are consistently identified as barriers to NCLEX success. In fact, the one most consistently reported as impacting NCLEX success is English as a second language (ESL). See Chapter 6 of this book for further discussion of the student with ESL.

Academic Factors

Academic factors are also characteristics an individual student brings to the learning environment. Academic factors are frequently studied for their effect on NCLEX success. Academic predictor variables often researched include admission scores, standardized test scores, GPA upon admission, high school rank, grades in prerequisite science courses, grades in upper division nursing courses, nursing theory course grades, and NCLEX predictor test scores (Barkley, Rhodes, & DuFour, 1998; Crow, Handley, Morrison, & Shelton, 2004; Daley, et. al., 2003; Gallagher, Bomba, & Crane, 2001; Lauchner, Newman, & Britt, 1999; Newman, Britt, & Lauchner, 2000; Nibert, Young, & Adamson, 2002; Roncoli, Lisanti, & Falcone, 2000; Yin & Burger, 2003).

A review of the literature reporting these academic variables affecting NCLEX success is extremely inconsistent. The results vary from study to study and often contradict each other. **One** factor that remains consistent across studies is the grades earned in nursing courses. Studies consistently indicated that the best predictor for NCLEX success is the number of grades higher than a C earned in nursing theory courses. This is followed by the number of high grades in nursing courses, then number of high grades in science courses (Oermann & Gaberson, 2006). As the number of C grades increased, the risk for NCLEX failure increased. The predictive ability of failure is extremely high when a student earns more than three C grades in nursing theory courses (Barkley, Rhodes, & DuFour, 1998).

Faculty should monitor the number of C grades the student earns in nursing courses. The specific percentage students earn makes a difference, so specific percentages should be monitored. Is the course grade a high C or a low C? If a C ranges from 78% to 83%, a student who consistently earns 83% as a C grade is much better positioned for NCLEX success than the student who consistently earns a 78%.

As faculty monitor the C grades, students must be alerted to the possibility of being at-risk for NCLEX failure. Strategies for remediation can be offered at the time the C grade is earned rather than waiting until the end of the program when NCLEX review is typically conducted.

Additionally, faculty may reconsider the grading scale used in the nursing program. Tracking student grades as they relate to success on NCLEX is important data for determining the lowest grade a student can earn as a passing grade in a nursing course. For example, a program's policy is the student must earn a C and establishes a 75% as the lowest C. Tracking specific percentages that students earn in all nursing courses may reveal that those who fail NCLEX earned between 75% and 78% in nursing courses. This data may indicate a need to raise the passing percentage for nursing courses to 78%.

Using the students' nursing course percentage grades also provides data for a proactive approach to remediation. Because studies indicate that students with fewer C grades pass NCLEX at a higher rate, remediation may best be implemented for students with a C grade of any percentage. One study indicated that a student with no C grades or below had a 97% pass rate on NCLEX; those students with just one C grade or below had an 84% pass rate. Those with three or more Cs, Ds, or Fs had a 51% pass rate (Beeson & Kissling, 2001). Based on these very specific findings, the best remediation plan should include remediation for students who earn a C grade, even if their actual percentage is at the high end of the C grade. Therefore, if a student earns an 83% on a test, even though this is a high C grade and at the passing level, immediate remediation is likely most helpful. This proactive approach as the student progresses through the nursing program provides just-in-time remediation in small increments, which is less overwhelming for the student than to wait until the end of the nursing program when a predictive examination indicates many areas of low scores.

Students Repeating a Nursing Course

As indicated in the previous section, students who earn a D or an F in a nursing course are at high risk for NCLEX failure. Most nursing programs have a readmission policy that allows students to retake nursing courses. Supporting students who repeat a nursing course is extremely important. Tutorial assistance either before or when concurrently enrolled in the nursing course should be employed so the student will earn a grade higher than C when the course is repeated (Washington & Perkel, 2001).

If there is a pattern that indicates that many students need to repeat a particular nursing course, faculty must evaluate the situation. This course may be a curriculum "choke point" that needs close scrutiny. Faculty may consider teaching methodologies and evaluation strategies used in the course and revise the course accordingly.

Teaching Strategies Related to Student Characteristics

It is helpful to use a tool that assesses student characteristics. Such a tool is the *Start Right in Nursing School™* program from College of DuPage. This is a self-assessment tool that gathers information about a number of student characteristics. Once these characteristics are known, the faculty and student can work together to develop strategies that promote learning.

Learning Styles

When developing teaching strategies, faculty should consider the results of the students' learning style inventories, and plan instruction to teach to a variety of learning styles. Faculty work with students to identify each student's individual preferred learning style and best ways to study based on that preferred style.

Difficult Content

Faculty should also make efforts to note areas of content students indicate they have the most difficulty learning. Areas of content in which many students require remediation may indicate a need to teach this material using different teaching strategies. Or, make available other means for students to study that same material, such as computer-assisted instruction or case studies.

English as a Second Language (ESL)

Incorporate an assessment of language proficiency, reading level, and reading comprehension as part of a pre-nursing assessment for potential nursing students or for counseling newly admitted students to the nursing major.

Several teaching strategies enhance learning for the student with ESL. Students may benefit from development of a vocabulary notebook to catalogue and further explain English words new to them. Exposing students with ESL to vocabulary via a variety of contexts to clarify and explain meaning further may be accomplished via computer-assisted instruction (CAI). Study groups offer a vehicle of exposure to the English language and the opportunity to clarify understanding of the meaning and significance of content (Malu & Figlear, 1998; Sims-Giddens, 2000). See Table 6.6 for an overview of insights about teaching students with ESL offered by Caputi, Engelmann, & Stasinopoulos (2006).

Testing/Evaluation Techniques Related to Student Characteristics

Many students suffer from test anxiety. Identifying test anxiety upon admission to the nursing program is extremely important so a plan of action can be developed. Students should receive assistance in ways to allay test anxiety. In some cases, referrals to external resources may be indicated to provide students with necessary support. Working through test items during classroom sessions often helps students feel empowered with the skill to answer test questions, relieving some test anxiety. To promote active self-involvement to improve testing, students can use the *Student Self-Checklist for NCLEX Success*. This tool helps students track their performance and take responsibility for remediating weak areas. The *Student Self-Checklist for NCLEX Success* can also be accessed on the CD-ROM accompanying this book.

Developed by Dr. Caputi, the *Student Self-Checklist for NCLEX Success* tool incorporates many student characteristics that can result in either success or failure on NCLEX. The items listed on the tool consist of both academic and non-academic factors. Some non-academic factors that affect the student's ability to pass NCLEX include test anxiety, test-taking skill, and the student's own personal perceptions about the ability to pass (Mills, Wilson, & Bar, 2001). Addressing these issues as the student proceeds through the program provides time for dealing with them.

Figure 9.2 – Student Self-Checklist for NCLEX Success

Success Activity	Funda-mentals	Med/Surg 1	Maternal-Child	Mental Health	Med/Surg II	Critical Care	Integrated Concepts
Earned 85% or higher on each exam							
Answered Application/Analysis questions correctly							
Remediated areas of content with a test score <85%							
Analyzed test-taking strategies							
Eliminated test anxiety							
Used stress reduction techniques during tests							
Eliminated negative self-talk before & during exams							
Took responsibility for studying for each test							
Took responsibility for my own learning							
Developed a study schedule for classroom exams							
Developed a study schedule for remediation after exams							
If repeating a nursing course, arranged for a tutor							
Completed case studies r/t course content							
Completed review in NCLEX review books r/t course content							
Completed 500 NCLEX review questions r/t course content							
Developed concept maps on difficult content							
Learned all pharmacology r/t course content							
Scored high on critical thinking exercises in clinical area							
Practiced prioritizing/delegating r/t course content in clinical area							
Scored high on standardized exam r/t course content	/////						
Scored at passing level on exit exam			/////		/////	/////	

©2006, Linda Caputi, Inc. Used with permission.

As the student completes the tool throughout the nursing program, the student develops a degree of self-awareness and self-responsibility related to study habits and testing. In one study, students who pass NCLEX on the first attempt are those who report taking responsibility for learning and being proactive in NCLEX test preparation. Those who did not pass on the first attempt perceived their lack of success was the responsibility of others and were less able to manage stress (Eddy & Epeneter, 2002). Use of the tool helps establish the positive characteristics identified for success in nursing courses and establishes this as a mindset for preparation for the NCLEX. Students learn to take an active role for NCLEX success from the very first nursing course. They take responsibility for developing a study schedule, seeking remediation, and working on test anxiety. Faculty are present to help students or refer students to others for help, but students learn that the responsibility for seeking help and engaging in helping behaviors lies within themselves. The goal is to empower students, not only for success on NCLEX, but for success throughout the nursing program.

Faculty can use the tool in Figure 9.2, *The Student Self-Checklist for NCLEX Success*, to help students in other ways as well. When reviewing student entries on the checklist, elicit from the student concrete examples that describe how the student took responsibility for learning. For example, a student might indicate twelve hours per week are spent studying content presented in the classroom. Studying takes the form of making flash cards, creating a concept map, or listening to a recording of the lecture. Faculty may identify methods that many students use for studying and incorporate those methods into their classroom teaching. For example, if students find constructing concept maps helpful, faculty may want to include concept mapping as a teaching strategy.

Allowing students ample time for testing is important. Consider the number and style of items in relation to the amount of time allotted for testing. If an item stem is lengthy, students will need more time to complete that item. Use of a standard English dictionary during testing for students for whom English is a second language should be considered.

Faculty may ask students to complete a test item query form after they review a test. Use of a test item query form provides an objective approach to test review and provides faculty with insights about student interpretation of particular test items. The test item query form enables a safe approach to discussion of test items that is non-threatening for both students and faculty. Rather than a potentially confrontational encounter between students and faculty, the tool requires that students provide literature to support their rationale that the keyed answer is not correct. Students should be instructed to bring their textbooks or any articles they have read in preparation for the test review. By allowing students a voice in their test review, faculty demonstrate respect for students and provide another avenue of learning after testing is complete. Faculty benefit as well, with knowledge of necessary item revision for future course modifications and test development. See Figure 9.3 for a sample test item query form.

Figure 9. 3 – Student Test Item Query Form

Student Test Item Query

Name: _____

Test Date: _____

Item number on test:

Rationale why I believe the keyed answer is not correct:

References: (Cite two published references that support why you believe the keyed answer is incorrect.)

What I believe to be the correct answer (provide rationale for your answer):

The Student Test Item Query may be accessed on the CD-ROM accompanying this book.

Thinking Skills

In an editorial about evidence-based practice, Tanner (1999) discusses two habits all students should develop, questioning why something is to be done and seeking the evidence that supports that action. Such habits exemplify critical thinking and must be nurtured in nursing students. The development of critical thinking skills in nursing students necessitates faculty thinking about *how* to teach as opposed to *what* to teach (Diekelmann, 2002; Ironside, 2004; Valiga, 2003).

With the common goal of providing safe and effective care to clients, an invitational forum sponsored by the National Council of State Boards of Nursing (2006c) explored evidence-based elements of nursing education in relation to the Institute of Medicine's five competencies, and cited the report, *Health Professions Education: A Bridge to Quality* (2003). These competencies include:

- provide patient-centered care
- work in interdisciplinary teams
- employ evidence-based practice
- apply quality improvement
- utilize informatics

Competencies of providing patient-centered care and employing evidence-based practice were found to have better outcomes when critical thinking is integrated in the curriculum. In addition, research findings indicated graduates experienced less difficulty with assignments when afforded the opportunity to analyze multiple types of data when making client decisions (National Council of State Boards of Nursing, 2006d).

In an effort to determine if the NCLEX examination could benefit from innovations in testing, a survey of the state boards of nursing was conducted to identify important attributes for entry-level RNs (National Council of State Boards of Nursing, 2006d). The five most important attributes are listed in order of rank:

1. Application of knowledge to practice
2. Critical thinking
3. Ethical/Moral standards of practice

Chapter 9: A Model for NCLEX® Success

4. Competence in performing clinical skills
5. Effective communication skills (oral, written, electronic & therapeutic)

The five most important attributes identified for entry-level LPN/LVNs are listed in order of rank:
1. Application of knowledge to practice
2. Competence in performing clinical skills
3. Critical thinking
4. Ethical/Moral standards of practice
5. Effective communication skills (oral, written, electronic & therapeutic)

The results of this survey highlight the importance of critical thinking for entry level nurses. The development of thinking skills in nursing students is of paramount importance for safe, competent practitioners.

Teaching Strategies Related to Thinking Skills

Faculty can design strategies to promote thinking skills. Several teaching strategies have been used to foster critical thinking in nursing students and include concept maps, role-play, case studies, computer-assisted instruction, assignments provided in advance to use in class to augment discussion, reflective writing, journaling, questions to engage students in discussion, and assignments that encourage thoughtful approaches to content (Walsh & Seldomridge, 2006).

Of key importance is the learning climate. To evoke thinking skills in students, the learning environment must be such that students and faculty interact together to extract meaning from experience. If faculty are to assist students in their thinking process, faculty must be able to determine what and how students are thinking.

Faculty should understand and use knowledge about how students develop critical thinking skills related to nursing content. Knowledge of how students develop critical thinking in nursing enables faculty to use teaching strategies that best meet the needs of the students. For example, beginning nursing students are in the "right from wrong" stage of critical thinking. These beginning students learn content by applying rules (McGovern & Valiga, 1997). During this stage, faculty assist students to learn critical thinking by explaining what thinking skills constitute critical thinking, then providing examples of those thinking skills applied to nursing. For example, beginning students learn the normal ranges of vital signs. They often want to apply those ranges to all client situations. They do not understand that a blood pressure of 100/60 may be perfectly acceptable for some clients (Caputi, 2003). To help students develop beginning critical thinking skills at this level, faculty can use post-conference in clinical to direct students to discuss their clients' vitals signs. During the discussion the students compare and contrast their findings and discuss why some vital signs, although out of range of normal, are acceptable. This kind of teaching strategy assists students to begin thinking critically about their assessment findings.

As students move through the phases of developing critical thinking, faculty provide teaching strategies that continuously challenge students' thinking. Examples of clinical teaching techniques include questioning students at continuously higher levels and teaching students to use available resources to answer questions rather than the teacher providing answers for them.

Other critical thinking strategies relate specific classroom content to clinical experiences. Creating awareness in students regarding the relationship of content to their clinical learning is helpful. Invite students to discuss clinical experiences, either past or present, and discuss how these experiences relate to the topic of discussion. Guide students to make these associations. Bring student clinical experiences to life in the classroom. Ask students to bring an example of a client situation from the clinical setting with a diagnosis related to the content of study. Students should be instructed to bring all data collected about that client. For example, when teaching in the classroom and discussing hypertension, ask the student who cared for a client who required renal dialysis as a result of uncontrolled hypertension to provide a short case presentation about the client. Explore with the students any factors that put this client at risk for developing hypertension. Ask the students focused questions such as, what is the relationship between renal failure and hypertension and what are the chief concerns for this client? Work with students to identify and prioritize nursing interventions. Ask the student who cared for the client to state the most important nursing intervention provided during the clinical experience. Also explore what the students do not understand. Pointedly ask students what seems confusing or what questions would they have if they were the client? This provides an opportunity for faculty to discern learning needs and provides a safe environment in which to pose questions.

Develop case studies to provide a realistic picture of the variables students need to consider when they learn about the care of clients. Ask students to prioritize the interventions in the case study and identify which nursing tasks can be delegated to a licensed practical nurse or a nursing assistant. Faculty may turn to clinical experience or journal articles to gather data to write their own case studies. Alternatively, case studies may be found in texts or instructional aids accompanying texts. The *Critical Thinking Tutorial* and *Critical Thinking Case Studies and More* software programs offered by College of DuPage Press may be used in class or independently viewed by students. These case studies include a critical thinking advisor that demonstrates application of critical thinking theory to client care.

Concept mapping fosters critical thinking (Caputi & Blach, in press). As students advance to higher level nursing courses, replace traditional five-column care plans with concept map care plans. Establish student groups to construct the concept map care plan to promote cooperative learning while fostering critical thinking. Students then present the concept map to other student groups and explain how they came to understand relationships among the sub-concepts. Verbal presentation is especially helpful. As students present the concept map, faculty are able to discern the connections students may or may not have discovered. This allows faculty to lead students to make associations among the data.

Use a variety of critical thinking tools to enlighten students in the process of critical thinking (Caputi, 2004). For example, students may complete a tool for a client with a particular condition or disease state that directs the students in their data collection and knowledge development. One example is a critical thinking tool students complete for the client with congestive heart failure. The tool directs students to think about factors that are of primary importance, the clinical manifestations of congestive heart failure, the lab values of concern, the medications currently prescribed, and any special teaching needs. The tool further prompts students to think about the most important concern relative to the client. Students should then compare and contrast their tools, focusing on differences such as the clinical manifestations for a client with right-sided heart failure and a client with left-sided heart failure. Such tools provide a focus for students to know what to address in clinical practice and offer a way to think about their thinking while they are performing in the role of the nurse (Caputi, 2004; Engelmann and Caputi, 2005).

Skilled thinking in nursing requires reflecting on the thinking process as the nurse is thinking. Novice nurses have difficulty with the skill of reflective thinking. To help develop self-awareness of thought processes while providing nursing care, provide students with reflective activities. Ask students to reflect on their response to a particular situation and how they view their actions. Function as a facilitator and use feedback and questioning to encourage students to reflect on their experiences (Zygmont and Schaefer, 2005). For example, after students obtain report on assigned clients, the second consecutive day of care ask the students what, if anything, they will change in providing care for their clients from the previous day. Process with the students their rationale for why they would or would not make changes to their plan of care.

Testing/Evaluation Techniques Related to Thinking Skills

Faculty should keep in mind the best methods to use to evaluate activities designed to promote thinking skills. These methods include critical thinking test items, concept maps, and critical thinking tools.

Critical Thinking Test Items

When designing test items, use published guidelines for writing critical thinking test items. Morrison, Nibert, and Flick (2006) provide guidelines for this task. Some of these guidelines include:

1. Faculty should be familiar with their school's curriculum design, philosophy, and objectives. The overall curriculum is designed to affect certain outcomes. Critical thinking should be one of these outcomes. Faculty design instructional methods to meet particular competencies. Evaluation tools are designed to determine the effectiveness of the instructional methods (Morrison, Nibert, & Flick, 2006).
2. Write critical thinking test items. Students must be able to apply course content to clinical practice; therefore, test items should focus on patient situations and must ultimately be written at the application or analysis cognitive level. Students must also be able to engage in multilogical thinking. Such thinking necessitates knowledge of several facts, or a number of steps in the thinking process, to answer the question. Questions that ask what is the best or the highest priority require the student to think critically and require a high degree of discrimination, an important component of a critical thinking test item (Morrison, Nibert, & Flick, 2006).
3. Use a test blueprint designed for critical thinking tests. The test blue-

print provides a method for systematically selecting test items and is the first step in test assembly. The test blueprint categorizes test items according to course objectives, steps in the nursing process, NCLEX test plan categories, and cognitive levels (Morrison, Nibert, & Flick, 2006). Identifying the step in the nursing process addressed by the question ensures the test item has a nursing focus. See Figure 9.4 for a sample test blueprint. This test blueprint is included on the CD-ROM accompanying this book.

Concept Maps

Evaluation of concept maps provides feedback on the student's thinking skills. Because concept maps are used for many purposes, they are graded according to the expectations outlined in the assignment. Concept map care plans may be graded by determining the relationships among sub-concepts that address assessment data, short, and long-term goals, nursing diagnoses, nursing interventions, and teaching components (Couey, 2004). Grading a concept map constructed for the purpose of explaining client education related to a particular pathophysiology requires the student to demonstrate very different links between and among sub-concepts than a concept map focused on direct client care.

Critical Thinking Tools

Critical thinking tools provide ideal material for summative evaluation of critical thinking. For example, students complete a critical thinking tool through a clinical rotation. They are given feedback as a formative evaluation strategy. Then, at the end of the clinical rotation, the same tool is used but for summative evaluation purposes. Although the same tool is used, the students apply the critical thinking processes required to complete the tool to a new client situation demonstrating transfer of thinking skills. Having experienced the context in a similar situation, students are able to relate the thinking process to a new situation.

Critical thinking tools can be used throughout the program, even with beginning nursing students. For example, beginning students may require practice with gathering complete and accurate information prior to performing client care. A tool such as the one in Figure 9.5 may be used.

After students have practice using this tool on several occasions and receiving feedback from the teacher, the tool may then be used to evaluate the student's

Figure 9.4 – Sample Test Blueprint

Test Blueprint

Question	Course Objective	Step in the Nursing Process	NCLEX® Category	Cognitive Level
1		Assessment	1	Application
2		Diagnosis	3	Analysis
3		Intervention	4	Knowledge
4		Diagnosis	8	Comprehension
5		Diagnosis	2	Application
6		Assessment	1	Analysis
7		Intervention	1	Analysis
8		Intervention	5	Analysis
9		Diagnosis	6	Application
10		Diagnosis	6	Knowledge
11		Evaluation	8	Application
12		Assessment	1	Application

Key:
NCLEX Category
1. Management of Care
2. Safety and Infection Control
3. Health Promotion & Maintenance
4. Psychosocial Integrity
5. Basic Care & Comfort
6. Pharmacological & Parental Therapies
7. Reduction of Risk Potential
8. Physiological Adaptation

©Linda Caputi, Used with Permission

ability to collect the necessary information and answer the questions noted on the tool. This tool is included on the CD-ROM accompanying this book.

Figure 9.5 – Collecting Data for Client Care

On a separate sheet of paper, answer the following:
1. Client information:
    Age:
    Reason for admission:
    Date of admission:
    Diagnostic procedures:
    Surgical procedure:
    Diet:
    Activity:
2. Medications:
    Drug:
    Reason why it was prescribed:
    Therapeutic effects expected:
    Adverse effects to monitor:
(Complete for all medications prescribed.)
3. Client history:
    Important information from history:
    From the history, the most important data impacting this
        hospitalization is:
4. Diagnostic tests:
    Name of test:
    Why was this test ordered?
    (Complete for each test ordered.)
5. Problems occurring for this client during the preceding 24 hours:
    How were the above problems handled?
6. Was the physician called for any reason? If so, why?
    What information was gathered prior to notifying the physician?
    What actions were taken?
7. Potential problems that could occur for this client:
    Interventions to prevent the potential problems:
8. Look at the client's nursing care plan:
    List the nursing diagnoses:
    Prioritize the nursing diagnoses:
    How did you determine the order of prioritization of the nursing diagnoses?
    What are the interventions for the top two nursing diagnoses?
    Prioritize these interventions:
    Which of these interventions can be delegated and to whom?

> 9. Look at the shift report sheets for the past 24 hours. Based on those report sheets, what is the MOST IMPORTANT nursing intervention for you to carry out this shift?
> 10. If the physician came in at this moment and discharged this client, what are the most important teaching instructions for this client?
> 11. What if............................
> (Ask me to complete this question for you to answer.)
> Here the teacher poses a "what if" question based on the information the student collected.

©Linda Caputi, Used with Permission

NCLEX Review Books

Use of NCLEX review books and computer programs with practice questions provide students with exposure to NCLEX-style questions from a variety of perspectives, some of which will be different than those offered by the course faculty. Faculty may select a few questions for each class period and instruct students on how to answer application and analysis questions. This practice may be continued throughout the program so students gain practice with NCLEX-style items. Faculty are cautioned to evaluate the test items in the NCLEX review book to ensure they are written at the application or analysis levels.

The following item may be used to exemplify a test item written at the analysis cognitive level. Faculty would use this item when discussing hyperthyroidism and explain that the student would need to understand multiple concepts to answer the question.

Test Item: Which assessment data would the nurse assign the highest priority when caring for a client who has undergone a thyroidectomy?
  A. Amount of fluid intake
  B. Hourly urine output
  C. Level of consciousness
  D. Ease of respirations

Rationale: Respiratory distress presents the greatest potential for risk of complications for a client who has undergone a thyroidectomy due to the potential for tetany or swelling (Ignatavicius & Workman, 2006); therefore, option D, ease of respirations, represents the assessment data of the highest priority. In answering this question, the student must know what complications are possible following a thyroidectomy and determine which data represents the complication that poses the greatest threat to the client. To answer this item correctly, students apply knowledge of airway, breathing, and circulation as priorities of care. Students also apply knowledge of the edema of the surgical site and its close proximity to the trachea and parathyroid gland injury resulting in tetany, both of which can interfere with respiratory function. Students must carefully weigh each distracter as the other assessment data would be appropriate to collect for this client; however, distracters A, B, and C are not the highest priority.

Nursing Knowledge

A key role faculty play in student success is guiding students through the process of attaining nursing knowledge. Students must be vested in this process. Faculty must empower students to be proactive in their learning of nursing knowledge (Stark, Fiekema, & Wyngarden, 2002).

Overall, faculty must provide teaching that prepares a practitioner for the role of the nurse in the 21st century. Curriculum is planned with this goal in mind within the program's organizing framework based on the program's philosophy and learning outcomes. Faculty select textbooks that best support their program's learning outcomes.

The textbooks are then augmented with other sources of nursing content to ensure up-to-date information. The National Council of State Boards of Nursing (NCSBN) provides two documents that can be used for this purpose. One is the *Report of Findings from the 2005 RN Practice Analysis: Linking the NCLEX-RN Examination to Practice* (Wendt, & O'Neill, 2006) which will be referred to in this chapter merely as the practice analysis. The other is the *National Council of State Boards of Nursing Detailed Test Plan for the NCLEX-RN Examination* (National Council of State Boards of Nursing, 2006e) referred to in this chapter as the NCLEX test plan. A final source of information for faculty is information published by national organizations, such as the National League for Nursing and the American Nurses Association.

Practice Analysis

The NCSBN publishes the practice analysis every three years. This document is based on survey research conducted to discover the activities performed by newly licensed nurses during their first six months of practice. A panel of subject matter experts reviews the compiled list of 150 activities included on the survey. New graduates complete the survey, ranking the activities according to the frequency in which they engaged in that activity. The practice analysis is used to help evaluate the validity of the NCLEX test plan (Wendt & O'Neill, 2006).

Faculty can use the practice analysis when making decisions about what content to include in instruction. A major issue facing faculty is what to teach and what not to teach. Faculty consistently remark that it is impossible to teach everything. The practice analysis can provide guidance. For example, faculty would ensure inclusion of content related to maintenance of client confidentiality, principles of infection control, and vital sign assessment in all areas of nursing content because these are activities with the highest number of respondents reporting performance related to their work activities. In contrast, faculty may address to a much lesser extent the activities of microderm-abrasion, botox, and laser treatments as these activities were reported to apply to the work settings of the lowest numbers of participants (Wendt & O'Neill, 2006).

The NCLEX Test Plan

The NCLEX test plan derives from the practice analysis. Therefore, the test plan represents the knowledge and thinking skills a newly licensed nurse will need. The test plan provides a breakdown of categories with related percentage of questions from each category.

The test plan uses a client needs framework and is composed of four major categories. Four processes are integrated into the four categories of the test plan and include nursing process, caring, communication and documentation, and teaching and learning. Test items comprise a certain percent of the test for each client needs category and subcategory based on the findings from the practice analysis. Distribution and percentage for each category and subcategory of client needs are listed in Table 9.1 (National Council of State Boards of Nursing, 2006e).

Included in the NCLEX test plan published by the NCSBN are specific objectives for each subcategory. This information is extremely helpful for faculty

Table 9.1 – Distribution and Percentage for Categories on the NCLEX-RN Test Plan

Categories of the NCLEX	
o Safe, Effective Care Environment	
▪ Management of Care	(13-19%)
▪ Safety and Infection Control	(8-14%)
o Health Promotion and Maintenance	(6-12%)
o Psychosocial Integrity	(6-12%)
o Physiological Integrity	
▪ Basic Care and Comfort	(6-12%)
▪ Pharmacological and Parenteral Therapies	(13-19)
▪ Reduction of Risk Potential	(13-19%)
▪ Physiological Adaptation	(11-17%)

when considering content to cover and for students studying for the NCLEX. Although faculty should not frame the entire nursing program curriculum based on this publication, the objectives included in this document should be referenced often. Faculty ensure that, in addition to other content taught, these objectives are addressed.

Information from National Organizations

    Information in textbooks is typically a few years old when a new edition is released. Therefore, faculty must stay up-to-date on important content related to the areas they teach. Faculty should monitor nursing specialty organizations to ascertain the latest information that is important for entry-level nurses. Emphasizing information which is important to the entry-level nurse is critical. Faculty must teach to the level of their students; it is important to be discerning when considering new information.

    In addition to nursing specialty organizations, general healthcare organizations are also extremely helpful. Organizations such as the Centers for Disease Control and Prevention (CDC) and the Joint Commission on the Accreditation of Healthcare Organizations (JCAHO) provide helpful insights. Use of morbidity and mortality statistics from the national and state levels provides another source of information.

Faculty may find that with all the demands of teaching, there is limited time to continuously follow the publications of these organizations. A helpful tactic is to assign individual faculty to monitor websites or other resources of a specific organization, then report to the full faculty any new information. In this way, faculty share the work of updating content without becoming overwhelmed by the task.

Teaching Strategies Related to Nursing Knowledge

While it is essential that faculty provide content, that content should not be covered at the expense of engaging students in thinking. Success on the licensure examination requires that students know content, and apply critical thinking and clinical decision making using that content. Many of the objectives listed in the NCLEX test plan refer to these thinking skills. Using those objectives, faculty can plan a variety of teaching strategies to incorporate this content. For example, Emergency Response Plan is a subcategory of Safety and Infection Control. There are four objectives under this subcategory. When students are assigned to the Emergency Department for a clinical assignment, they may share in post-conference how that department addresses an emergency response plan. The group might then role play or develop a case study that incorporates an emergency response plan and clinical decisions related to client care during an emergency.

Students must learn the lesson of staying current in nursing knowledge, just as faculty do. One approach to teaching this lesson is to emphasize evidence-based nursing practice. Evidence-based nursing practice requires students to consult journals and credible websites to determine best practice. Assign students to research the nursing care of the population of clients on the unit they are assigned. When the student provides care, the student should compare and contrast the care provided with that found in the student's research. This work is then discussed in post-conference. Topics may include the latest practice protocols, new diagnostics tests, and current pharmacological treatments.

Testing/Evaluation Techniques Related to Nursing Knowledge

Traditional four-option, multiple choice tests are standard in nursing education programs. Faculty **must** know how to write quality tests. There are two components faculty should consider for developing quality tests – quality test items and scientific test analysis (Morrison & Walsh-Free, 2001).

Quality Test Items

Quality test item development involves writing rationales for each test item, writing questions at the application or above cognitive level, requiring the student to use multilogical thinking to answer the question, and requiring a high level of discrimination to choose from plausible alternatives (Morrison, Nibert, & Flick, 2006). Quality test items flow from a test blueprint that is based on the objectives of the course and reflect the nursing process. Test items must be carefully crafted to reflect this content and measure the construct being tested. For example, test items about prioritization and delegation skills written to test student application of these particular skills ask which intervention the nurse should perform first, or which task may be delegated to a nursing assistant. Such questions place the student in the role of the nurse managing client care to answer the question.

Scientific Test Analysis

Testing policies for the nursing program should stipulate that all tests undergo scientific test analysis. An overall test analysis is used to determine the reliability and validity of each test. Teacher-made tests should be evaluated for reliability, which refers to consistency of test scores, and validity, the extent to which the test measures what it is supposed to measure. The point biserial correlation coefficient, a measure of a test item's ability to discriminate between high achievers and low achievers, based on the test as a whole, and item difficulty should be obtained for all test items (Morrison, Nibert, & Flick, 2006).

The test analysis data is also used to determine if the tests developed by faculty are well-constructed and fairly assess student achievement. Writing tests that are not too easy or too difficult is extremely critical in test construction. Either type of error results in test data that is not dependable as a measure of the student's ability to pass NCLEX.

Test data should be stored using a systematic approach and include the test blueprint, the test analysis summary, the distribution of scores and grades on the test, a copy of the keyed test, and a copy of the test with rationales listed. Faculty feedback about how to improve items should also be noted (Morrison, 2005).

Preparing Students to Test Well

Testing well is a skill that faculty help students develop. Faculty should provide examples of test items that address each cognitive level and the background information necessary to understand and answer critical thinking, multiple choice test items. To develop student awareness of critical thinking test items, faculty explain test items that require multilogical thinking, or knowledge of more than one fact to answer the question, and a high level of discrimination to choose the correct answer from alternatives (Morrison, Nibert, & Flick, 2006). Providing students practice with test items and feedback on their performance enhances student confidence when taking examinations.

Standardized Testing

Tests written by an outside source can provide valuable information relative to a student's mastery of content. It is critical to keep in mind that the objective of standardized testing is to identify student needs so interventions may be employed as soon as possible. A comprehensive assessment plan in place throughout the nursing program provides the necessary foundation for passing NCLEX-RN (Spector & Alexander, 2006). However, a comprehensive assessment plan must include a strategy for remediation. Students should not be evaluated as achieving a below-standard grade then left on their own to remediate. Most students will choose not to engage in any remediation efforts. Remediation must be available for students. Consequences must be employed if remediation is not completed.

As a check on curriculum, faculty should compare scores on standardized examinations with students' GPAs. If students with high or above average GPAs are not scoring well on the standardized exams, faculty need to question why this might occur and evaluate their teaching, testing, grading methods, and expectations. If there is incongruency between results on an exit exam, for example, and the student's performance while in the program, the school should review its curriculum (Spector & Alexander, 2006).

Exams may be administered at the conclusion of a course to measure a student's ability to meet specific course objectives. Identification of content in which students obtained low test scores provides faculty with information to plan review of that material. Testing at the conclusion of a course provides feedback about student knowledge gaps prior to the student moving on to the next course and well in advance of an exam taken at the conclusion of the program.

Exams may also be administered near the conclusion of the program, as students prepare for NCLEX. Such exams, taken as students exit the program, provide a final check on student preparedness for the licensure exam (Morrison, 2005).

Progression Policies and Use of Benchmarks

Individual schools must establish a policy to address how they will use the results of the standardized exams they administer. For example, will the exam results be used only to evaluate curriculum? Will the exam score constitute a certain percentage of the student's course grade? Will the exam results be used to provide feedback for students as they prepare for the next course or prepare for NCLEX? Or, will the exam results determine a student's ability to progress from one course to the next, one level to the next, or graduate from the program?

In one study, the consequences for students who did not achieve the designated benchmark after the permitted number of retests of the exit exam included (Nibert, Young, & Britt, 2003):
- an incomplete or failing grade in the capstone course
- denial of eligibility for graduation
- withholding approval of NCLEX-RN candidacy

In another study that looked at use of progression policies, NCLEX-RN pass rates improved in seven programs by 9 to 41% within two years of implementation of a progression and remediation policy (Morrison, Walsh-Free, & Newman, 2002).

Research Study – Using a Test to Predict NCLEX Success

To gain a sense of the percentage of nursing educators who are using predictor tests and how the results of the predictor tests are used, the authors conducted a survey. The survey was administered via a blind mailing to 199 randomly selected nursing faculty from all levels of undergraduate, pre-licensure, registered nurse programs. A total of 34 faculty completed the survey for a response rate of 17%.

Faculty were asked to respond to the following nine items about use of predictor tests to help predict NCLEX success for nursing students:

1. Do you administer a standardized nursing examination before graduation that can be used to predict the student's chances of passing NCLEX? Results: 33 of the 34 respondents reported using a standardized predictor test.
2. Please select all the standardized nursing examinations that you use as a predictor of NCLEX success. Thirty-two of the 33 respondents indicated the predictor test they used. One respondent reported using two tests, ATI and NLN and another reported using both Mosby and NLN. Table 9.2 lists the tests and the number of respondents using those tests.

Table 9.2 – Standardized Examinations Used As Predictors of NCLEX Success

Test	Number of Respondents
ATI	8
ERI	4
HESI	12
Mosby	3
NLN	3
Arnett	4

3. How do you use the results obtained from the standardized predictor exam? See Table 9.3 for a listing of responses to this question.

Responses indicate faculty use the results of the predictor test for assessment purposes, to identify weak areas requiring further study or remediation, for review or remediation purposes, and as part of course completion and progression.

4. Must your students obtain a certain score on the standardized predictor exam to qualify for graduation? Results: Ten of the 22 respondents to this question require students to obtain a certain score.
5. What percentage of students had delayed graduation as a result of failure to achieve a passing score on the standardized predictor exam in: 2002,

Table 9.3 – How Results Obtained From Standardized Predictor Tests Are Used

Do not use the results at this time. Simply present the results to the student and file a copy in the student's record. If we receive notice that the student did not pass NCLEX-RN, we pull the student file and review the HESI results to see if the NCLEX-RN results match the prediction.

Students receive an incomplete grade in course, do remediation, and retake test.

Help students identify areas of weakness.

The results are given to students to help identify their weak areas and give a focus for study. They are used by faculty to see how the class as a whole did and what areas of the curriculum could be strengthened.

If the student does not reach the minimum percentile designated, then that student must remediate via a specific plan and if not successful a second time they are excused from the program.

They are used to determine if students are eligible to graduate from the program.

We have incorporated the HESI into a role transition/leadership course and students must score a 900 to pass the course (they get three tries).

To recommend remediation.

Student feedback and course assessment.

As an exit exam for completion of the final course. And as an evaluator of our curriculum. We only started this in spring 04. In spring 04, anyone who scored below 850 had to pass the RNCAT exam, which they all did very readily. This year (2005) all who fail (25/90) have to pay to retake the HESI. We are still negotiating the process for the people who are not successful on their second attempt.

Schedule those who score below level predictive of NCLEX pass for a review course.

To advise the student/graduate and to look at the curriculum for weaknesses.

I used HESI results to revise course content.

Decided not to due to inconsistencies noted.

Specified score required prior to submission to state completion of curriculum. Option if unable to achieve required score of taking a review course identified by our program with notification from the review course that participant is ready for NCLEX. Assessment and curriculum revision.

We use ATI testing periodically throughout the program. We will graduate our first class in 2006. Will use to modify courses based on results.

We have only begun using the HESI this year. Prior to that time, we used the Mosby Assess Test. Currently, we use the HESI results to make suggestions to our students about the level of preparation that we would recommend prior to their taking the NCLEX. We have implemented a paper in our leadership course which requires the student to develop a plan for NCLEX preparation based upon their HESI results.

We use them as a part of program progression and course completion.

Program evaluation and student assessment and advising.

Based on student's score, students are assigned a number of test questions to complete.

To gather information so we can begin to predict success on NCLEX.

Only to predict success, possible curriculum changes with new material added to theNCLEX, and areas to identify as needing review.

To identify areas of weakness, then we institute a remediation program if needed.

For review of weak areas.

For remediation.

To determine the level of intervention for the student's NCLEX success plan.

To review with the student areas of weakness.

Given to students to review.

Collecting data to determine if the test is predictive.

Advisory.

> Exit exam must be passed at national average to graduate.
>
> We counsel students regarding weak areas and encourage them to use a review book and/or sign up for a review class.

(All text in the above table is drawn from a survey and is presented verbatim.)

2003, and 2004? Only nine respondents answered this question. Results: Five of nine respondents indicated they had students who were delayed in graduation. The other four respondents reported no delay in graduation due to failure to achieve a passing score on the predictor exam.

6. What percentage of students never graduate as a result of failure to achieve a passing score on the standardized predictor exam? Results: All 13 respondents to this question indicated 0% never graduate as a result of failure to achieve a passing score on the predictor exam. Three respondents qualified their response stating this was the first semester or year of implementation and data are not yet available.
7. Is remediation provided if the student fails to obtain the established passing score on the standardized predictor exam? Twelve of 13 respondents provide remediation for students who do not obtain the established passing score on the predictor exam.
8. Please describe the type of remediation that you offer to students who do not obtain the established passing score on the standardized predictor exam. See Table 9.4 for a listing of the type of remediation offered for students.
9. What was your first time pass rate on NCLEX? See Table 9.5 for a listing of pass rates comparing three years in succession as reported by each school.

The details of how the survey was written and administered, the total survey, and the complete results can be found on the CD-ROM accompanying this book.

Table 9.4 – Type of Remediation Offered to Students

The student is to print out areas that they were unsuccessful in on the exam and read/study those areas. The student then must pass the unproctored test with 100% before being allowed to retake the proctored test.

Students remediate on their own with NCLEX review books and the ATI remediation.

NCLEX software, literature, videos.

ATI modules.

We use institutional version of NCLEX 3000.

Additional tutoring by the faculty in each content area.

Our students review in an organized manner the entire last semester of their senior year with completion of at least 100 questions with an attained score of 85% on each 100 questions. For example, 100 questions in Fundamentals, 100 questions in Maternity, etc.

Student meets with the faculty administering the standardized test for the course. They review the student's test results and emphasize areas of need. The student takes the practice test and completes it at 80%, then retakes the standardized test. If failed a second time, a meeting with the course coordinator and review precedes the third attempt. The student would then receive an "Incomplete" for the course and have the next semester to repeat the test until the 60th percentile is reached.

NCLEX prep courses, computer and physical.

Individual advising by faculty, peer study with other students, established guidelines prepared by faculty to assist with remediation. Use of additional software "review courses" to practice NCLEX test taking.

Software and tutoring.

Table 9.5 – Listing of Pass Rates

2002	2003	2004
87%	92%	88%
100%	100%	92.31%
73%	92%	88%
>95% (have two classes)	>95% (have two classes)	100% 4-Dec
89%	92%	98%
I'm not sure	I'm not sure	I'm not sure
100%	100%	100%
95%	92%	90%
?	?	90%
87	91	95
98%	92%	93%
95%	90%	80%
92%	88%	90%
86%	72%	72%
57%	33%	?
not available	not available	not available
n/a	n/a	n/a
91%	94%	88%
100	100	93
84%	95%	95%
94%	77%	96% (one semester so far)
70%	60%	50%
N/A	N/A	N/A
94%	96%	94%
100%	100%	100%
100%	100%	93%
100%	96.70%	93%
92.5	93.9	92.13%
not used in 2002	not used in 2003	not used in 2004
I do not know that information	same response	same response
data not available at this moment	data not available at this moment	data not available at this moment
92%	78%	86%
70	74	76
100%	95%	95%

Pulling It All Together

At the completion of the nursing program consider offering an end-of-the-program NCLEX preparation course. Identify measures to address the three major components of the Caputi model: student characteristics, thinking skills, and nursing knowledge. Chapter 10 covers the topic of an NCLEX success course.

A Hypothetical Nursing School Example

Hypothetical Nursing School (HNS) faculty expanded their Student Success Program to address the needs of the student at-risk for NCLEX failure. Interventions were planned based on application of the components that comprise the Caputi Model for NCLEX Success.

Student Characteristics

To address the student at-risk for NCLEX failure, HNS faculty implemented a policy requiring all students to complete and maintain ongoing self-assessment through use of the *Student Self-Checklist for NCLEX Success*.

As part of their Student Success Program, HNS faculty agreed to use the information recorded on the *Student Self-Checklist for NCLEX Success* in conjunction with the information already gathered by the *Checklist of Positive and Negative Factors* and the *Start Right in Nursing School: A Self-Assessment Tool* ™ to identify variables with the potential to affect NCLEX success.

Faculty met individually with students twice during each term and assessed student progress through review of the *Student Self-Checklist for NCLEX Success*. This information was compared with previously collected data. Students experiencing difficulty were referred to the Retention Specialist for further assessment and intervention. Content areas identified as problematic by students were flagged and referred to the Curriculum Committee for further exploration.

Based on a need identified by more than half of the students, the Retention Specialist designed a one-hour seminar focused on stress-reducing measures and suggestions for study plans/schedules that make use of time management skills. The seminar was offered to all students who self-identified they needed help to reduce stress and design a study plan/schedule as well as students referred by faculty.

Teaching Strategies Related to Student Characteristics

Faculty decided to award five points at the end of each course for students who completed the *Student Self-Checklist for NCLEX Success*. To receive all the points, students were required to submit proof of the strategies they implemented to address the success activities listed on the tool.

To help reduce stress associated with testing, faculty created study guides to focus students in their preparation for testing. The study guides provided direction specific to the topic being tested.

Testing/Evaluation Related to Student Characteristics

Faculty increased the amount of time allowed for multiple-choice testing. They plan to track performance for those students who previously reported insufficient time for testing to determine reduced test anxiety and improved test performance resulting from the increased time.

Students for whom English is a second language or who worked more than 20 hours per week were monitored closely by the Retention Specialist. The Evaluation Committee planned to correlate the results of NLCEX performance with these two variables.

Thinking Skills

A more student-centered approach to teaching and learning was adopted by HNS faculty to foster student thinking skills. Faculty realized they wanted to stimulate more active and reflective learning on the part of students. To accomplish this transition, HNS faculty restructured classes to allow time to process information from the previous class before moving forward with new concepts, decreased the amount of time spent lecturing during class time, and used case studies and structured opportunities throughout class to pose and answer questions.

HNS faculty designed a one-credit hour course to address testing issues related to NCLEX. The course provided an overview of the NCLEX test plan, the elements of critical thinking in multiple choice test items, and practice taking NCLEX-style test questions. All students were required to take this testing success course during the second term of the program. The faculty believed early scheduling of the course would help students not only on NCLEX, but also pass exams administered in the nursing program.

Teaching Strategies Related to Thinking Skills

Students were encouraged to discuss client care situations related to class content. Faculty directed the discussion and posed questions to highlight important points to provide a more complete picture of the client with a particular condition. Students worked in small groups to answer the questions, then discussed them with the larger group. For example, the following questions were posed to involve the students in the thinking about a client who required renal dialysis:

- why did the client require dialysis?
- what were the lab values for the client?
- what communication might you have with other healthcare providers about the needs of this client?
- how would you manage care of this client along with other assigned clients?
- what stands out most about this client?

All faculty implemented use of critical thinking tools to guide students in their thinking during clinical. Concept maps were also assigned. As an additional element to their concept map assignments, students were asked to prioritize their nursing interventions and indicate which interventions could be delegated and to whom.

The Critical Thinking Tutorial and *Critical Thinking Case Studies and More* programs were purchased by HNS. The tutorial was used to introduce the concept of critical thinking, and individual case studies were used throughout the curriculum to address various course topics.

Testing/Evaluation Related to Thinking Skills

Course points were restructured and additional objectives were added to reflect the new assignments faculty designed. Previously, multiple choice tests almost exclusively determined a student's grade. Faculty provided guidelines and the point distribution for each test and assignment, which included classroom tests, a concept map, a reflection paper, and completion of the *Student Self-Checklist for NCLEX Success*. However, the student must achieve a passing score on the objective tests prior to the inclusion of grades from the additional assignments.

To encourage ongoing use of NCLEX review texts, the last 10 minutes of every class were devoted to discussion of test items the students selected from their NCLEX review texts. This strategy served as a further check on a student's ability to understand a particular concept or approach to client care.

Nursing Knowledge

The Nursing Curriculum Committee was charged with the task of determining key factors to consider regarding content to include in the curriculum. HNS faculty compared information from the practice analysis and the NCLEX test plan to the school's *NCLEX Program Reports*. HNS faculty determined previous students experienced difficulty in the test plan category of Safe and Effective Care Environment and implemented review of infection control and safety measures for all students. Pharmacological and parenteral therapies were also noted to be problematic test plan categories for the previous class. Faculty decided to augment instruction about pharmacology by adding a one-credit hour course to address the role of the nurse in managing pharmacological interventions. All students will take this course in the second term of the program.

Teaching Strategies Related to Nursing Knowledge

HNS faculty added objectives to their clinical evaluation tool that addressed student awareness and use of agency protocol, client safety measures, and infection control practices. Faculty used clinical conference time to address special concerns related to management of client care and pharmacology, such as caring for the client who has a patient-controlled analgesia device.

During clinical conference, faculty processed relationships among variables related to client care using concept mapping. Concept maps presented during clinical conference were brought to class for augmentation of content addressed in class.

To address clinical judgment and decision making, faculty established mock courts of law. Students played roles of lawyer, nurse, client, physician, or other healthcare provider to explore how decision making by the nurse impacts the well-being of the client and the nurse's ability to continue in professional practice. The rest of the class served as the jury.

HNS faculty assigned students to shadow a nurse in the practice setting for one day. The student made observations about the nurse's actions and recorded them for later discussion. Students and faculty processed this activity together, discussing the role of the nurse, decisions the nurse made, and the implications for nursing practice.

Testing/Evaluation Related to Nursing Knowledge

HNS faculty decided to require students who earned less than a B- on their exams to meet with the Retention Specialist to review their test performance using the LLUSN-LAP analysis tools. HNS faculty mandated students repeating a course arrange for a tutor through the Student Assistance Department at the college.

HNS faculty also provided test reviews. Students were allowed to complete and submit the test item query form as a point of discussion about test items. Faculty used the information collected in conjunction with test item analysis.

In accordance with their goal to increase NCLEX pass rates by 5%, HNS faculty implemented specialty course exams and an end-of-the-program predictive exam administered by an outside entity. All exam results will be tracked and used in conjunction with the *Student Self-Checklist for NCLEX Success*. All specialty exams will constitute 10% of the course grade. The predictor exam will constitute 5% of the final course grade.

The Evaluation Committee will track results from the predictor tests in relation to NCLEX pass rates. Recommendations regarding possible establishment of a progression policy will be considered for the next year.

The Evaluation Committee plans to evaluate future *NCLEX Program Reports* for improvement in the areas of client safety and infection control, and pharmacological and parenteral therapies.

Closing Thoughts

Both students and faculty must adapt a proactive approach if they are to have a positive impact on NCLEX success. This proactive approach involves a realistic appraisal of the students' academic and non-academic strengths and weaknesses, identification of students' needs, and planned interventions that start from the beginning when students enter the nursing program and conclude upon graduation. Providing students with the necessary resources and guidance to address these variables are essential for a positive outcome on NCLEX. Through advance planning and strategies in place in the Student Success Program, faculty have the ability to make a critical difference in their students' outcome on NCLEX.

Learning Activities

1. Select and implement a new teaching strategy to foster critical thinking skills in the clinical setting.
2. Use the Test Item Query tool or a similar tool to provide a mechanism for student feedback about test items during a test review. What additional information did you learn about test items you wrote based on this feedback? Did students test better on subsequent tests after implementation of test review?
3. Develop a tool for tracking student grades through the program. Determine the relationship of the students' grades in nursing courses and their success on NCLEX.

References

Arathuzik, D., & Aber, C. (1998). Factors associated with National Council Licensure Examinations – Registered Nurse success. *Journal of Professional Nursing, 14*(2), 119-126.

Barkley, T. W. Jr., Rhodes, R. S., & Dufour, C. A. (1998). Predictors of success on the NCLEX-RN among baccalaureate nursing students. *Nursing and Health Care Perspectives, 19*(3), 132-137.

Beeman, P. B., & Waterhouse, J. K. (2003). Post-graduation factors predicting NCLEX-RN success. *Nurse Educator, 28*(6), 257-260.

Beeson, S., & Kissling, G. (2001). Predicting success for baccalaureate graduates on the NCLEX-RN. *Journal of Professional Nursing, 17*(3), 121-127.

California Board of Registered Nursing. (2000, December). *Executive summary NCLEX-RN Task Force report: The problem and the plan.* Retrieved May 30, 2006 from http://www.rn.ca.gov/forms/pdf/taskforce00.pdf.

Caputi, L. (2004). Operationalizing critical thinking. In L. Caputi & L. Engelmann (Eds.), *Teaching nursing: The art and science, Vol 1 & 2,* Glen Ellyn, IL: College of DuPage Press.

Caputi, L. (2003). *The Critical Thinking Tutorial.* (software). Glen Ellyn, IL: College of DuPage Press.

Caputi, L., & Blach, D. (in press). *Integrating concept maps into a nursing curriculum.* Glen Ellyn, IL: College of DuPage Press.

Caputi, L., Engelmann, L., & Stasinopoulos, J. (2006). An interdisciplinary approach to the needs of non-native speaking nursing students: Conversation circles. *Nurse Educator, 31*(3), 107-111.

Couey, D. (2004). Using concept maps to foster critical thinking. In, L. Caputi, & L. Engelmann (Eds.), *Teaching nursing: The art and science, Vol 1 & 2,* Glen Ellyn, IL: College of DuPage Press.

Crow, C. S., Handley, M., Morrison, R. S., & Shelton, M. M. (2004). Requirements and interventions used by BSN programs to promote and predict NCLEX-RN success: A national study. *Journal of Professional Nursing, 20*(3), 174-186.

Daley, L. K., Kirkpatrick, B. L., Frazier, S. K., Chung, M. L., & Moser, D. K. (2003). Predictors of NCLEX-RN success in a baccalaureate nursing program as a foundation for remediation. *Journal of Nursing Education, 42*(9), 390-398.

Diekelmann, N. (2002). Pitching a lecture and reading the faces of students: Learning lecturing and the embodied practices of teaching. *Journal of Nursing Education, 41*(3), 97-99.

Eddy, L. L., & Epeneter, B. J. (2002). The NCLEX-RN experience: Qualitative interviews with graduates of a baccalaureate nursing program. *Journal of Nursing Education, 41*(6), 273-278.

Endres, D. (1997). A comparison of predictors of success on NCLEX-RN for African American, foreign-born, and white baccalaureate graduates. *Journal of Nursing Education, 36*(8), 365-371.

Engelmann, L., & Caputi, L. (2005). Ideas to develop critical thinking in the classroom and clinical. In, L. Caputi (Ed.), *Teaching nursing: The art and science, Vol 3,* Glen Ellyn, IL: College of DuPage Press.

Gallagher, P., Bomba, C., & Crane, L. (2001). Using an admissions exam to predict student success in an ADN program. *Nurse Educator 26*(3), 132-135.

Higgins, B. (2005). Strategies for lowering attrition rates and raising NCLEX-RN pass rates. *Journal of Nursing Education, 44*(12), 541-547.

Ignatavicius, D., & Workman, M. L. (2006). *Medical-surgical nursing: Critical thinking for collaborative care*. St. Louis: Elsevier.

Ironside, P. (2004). Covering content and teaching thinking: Deconstructing the additive curriculum. *Journal of Nursing Education, 43*(1), 5-12.

Lauchner, K. A., Newman, M., & Britt, R.B.(1999). Predicting licensure success with a computerized comprehensive nursing exam: The HESI exit exam. *Computers in Nursing, 17*(3), 120-127.

Malu, K., & Figlear, M. (1998). Enhancing the language development of immigrant ESL nursing students: A case study with recommendations for action. *Nurse Educator, 23(*2), 43-46.

McGovern, M, & Valiga, T. (1997). Promoting the cognitive development of freshman nursing students. *Journal of Nursing Education*, 36(1), 29-35.

Mills, L. W., Wilson, C. B., & Bar, B. B. (2001). A holistic approach to promoting success on NCLEX-RN. *Holistic Nurse, 19*(4), 360-374.

Morrison, S. (2005). Improving NCLEX-RN pass rates through internal and external curriculum evaluation. In M. H. Oermann & K. T. Heinrich (Eds.), *Annual review of nursing education, Vol 3,* New York: Springer.

Morrison, S., & Walsh-Free, K. (2001). Writing multiple-choice test items that promote and measure critical thinking. *Journal of Nursing Education, 40*(1), 17-24.

Morrison, S., Walsh-Free, K., & Newman, M. (2002). Do progression and remediation policies improve NCLEX-RN pass rates? *Nurse Educator, 27*(2), 94-96.

Morrison, S., Nibert, A., & Flick, J. (2006). *Critical thinking and test item writing*.Houston, TX: Health Education Systems, Inc.

National Council of State Boards of Nursing (2004). *NCLEX-RN examination: Test plan for the national council licensure examination for registered nurses*. Chicago: Author.

National Council of State Boards of Nursing (2005). *NCLEX-PN examination: test plan for the national council licensure examination for licensed practical/vocational nurses.* Chicago: Author.

National Council of State Boards of Nursing (2006a). Retrieved July 13, 2006, from http://www.pearsonvue.com/nclex/#tutorial.

National Council of State Boards of Nursing (2006b). Retrieved July 10, 2006, from http://ncsbn.org/pdfs/NCLEX_Stats_Fact_Sheet.pdf.

National Council of State Boards of Nursing (2006c). *Report of the Invitational Forum.* Chicago: Author.

National Council of State Boards of Nursing (2006d). *The Threshold of Regulatory Excellence: Taking up the challenge.* Chicago: Author.

National Council of State Boards of Nursing (2006e). *NCLEX-RN examination: Test plan for the national council licensure examination for registered nurses.* Chicago: Author.

Newman, M., Britt, R. B., & Lauchner, K.A. (2000). Predictive accuracy of the HESI exit exam. *Computers in Nursing, 18*(3), 132-136.

Nibert, A., Young, A., & Adamson, C. (2002). Predicting NCLEX success with the HESI exit exam: Fourth annual validity study. *Computers in Nursing, 20*(6), 261-267.

Nibert, A. T., Young, A., & Britt, R. (2003). The HESI exit exam: Progression benchmark and remediation guide. *Nurse Educator, 28*(3), 141-145.

Oermann, M. H., & Gaberson, K. B. (2006*). Evaluation and testing in nursing education.* (2nd Ed.) New York: Springer.

Poorman, S. G., & Webb, C. A. (2000). Preparing to retake the NCLEX-RN: The experience of graduates who fail. *Nurse Educator, 25*(4), 175-180.

Roncoli, M., Lisanti, P., & Falcone, A. (2000). Characteristics of baccalaureate graduates and NCLEX-RN performance. *Journal of New York State Nurses Association, 31*(1), 17-19.

Siktberg, L., & Dillard, N. L. (2001). Assisting at-risk students in preparing for NCLEX-RN. *Nurse Educator, 26*(3), 150-152.

Sims-Giddens, S. S. (2000). Graduation and national council licensure examination pass rate of Mexican-American undergraduate nursing students. (Doctorial dissertation, Northern Arizona University 2000), 89.

Spector, N. (2006). Evidence-based health care in nursing regulation. Retrieved November 10, 2006, from https://www.ncsbn.org/Evidencebased_NSpector.pdf.

Spector, N., & Alexander, M. (2006). Exit exams from a regulatory perspective. *Journal of Nursing Education, 45*(8), 291-292.

Stark, M., Feikema, B., & Wyngarden, K. (2002). Teaching strategies. Empowering students for NCLEX success: Self-assessment and planning, *Nurse Educator, 27*(3), 103-105.

Tanner, C. (1999). Editorial. *Journal of Nursing Education, 38* (3). 99.

Tanner, C. (2006). Guest editorial. *Journal of Nursing Education, 45*(8), 291.

Valiga, T. (2003). Teaching thinking: Is it worth the effort? *Journal of Nursing Education, 42*(11), 479-480.

Walsh, C. M., & Seldomridge, L.A. (2006). Critical thinking: Back to square two. *Journal of Nursing Education, 45*(6), 212-219.

Wendt, A., & O'Neill, T. (2006). *Report of the findings from the 2005 RN practice analysis: Linking the NCLEX-RN examination to practice.* Chicago: National Council of State Boards of Nursing (NCSBN), Inc.

Washington, L. J., & Perkel, L. (2001). NCLEX-RN strategies for success: A private university's experience. *The ABNF Journal, 12*(1), 12-16.

Williams, D., & Bryant, S. (2001). Preparing at-risk baccalaureate nursing students for NCLEX success. *Kentucky Nurse, 4*(1), 17-18.

Yin, T., & Burger, C. (2003). Predictors of NCLEX-RN success of associate degree nursing graduates. *Nurse Educator, 28*(5), 232-236.

Zygmont, D. M., & Schaefer, K. M. (2005). Making the transition from teacher-centered to student-centered instruction: A journey taken by two educators. In M. H. Oermann & K. T. Heinrich (Eds.), *Annual review of nursing education, Vol 3*, New York: Springer.

Chapter 10: An NCLEX® Success Course

The final element of a Student Success Program is the development and implementation of a carefully designed course to focus students for NCLEX success (Mills, Wilson, & Bar, 2001; McQueen, Shelton, & Zimmerman, 2004). NCLEX pass rates improve with an NCLEX success course (Frith, Sewell, & Clark, 2005). The goals of the course are to support, motivate, test, remediate, and guide students so they will have an excellent chance of passing the NCLEX on the first attempt.

This chapter presents issues and considerations for planning an NCLEX success course. The purpose of the chapter is to present a structured approach to prepare students for licensure, both academically and mentally. The chapter concludes with research studies that provide additional ideas that can be used when planning your own NCLEX success course.

Planning an NCLEX Success Course

When planning an NCLEX success course, consider issues such as credit hours, when to offer the course, which students should take the course, and what to include in the course. Finally, specific learning activities are planned.

An NCLEX success course can range from one to three credit hours. The course is typically taught in the last term of a nursing program. The timing of the course should be when students have had most of the nursing content and when enough time remains to provide remediation.

It may be tempting to require only students who score below a set standard on a predictor test to take the NCLEX success course. However, this may be counterproductive. Students who are not required to take the course may decide they are ready to take NCLEX and not engage in any review. This is a mistake. All students should be required to take the course.

Chapter 10: An NCLEX® Success Course

When deciding what learning strategies to include in the course, there are four important areas to consider. These four areas can be used as an organizing framework for the content of the course. These include:
1. Remediating content
2. Testing
3. Building confidence
4. Developing a plan for after graduation and before taking NCLEX

What to Include in the NCLEX Success Course

To determine what to include in the NCLEX success course, use the four areas listed in the previous section as a guide. These include remediating content, testing, building confidence, and developing a plan for after graduation and before taking NCLEX.

Remediating Content

The optimal way to determine what content should be reviewed for each student is to administer a predictor exam. A predictor exam is often referred to as an exit exam because it is administered near the end of the student's course of study for the purpose of evaluating knowledge of content necessary for success on the licensure exam. There are many such tests on the market from companies such as Assessment Technologies Institute (ATI), Educational Resources, Inc. (ERI), and Elsevier offering the Health Education Systems, Inc. (HESI) exams, and from organizations such as the National League for Nursing (NLN). A quick search on the internet leads to more information about these products.

After a thorough evaluation of the available products, faculty should select the predictor exam that best meets their students' needs. When reviewing testing products, keep in mind the following:
1. What research is available about the accuracy of the predictions made by the exam?
2. What technical support is available and how reliable is that support?
3. Does the company have remediation materials available?
4. If remediation materials are available, does the predictor exam direct students to specific materials based on their test results?

These are important questions to ask regarding a predictor exam. The answers will be helpful when planning the course.

Prior to administration of the predictor exam, faculty should decide whether the exam results will be used for assessment purposes only, a course grade, or in conjunction with a progression policy. The policy should stipulate the required score, and the number of times and under what conditions a student may retest.

Upon completion of the predictor exam, faculty should meet with students to discuss exam results and learning goals. The following approach is offered to address both individual and group learning needs identified by the predictor exam.

Individual Remediation

Faculty meet with each student to review the results of the predictor exam and develop a systematic plan for reviewing nursing content. The student should focus on weak areas first, then move to other areas as time permits. Depending on the materials available, students plan how they will study. They may use:

1. Their textbooks
2. Materials provided by the testing company
3. Computer-assisted instruction
4. Case studies related to their identified content areas
5. NCLEX review books with practice questions
6. Study groups consisting of students working on the same content areas

NCLEX review books can be extremely helpful for remediation of content. Choosing a book that has content review as well as test questions is ideal. Answering practice questions related to weak areas as identified on the predictor test is mandatory. Students can be assigned to answer NCLEX review book questions relating to each weak area until they earn a specific score. For example, the faculty may request the student to continue answering questions until a score between 85 and 100% is obtained. Faculty meet with students once a week to review their performance on the practice questions and clarify any misunderstandings.

Faculty should encourage peer study groups (DeCicco, 2001). Study groups can be initiated by faculty or by students. For example, if a number of students scored poorly on a particular area, faculty can ask if students would like to join a group at a certain time and in a certain location to study that topic. Faculty can then be available to answer questions. Or, students may form these study groups on their own without the teacher present. Many students find study groups helpful in developing a support group with a common goal.

Group Remediation

Faculty study the aggregate scores of the predictor exam to determine content in which many students earned low scores. Class sessions are planned to review this content for all students.

During group remediation, use case studies to apply knowledge to new situations (Frith, Sewell, & Clark, 2005). Use simulated clinical situations for making decisions about appropriate client care. Taking a "non-lecture" approach can better foster critical thinking, problem solving, and decision making – all important cognitive skills needed to pass NCLEX.

The aggregate data from the predictor exam is also used for curriculum revision and improvement. If many students score low on a particular content area, new approaches to teaching that content are in order.

NCLEX Review Course

Many schools incorporate an NCLEX review course into their NCLEX success course. An NCLEX review course is different than the remediation designed for the NCLEX success course. An NCLEX review course provides a different perspective on the content and another chance to interact with the material. The more perspectives on a topic, the greater the chance the student will understand the material. An NCLEX review course also provides another opportunity for students to determine what areas of content they need to study.

Another important reason to mandate an NCLEX review course is because the predictor exam cannot test everything. Content not tested may have been content students had learned many semesters earlier (Siktberg & Dillard, 2001). A comprehensive NCLEX review course will touch on all these areas.

Incorporating an NCLEX review course into the NCLEX success course renders the review course mandatory because it is part of a required nursing course. If the review course is not mandatory, many students will not take one.

Faculty have options regarding the NCLEX review course. They may choose to teach the course themselves, or arrange an independent company to conduct the review course. Online reviews are also offered by several sources (James,

2006). The cost of the review course is part of the tuition for the NCLEX success course.

Critical Thinking

Incorporate into the remediation process practice with critical thinking activities (Siktberg & Dillard, 2001). Include content that requires students to prioritize and delegate nursing care. Use case studies to encourage critical thinking. Use concept maps to review content and connect nursing interventions to pathophysiology.

Faculty/Student Meetings

As previously mentioned, throughout the course, students meet with faculty to track how their remediation and practice testing is progressing. Weekly meetings with students are best. The student and faculty review the student's individual study plan and determine if the student is on track. These meetings are extremely important to ensure the study plan is being followed as well as clarifying any misunderstandings the student may have. Tracking the student's scores on NCLEX practice exams as part of their study plan provides objective data about the student's progress.

Administering a Second Predictor Exam

As part of the remediation process, a second predictor test is administered near the end of the course to determine if students have improved in their mastery of the content and critical thinking skills. This second predictor test can be used in the same manner as the first, to determine areas of weakness that require further study. Some schools mandate the student must earn a specific score on this second exam to graduate and take the NCLEX. This is an important decision for faculty to make with careful consideration of all the repercussions of that decision.

Testing

Although students should have been exposed to NCLEX-style test questions throughout the nursing program, including test-taking skills in the NCLEX success course is helpful. Eddy and Epeneter (2002) interviewed students after taking NCLEX and most stated they felt they were unprepared to answer NCLEX-style questions, and that nothing had prepared them for this experience. Therefore, including instruction on how to take NCLEX-style questions as part of this course is important. For example, faculty might pose a test item that requires students to prioritize the nursing interventions they would perform.

A class session should review how to dissect questions to determine exactly what is being asked, how to accurately read the stem and distracters, and how to focus on the main idea presented in the question. During class, ask students to identify appropriate test-taking strategies; have them explain how they worked through questions. This provides an opportunity to identify student errors and correct any misunderstandings in their approach to answering test questions. Specifically instruct students to do the following:

- pay attention to key words and concepts such as age, sex, and marital status.
- identify the key element of the question which will be a problem, such as a disease, symptom, or behavior.
- look for details of the problem. For example, is the question asking for nursing actions, client symptoms, or family responses?
- when reading a test item, ask what the question is asking. Does the question ask about a specific aspect of nursing care, such as assessment, planning, implementation, or evaluation?

Students should plan to take between 4,000 and 5,000 practice NCLEX-style questions. They should spread the questions over all areas of content including children's health, women's health, adult health, mental health, and pharmacology. Establish 85 to 100% as a passing score for these practice tests (Siktberg & Dillard, 2001). Require students to develop a "look-up" list of specific content for areas where they scored low on these practice tests. Students should plan specific study strategies to learn this content.

Also include psychological issues related to testing, such as test anxiety and negative self-talk (Frith, Sewell, & Clark, 2005). Teach students relaxation strategies such as deep breathing, stretching, and visualization techniques to deal with test anxiety (Mills, Wilson, & Bar, 2001).

Building Confidence

Employ tactics that require students to be responsible for their study for NCLEX. Students who pass NCLEX on the first attempt accept responsibility for learning and are proactive. Those who do not pass often believe their lack of success was the responsibility of others (Eddy & Epeneter, 2002).

Encourage students to take control and create a study schedule and be responsible for sticking to it. They should plot out their schedule on a calendar, recording when case studies and specific numbers of practice questions will be completed. They should review this calendar each week to ensure the timeline is being met. Persistence in study and review breeds knowledge and confidence when taking the NCLEX exam. Students should pace their study so their work is spread out over the course of the semester and not wait until the day before taking a follow-up predictor exam.

Providing information about the NCLEX exam helps students feel familiar with what to expect on the day of the test. Provide students with the National Council of State Boards of Nursing website address (ncsbn.org) and direct them to the candidate tutorial and NCLEX review.

Implement strategies to destroy negative self-thoughts about ability to succeed on NCLEX. Ideally, such strategies would have been implemented throughout the students' time in the nursing program. A lack of emotional distress is positively correlated with NCLEX success (Mills, Wilson, & Bar, 2001). Inviting a counselor to conduct sessions on positive self thought, cognitive restructuring related to negative feelings about testing, and stress reduction is important to build confidence.

Invite previous graduates to speak to the current class about their experience preparing for and taking NCLEX. This puts a face on the NCLEX experience. Encourage students to prepare questions for the graduates and provide these questions to the speakers in advance. These graduates can share any measures that were effective as they prepared for NCLEX.

Developing a Plan for After Graduation and Before Taking NCLEX

Instruct students to put everything else on hold when studying for NCLEX. They should not plan any major life changes between graduation and taking the NCLEX. Faculty should also counsel students to begin to save money for the licensure application process, so students do not delay testing due to insufficient funds. Review for the exam must continue, even after they successfully complete an NCLEX success course in their nursing program. Review should occur in an organized way so students do not overlook any content needs.

Some students work best with a study partner or study group which provides a support for their study and ensures they stay on track. Studying with other graduates can provide a sense of empowerment and commitment for some students. Following is a possible plan for studying with another student or with a group of students (Eddy & Epeneter, 2002):

1. Develop a schedule for study.
2. Meet twice a week reviewing questions from an NCLEX review book.
3. Each person answers the question, then discusses their rationales before looking up the correct answer and rationale in the book.
4. Use a variety of NCLEX review books.
5. Talk with each other about stress related to the NCLEX and discuss possible relaxation techniques.

Students are encouraged to study a substantial number of hours, particularly in the week before the exam. The more hours a student studies, the greater the chance of passing. Many students study an average of 65 hours between graduation and taking the NCLEX. It is particularly important to study the week prior to taking the exam (Beeman & Waterhouse, 2003).

Many graduates seek full-time employment immediately after graduation, reducing the amount of time available for study. They often believe the information they are learning in their nursing positions takes the place of studying for the NCLEX. Graduates must be cautioned that learning new nursing material on the job does not substitute for reviewing content for the NCLEX (Beeman & Waterhouse, 2003). Graduates must study for the exam. Taking time to study and not working the week prior to taking the NCLEX is the best approach. Engaging in intense studying the week before the exam is helpful.

Students should be advised to carefully plan for the day of testing. They should drive to the testing center and visit the site. This helps allay anxiety about traveling to the site and finding the room where the test will be administered. Students should be advised to get a good night's sleep the evening before the exam, eat a good breakfast the day of the exam, and keep that day free from other concerns (Stark, Feikema, & Wyngarden, 2002).

Students should be advised to take the exam as soon as possible after finishing nursing school, but not until they believe they are ready. When taking the NCLEX exam, students should be advised to not rush through the test. They should know that if they pass or if they fail, they will answer 50 to 55% of the questions correctly in each category. Finally, students should perform a realistic self-appraisal before taking NCLEX. If personal situations change, students should consider rescheduling testing to a more optimal time.

Evaluating the NCLEX Success Course

There are several objective measures faculty can use to evaluate the NCLEX success course. To determine if remediation strategies were effective, compare scores on the initial predictor exam with subsequent testing to determine if scores improved. Consider how many students did not meet the acceptable passing score on the second or subsequent predictor tests. If a large number of students did not pass on subsequent testing, investigate reasons why. Perhaps the approach to remediation needs to be revised.

The ultimate evaluation of the NCLEX success course is performance on the NCLEX. Was the pass rate higher for students who took the NCLEX success course than for students who did not take the NCLEX success course? Is the NCLEX pass rate higher than in years when an NCLEX success course was not offered?

Finally, student evaluation of the course provides a less objective, but equally valuable, evaluation of the course. It is important to have students report on their level of confidence when taking the NCLEX, and if they believe the NCLEX success course contributed to their success or failure.

What Faculty Can Learn from Students about NCLEX Success

A valuable source of information about preparing students for the NCLEX is students themselves. Graduates who have recently taken the NCLEX can provide insights that are not available from any other source. *The NCLEX Experience: Interview Protocol* developed by Eddy and Epeneter (2002) provides a perspective from the graduate that may be used to make changes to both the NCLEX success course and the general nursing curriculum.

The interview protocol offers suggestions for the interviewer who talks with graduates who have taken the licensure exam. Figure 10.1 presents this interview protocol.

Chapter 10: An NCLEX® Success Course

Figure 10.1 – The NCLEX Experience: Interview Protocol

Directions to interviewer: Please read and absorb the questions as thoroughly as possible prior to beginning the interviews in order to decrease redundancy (i.e. re-asking a question that has already been answered). Some of the questions are followed by probes or examples, which only need to be used if the subject doesn't seem to understand the question.

Please record responses as thoroughly as possible. Prior to beginning the interview, explain the nature of the interview and how the responses will be used, (including for possible publication) as clearly as possible, and remind the graduate that participation is voluntary. Ask for their consent to be part of the study and record the date and time consent is given. Remind the interviewee that their responses will be kept completely confidential and that only group data will be reported. The original interview protocols will be kept in a locked file cabinet and will be destroyed once the data is analyzed.

Demographics:

Name_____ D.O.B._____
Consent attained? Yes___ No___ Date & Time of Consent_____
Number of weeks between graduation and sitting for exam _____

Questions about the exam itself:

1. How did you prepare for the NCLEX exam? Probe: review course, self study with review book, self study with computer program, EXAMCO, etc.
2. What were your feelings during the exam? Probe: confident? unsure? bored? panicked?
3. Did anything happen during the exam that affected your performance? Probe: noise level, hunger, other physical discomfort?
4. Why do you think you passed/didn't pass the exam on the first try? This question is <u>very</u> central to meaningful results from this study and should be given ample time.
5. What aspect of the NCLEX did you find the most difficult? Why? Probe: this could be either a part of the test OR a factor in the whole testing experience.

6. How long did you spend taking the exam? If you took the entire time allowed, did you answer all of the questions? Did you have as much time as you felt you needed to complete the exam?
7. Was there anything that particularly surprised you about the exam?
8. How many questions did you answer before the exam discontinued?

Questions about the relationship between nursing education and success or failure on the NCLEX:

9. How would you describe your test-taking abilities during the nursing program? Probe: What is your learning style? How well do you usually do on multiple choice questions?
10. How were your classroom experiences helpful or not helpful in preparing you for the exam? Probe: for example, anything specific in the way the courses were taught or organized?
11. How were your clinical experiences helpful or not helpful in preparing you for the exam?
12. Can you identify at least one thing that the nursing program could have done differently that would have helped you in the exam?
13. Can you identify one thing in your own behavior while a student that would have helped you in the exam? Probe: if you had it to do over again, what would you change about your study habits, outside activities, outside work, etc.
14. Were you surprised about your NCLEX results? Why or why not?
15. Is there anything else that you would like to tell us that could help us better understand how to help students be successful on the NCLEX?

College of DuPage Press and Drs. Linda Caputi and Lynn Engelmann wish to thank the authors, Linda Eddy and Beverly Epeneter for permission to print their tool, The NCLEX Experience: Interview Protocol (2002).

A copy of this interview protocol may be accessed on the CD-ROM accompanying this book.

Research Study – Helping Students Prepare for NCLEX

To gain a sense of the percentage of nursing educators who employ interventions to help students prepare for NCLEX and to learn what those interventions are, the authors conducted a survey. The survey was administered via a blind mailing to 205 randomly selected nursing faculty from all levels of undergraduate, pre-licensure, registered nurse programs. A total of 29 faculty completed the survey for a response rate of 14%.

Faculty were asked the following four questions about use of a review course to help students prepare for NCLEX:

1. Do you sponsor or offer an NCLEX review course before your nursing students take the NCLEX for the first time? Results: 76% of the 29 respondents offer an NCLEX review course.
2. When is the review course offered to your students? Results: 32% of the respondents offer a review course before graduation and 59% offer a review course after graduation.
3. Is the NCLEX review course mandatory? Results: 35% of the programs mandate a review course.
4. Describe the NCLEX review course you sponsor or offer to your nursing students. See Table 10.1 for a listing of comments shared by faculty describing their review course.

The responses noted in Table 10.1 suggest faculty believe it is important to offer a review course. The primary method of review identified in this study is a review course offered at the end of the curriculum that is comprehensive, with review of NCLEX-style test items. Of the 22 respondents, nine indicated the review course is offered by an outside review company or the review takes place at a different location.

Faculty were also asked the following two questions concerning collaboration with local healthcare organizations to facilitate NCLEX success:

1. Do you collaborate with local healthcare organizations to facilitate NCLEX success for your graduates? Results: 14% of the 29 respondents collaborate with healthcare organizations to facilitate NCLEX success.

Table 10.1 – How Faculty Describe an NCLEX Review Course

Description of NCLEX Review Course
Covers medical/surgical, pediatrics, mental health, maternal health, leadership, and community.

Kaplan, structured using multiple choice questions with a systems and nursing process focus.

Covers: adult health, child health, maternal/infant health, mental health, test taking strategies, and stress reduction. Structured: five days, seven hrs/day.

Covers all areas from fundamentals, medical-surgical, maternal-child, pediatrics, and pharmacology. Two day course in lecture type format.

MEDS Review course - offered free each semester to schools who sign on to use of LS/RN program - which we do. Content review followed by quizzes with review of answers - four days from 8am-4pm.

The course is performed from an outside source (I believe it is Meds—I am not sure because I am not involved in this process as I am only a first year instructor).

Kaplan review.

Guided test question review.

A review course that can be attended as a "live" course or can be viewed as a PowerPoint/CD presentation as a class. Course is comprehensive and approximately four days long as viewed by CD. This course is through Educational Resources, Inc.

This is the first year. We are doing a "pilot" review course at no cost. It will be three days of outlined review. There are questions during the course, but we have NCLEX review questions in our computer lab. Students review test-taking strategies especially for computer use and alternative questions.

All major specialty areas and mostly questions.

It usually is a four day course that covers the content presented in most review books.

We do the HESI and everyone is required to take that. The NCLEX review per se is offered at a reduced cost to students and is voluntary. I don't know anything about it in detail.

> Kaplan's Review courses with additional test review. College elective course.
>
> Students meet weekly with a faculty member and have completed homework (20 or more assigned questions from a review book) and then discuss their answers and reasons for the right and wrong answers.
>
> Two credits, one in fall semester and one in spring semester of senior year. Students have an NCLEX review book each semester and take weekly quizzes. In class students practice review questions on the computer.
>
> Over three days – offered at a different institution.
>
> The review course is a preplanned course by ATI. The faculty teach the course content prior to graduation. It is made up primarily of questions, answers are reviewed, why one is incorrect versus the other that is correct. The review is set for two full days and we provide lots of food.
>
> Covers total curriculum.
>
> Four days.
>
> CEU type course: eight hours; use ERI RN exam to model course; case studies and questions.

(All text in the above table is drawn from a survey and is presented verbatim.)

2. Describe the collaboration you have in place with local healthcare organizations to facilitate NCLEX success.

In this study, four of the 29 nursing programs responding to the survey report they collaborate with local healthcare agencies to facilitate NCLEX success. Two programs indicate that graduates are sponsored to take a class to prepare for NCLEX. One program uses clinical simulations and one program has established preceptorships, which has lent to an investment in the student as a future employee with job offers prior to graduation. Faculty were asked the following two questions about remediation for graduates who do not pass NCLEX:
1. Do you have remediation in place for graduates who do not pass NCLEX? Results: Six of the respondents have remediation in place.

2. Describe the remediation that is provided for graduates who do not pass NCLEX. See Table 10.2 for a listing of comments shared about remediation provided for graduates upon failure of NCLEX.

Table 10. 2 – Remediation Provided for Graduates Who Do Not Pass NCLEX

Description of Remediation Provided for Graduates Who Do Not Pass NCLEX
They can return to the college and have access to our computer lab which has many practice NCLEX exams.
Do the RN review course offered through Educational Resources, Inc.
We provide online and personal remediation for any student who chooses to take it.
Individualized study plans with college advisors.
For students we use the online review plus the mentor program and other software to assist students. This is also offered to those who fail.
Follow-up NCLEX review course.

(All text in the above table is drawn from a survey and is presented verbatim.)

Of the six respondents who offer remediation for graduates who fail NCLEX, three offer individualized assistance. All six implement some type of study, either through review of NCLEX practice items or an NCLEX review course.

Faculty were asked the following two questions about graduates at risk for not passing NCLEX on the first attempt:
1. What factors do you believe put a graduate at risk for not passing the NCLEX on the first attempt? See Table 10.3 for a listing of comments about the reasons graduates are at risk for not passing NCLEX on the first attempt.
2. Of the factors you listed, what do you feel is the NUMBER ONE reason graduates are at risk for not passing the NCLEX on the first attempt? See Table 10.4 for a listing of the NUMBER ONE reason faculty believe

Table 10.3 – Factors That Place Graduates At Risk for Not Passing NCLEX on First Attempt

Factors That Place Graduates At Risk for Not Passing NCLEX on First Attempt

Missing classes, poor exam performance.

Poor reading comprehension, test anxiety, too much going on in their lives at time they take it, history of learning disability, poor performance on other standardized tests, and lacking computer skills.

Just passing general education courses (C grade) and nursing courses (C+ grade) throughout the nursing program. Score below 35 on NLN Achievement Tests. Score below 45 on Mosby Assess Test.

Waiting extended time to take the exam for the first attempt. Waiting to work until after the NCLEX is taken. Failure to take a review course.

Grade of C in nursing. ESL status.

Less than a 75 average in nursing courses. Working more than 20 hours per week. ESL. Family responsibilities. Waiting more than 3 months to take the exam.

Time from graduation to taking NCLEX. Overall scholastic performance in school.

Poor exam grades during school. Not academically endowed for passing. Poor academic history with low GPA.

Lack of language skills. Problems with abstract thinking in questions.

Difficulty with comprehension and/or difficulty with test-taking skills.

When English is the second language. Students who have previously failed a nursing course. The acceptance of an LVN/LPN education as equal to the generic nursing student education.

Poor performance on written exams (low GPA) and in clinical setting. Poor critical thinking. Outside stress.

Poor theory grades (borderline passing); ESL

Grades of a low C in most courses.

Students for whom English is not their first language, students who work full time or close to full time, and students who have performed marginally (Cs) all along in nursing courses.

Putting off taking the exam too long after graduation. Not preparing after graduation. Passing through the nursing program just at the passing level.

Anxiety, lack of focus. Not necessarily lack of knowledge!

Not preparing for test taking.

Grades of C in required nursing courses; poor ACT reading levels.

Personal stress around the time of the exam and just making it through school. This includes either working too many hours during the school year or having too many home responsibilities.

Inability to correctly read questions. Inability to prioritize with several answers being 'right'/over thinking the questions. Feeling overwhelmed/poor test-taking ability.

Grades at a C are at high risk for failure. Grades below a C do not pass. Students who are overconfident about their knowledge are at higher risk for failure. Students who have failed a medical-surgical nursing course are higher risk. Students who take it to "see where they fall" without preparation.

Poor science grades; less than 60th percentile on ATI tests; weak medical-surgical grades; low confidence; moving; marriage; and new job within 60 day period of board date.

History of one or more failures in pre-requisite science courses and a failure in a clinical nursing course.

Low GPAs. Students who repeat a nursing or science course.

Level of students coming in. Need for constant content review through testing.

Lack of adequate study prior to NCLEX. Poor academic performance during school.

English as a second language; reading comprehension problems as identified on the NET; having young children; working more than 10 hrs/week.

Poor academic performance; poor test-taking skills; and test anxiety.

(All text in the above table is drawn from a survey and is presented verbatim.)

graduates are at risk for not passing NCLEX on the first attempt.

Faculty indicate academic variables of low GPA, Cs in required nursing courses, poor science grades, poor test-taking skills, poor critical thinking skills, low scores on standardized achievement tests, and inadequate NCLEX preparation as reasons for NCLEX failure. Non-academic variables include

Table 10.4 – NUMBER ONE Reason Graduates are At Risk for Not Passing NCLEX on First Attempt

NUMBER ONE Reason Graduates are At Risk for Not Passing NCLEX on First Attempt
Poor exam performance.
Poor reading comprehension.
Just passing general education courses.
Failure to take a review course.
Grade of C in nursing.
Less than 75 average in nursing courses.
Student performance.
Poor exam grades during school.
Language skills.
Difficulty with comprehension.
English is not the primary language.
Poor critical thinking skills.
Narrow studying. They try to study the minimum. Some students will state that a C is passing and that is all they want.

Students with English as a second language.

Passing through the nursing program just at the passing level.

Lack of focus.

Not preparing for test taking.

Poor grades in required courses.

Not treating school as a full time commitment. Over-thinking questions.

Students who do not take the exam seriously and just go take it without preparation to "see where they fall."

Weak medical-surgical grades.

Failure in a clinical nursing course.

Students who repeat.

Constant remediation of content.

Lack of study for NCLEX.

English language/reading comprehension problems.

Poor academic performance.

(All text in the above table is drawn from a survey and is presented verbatim.)

English as a second language, test anxiety, waiting too long to take NCLEX, and outside stressors, such as work and family commitments.

In summary, faculty responded with a variety of NUMBER ONE reasons students are at risk for not passing NCLEX. These included poor academic performance, reflected by poor critical thinking skills, lack of focus, and earning Cs in nursing courses. Of the 29 responses, three respondents indicated problems with English language as a main factor for being at risk for NCLEX success.

Faculty were asked to share other comments about ways to prepare students for NCLEX success. See Table 10.5 for a listing of these comments.

Chapter 10: An NCLEX® Success Course

Table 10.5 – Ways to Prepare Students for NCLEX Success

Remediation after exams if scores less than 80%.

Mandatory test-taking and study skills workshop, which is presented in the first semester after admission. Test review sessions.

CAI on NCLEX review; NCLEX review book(s). Faculty designed course exams based on the NCLEX question format.

HESI examinations, ATI program, and computer examinations.

Use of computerized testing banks to supplement didactic course content.

Review classes - "mock" test which provides them with feedback on strengths and weaknesses. Encouraging practicing questions throughout nursing education.

Review sessions.

A preparatory course at the end of the last semester to review 3000 NCLEX questions.

Students who can articulate answers are sometimes unable to recognize choices. One-on-one sometimes is the only way to assist. Going over exams in a group is not always helpful to those at risk students.

We encourage students to do practice NCLEX-RN style questions throughout the program as they are studying. This year, we are requiring they pass an RN assessment exam in order to graduate. They will have to do remediation until they pass this exam.

Test items throughout the program are formatted to the NCLEX. Students continually tell us that the exams in our program were harder than the NCLEX, but most of all they felt prepared after graduating from our program.

Review test taking strategies especially for computer use and alternative questions. Make pilot review course mandatory.

Mosby assess test.

I encourage students to begin NCLEX preparation early. I have also seen a tremendous increase in student preparation for the NCLEX when they have to pass an exit exam to graduate from the nursing program. It has almost become the standard in Texas.

Since we have made the HESI mandatory, pass rates have improved. We have numerous on-line learning packages to assist students in preparing for the NCLEX. After they take the HESI, we recommend that they meet with a faculty coach to plan their preparatory strategies based on their HESI scores. This has resulted in a much improved pass rate.

Designing tests throughout the program with the same format as NCLEX. Providing practice tests. We are considering raising our pass rates for our courses. This would help our pass rates as it has with other colleges but it does not necessarily help the individual student. I would like to find a way to "force" the students to take NCLEX by a certain date after graduation. I do not like the fact that they schedule it themselves when they are "ready." I feel that there is way too much emphasis on this exam. It is a number and score as is the pass rate. There is much more to the profession of nursing and the pressure to get good "numbers" is overrated. We tell our students to assess the entire person not just the numbers, we need to do the same.

We use the Kaplan STAR test for formative evaluation.

Students are required to take ATI or other commercial tests and make the 60th percentile or they have to remediate by reviewing the ATI booklet, or their text, or both, and retake the exam to achieve the 60th percentile.

I find the MedsPub system very helpful and refer students to it frequently.

We are using a test program for prediction of success and remediation if the student does not make a predetermined score on the exam. We have just started, so unsure of the success.

Require exit interviews to assess student status at graduation and discuss NCLEX preparation.

We utilize the ATI tests and books to assist our students in preparation for course comprehensive finals and the ATI RN comprehensive exam. We strongly encourage them to take a review course before taking NCLEX and to also take the test as soon as possible after graduation.

The faculty are assigned to mentor and work with a small group of students. They monitor their online work and suggest appropriate faculty for special content help.

> Constant testing with rationales. Students need to learn strategies.
>
> Review sessions during the last term. Standardized exams with remediation throughout the program. Remediation of faculty constructed exams if test score is < than 75%. Critical thinking test items on every exam in the program.
>
> More practice with testing and typical case scenarios and questions.
>
> Mosby Assess test. ATI testing throughout the program.

(All text in the above table is drawn from a survey and is presented verbatim.)

The chief means identified to prepare students for NCLEX was to expose students to NCLEX-style test items and associated rationales on a regular basis throughout the nursing program. Faculty identified use of standardized tests, inclusion of critical thinking test items on every test, NCLEX review books, and NCLEX review courses as primary methods to prepare students for the licensure exam. In addition, faculty believe assistance in the form of a test-taking and study skills workshop provided early in the curriculum sets the stage for future success on NCLEX.

The details of how the survey was written and administered, the total survey, and the complete results can be found on the CD-ROM accompanying this book.

A Hypothetical Nursing School Example

Faculty at HNS planned an NCLEX Success Course for the final semester of their nursing program. The goal of the course supports their program goal of increasing their NCLEX pass rate by 5%.

Faculty reviewed all the predictor tests currently available on the market and determined they would use the HESI exam. With this decision made, the faculty developed an outline for the course:
- the course will be offered during the final semester of the nursing program.
- all students will take the HESI exit exam, meet individually with a faculty member, and develop a study plan.
- the course will meet two hours each week.

- during the first hour, content in the areas on the HESI exit exam where a majority of students scored poorly will be reviewed. Case studies, concept maps, and clinical scenarios will be used to present content. Critical thinking activities will be used.
- during the second hour, faculty will work with students answering NCLEX-style questions. Students will explain how they would dissect and answer a question. Students will work in small groups and present rationales for their answer choices. During this time, faculty will address test anxiety and relaxation techniques to use during testing. A member of the counseling staff will provide additional interventions for dealing with anxiety and promoting self-confidence and positive thinking. Students will also develop a plan of study to implement between graduation and taking the NCLEX.
- a four-day NCLEX review provided by an independent review company will be conducted near the end of the semester. The student must attend the review course to earn a passing grade for the course.
- a repeat predictor test will be given. The score on this predictor exam will count for 50% of the student's grade.
- the remaining 50% of the student's grade will be based on the number of NCLEX practice questions completed. Students must complete 3,000 questions to receive a C for this portion of their grade. They will receive a B if they answer 5,000 questions and an A if they complete more than 6,000 questions.

The HNS faculty will introduce this course in the next academic year. The course will be evaluated based on the change in the NCLEX pass rate, the difference in predictor scores from the beginning of the course to the end of the course, and student evaluations.

Closing Thoughts

This chapter presented an NCLEX success course as the final element of a Student Success Program. This is an extremely important component. Students who have been successful in a nursing program should have all the help necessary, and should expect, to pass the NCLEX exam.

Learning Activities

1. Study the available predictor exams on the market. Compare and contrast each test examining the research studies that support its effectiveness, the level of technical support offered, the type of reports the student and faculty receive, and the nature of the remediation materials available.
2. Design an NCLEX success course. Determine the number of credit hours and a week-by-week schedule of learning activities.
3. Survey local nursing programs to determine if they have an NCLEX success course as part of their nursing program. Interview faculty to determine what learning activities are included in their courses. Ask if their NCLEX scores have changed with the implementation of this course.

References

Beeman, P. B., & Waterhouse, J. K. (2003). Post-graduation factors predicting NCLEX-RN success. *Nurse Educator, 28*(6), 257-260.

DeCicco, C. H. (2001). Nursing students' perceptions of peer study groups. *Dissertation Abstracts International, 62-06B,* 201. (UMI No. AA1301622).

Eddy, L. L., & Epeneter, B. J. (2002). The NCLEX-RN experience: Qualitative interviews with graduates of a baccalaureate nursing program. *Journal of Nursing Education, 41*(6), 273-278.

Frith, K. H., Sewell, J. P., & Clark, D. J. (2005). Best practices in NCLEX-RN readiness preparation for baccalaureate student success. *CIN: Computers, Informatics, Nursing, 23*(6), 322-329.

James, E. (2006). NCLEX Success: Study groups, review courses and practice tests help prepare you. *Advance for Nurses, 4*(8), 29-30.

McQueen, L., Shelton, P., & Zimmerman, L. (2004). A collective community approach to preparing nursing students for the NCLEX RN examination. *ABNF Journal, 15*(3), 55-58.

Mills, L. W., Wilson, C. B., & Bar, B. B. (2001). A holistic approach to promoting success on NCLEX-RN. *Holistic Nurse, 19*(4), 360-374.

Siktberg, L., & Dillard, N. L. (2001). Assisting at-risk students in preparing for NCLEX-RN. *Nurse Educator, 26*(3), 150-152.

Stark, M., Feikema, B., & Wyngarden, K. (2002). Teaching strategies. Empowering students for NCLEX success: Self-assessment and planning. *Nurse Educator, 27*(3), 103-105.

Tables

Table 1.1 - Example Variables Influence Student Success	4
Table 1.2 - Variables Influencing Quality Assurance	6
Table 2.1 - Factors Interfering with Learning	24
Table 2.2 - Positive Factors	25
Table 2.3 - Summary of Select Studies Indicating Predictors of Success	26
Table 2.4 - Definition of the "At-Risk" Student	28-32
Table 2.5 - Number One Reason Students are At-Risk	32-35
Table 2.6 - Checklist of Positive and Negative Factors	40
Table 2.7 - Numbers of Students with Positive and Negative Factors from Hypothetical Nursing School	44
Table 3.1 - Example Point System for Selective Criteria Score	52
Table 3.2 - Criteria Commonly Used as Admission Criteria	54
Table 3.3 - Summary of Admission Criteria from 86 Schools of Nursing	58
Table 3.4 - Point System for HNS	73
Table 4.1 - Organizing Data to Plan Student Success — Checklist of Positive and Negative Factors	84
Table 4.2 - Student Learning Styles Assessment Survey Responses	91
Table 4.3 - Faculty Learning Styles Assessment	92-93
Table 4.4 - Success Program Components	96-97
Table 4.5 - Success Plan Specific to Nursing Students	97-98
Table 4.6 - Point in Curriculum Success Plan Offered	98-99
Table 4.7 - Point System for HNS	101
Table 4.8 - Student Data	103-105
Table 5.1 - Additional Factors that May Influence Success	124
Table 5.2 - Summary of Retention Specialist Activities	136-137
Table 6.1 - Student Critical Thinking Assessment Survey Responses	177-179
Table 6.2 - How Faculty Teach Critical Thinking	180-182
Table 6.3 - How Faculty Apply, Measure, and Evaluate Critical Thinking in Nursing Students	183-185
Table 6.4 - Clinical Experience Assessment and Documentation Tool	188-190
Table 6.5 - Faculty Insights from the Conversation Circle Experience	196
Table 7.1 - Program Outcomes	257
Table 8.1 - Abbreviations Related to Failing and Withdrawing from a Nursing Program	266

Table 8.2 - Percentage Required to Pass a Nursing Course	272
Table 8.3 - Number of Readmissions	277
Table 9.1 - Distribution and Percentage for Categories on the NCLEX-RN Test Plan	317
Table 9.2 - Standardized Examinations Used As Predictors of NCLEX Success	322
Table 9.3 - How Results Obtained From Standardized Predictor Tests Are Used	323-325
Table 9.4 - Type of Remediation Offered to Students	326
Table 9.5 - Listing of Pass Rates	327
Table 10.1 - How Faculty Describe an NCLEX Review Course	350-351
Table 10.2 - Remediation Provided for Graduates Who Do Not Pass NCLEX	352
Table 10.3 - Factors That Place Graduates At Risk for Not Passing NCLEX on First Attempt	353-354
Table 10.4 - NUMBER ONE Reason Graduates are At Risk for Not Passing NCLEX on First Attempt	355-356
Table 10.5 - Ways to Prepare Students for NCLEX Success	357-359

Figures

Figure 1.1 - The Merging of the Art and Science and Nursing Education — 12
Figure 1.2 - Graphic Representation of Methodologies — 13
Figure 1.3 - Elements of a Program Plan for Student Success — 14
Figure 2.1 - Relationship of Definition for At-Risk Student and Admission Components — 36
Figure 2.2 - Identifying Your At-Risk Student: The At-Risk Model — 42
Figure 3.1 - A Model for Developing an Admission Policy — 70
Figure 4.1 - Data Flow for Planning Your Student Success Program — 80
Figure 5.1 - Data Flow for Planning Your Student Success Program — 115
Figure 6.1 - Elements of a Student Success Program — 147
Figure 6.2 - Exam Analysis — 152-153
Figure 6.3 - Summary of Exam Techniques for Multiple Choice Questions — 153-154
Figure 6.4 - Exam Analysis Procedure — 155
Figure 6.5 - Learning Assistance Program Objective Exam Analysis Worksheet — 156
Figure 6.6 - LLUSN Learning Assistance Program Exam Analysis: Assessment and Intervention Protocol — 157-161
Figure 6.7 - Suggestions to Improve Exam Performance — 162-163
Figure 6.8 - Relating Theory to Practice — Encouraging Cognitive Leaps — 175-176
Figure 6.9 - Example Course Evaluation Tool — 204-206
Figure 7.1 - Rubric for Ranking Applicants to the Associate Degree Nursing Program — 239
Figure 8.1 - Theory Examination Advisement Tool — 268
Figure 8.2 - Skill Performance Deficiency Tool — 269-270
Figure 8.3 - Learning Content — 270-271
Figure 8.4 - Readmission Request Form — 279
Figure 8.5 - Leave of Absence Request Form — 280
Figure 8.6 - A Model for Developing a Readmission Policy — 289
Figure 9.1 - The Caputi Model for NCLEX Success — A Multifaceted Model — 298
Figure 9.2 - Student Self-Checklist for NCLEX Success — 303
Figure 9.3 - Student Test Item Query Form — 305

Figure 9.4 - Sample Test Blueprint — 312
Figure 9.5 - Collecting Data for Client Care — 313-314
Figure 10.1 - The NCLEX Experience: Interview Protocol — 347-348

Index

Academic advising 96, 149, 211
Academic assistance 151, 209, 212-213
Academic factors 24-25, 27, 39, 299
Academic load 23, 127, 240
Academic support 17, 130, 145-146, 209
Academic variables 25, 102, 297, 299, 355
Accommodations for testing 242
ACT 50, 52, 54, 57-58, 61, 251, 354
Active discussion 244-245
Active learning strategy 186
Administration 62, 74, 81, 112, 130-132, 136, 140, 215, 220-221, 237, 251, 259, 267, 296
Admission criteria 4, 9, 36, 38, 50-58, 61-68, 76, 78, 108, 115-116, 238, 261, 266, 281, 284, 288
Admission policy 41, 45, 50, 62, 64, 66-72, 75-76, 80-81, 141
Admission requirements 36, 50, 53, 58, 69, 74, 282
Admission testing 4, 237
Advance assignment 244-245
Advising 36, 51, 60, 72, 95-97, 99-100, 102-103, 133, 149-150, 195, 203, 209, 211, 214, 324, 326
Advising session 60, 72, 95, 97, 100, 103, 214
Alumni tutors 170, 240, 241
Analysis cognitive level 310, 314
Anatomy and physiology grade 73, 101

Application cognitive level 235, 259, 272-273, 310, 314, 319-320
ARNETT exam 236
Art 11-12, 222
Assessing critical thinking 176, 179, 186
Assessment and intervention protocol 152, 157
At-risk 9, 17, 21, 23, 28, 30-32, 36-39, 42-43, 45-46, 55, 59, 67-68, 71, 78-79, 95-97, 117, 141, 143, 145-146, 199, 209, 216, 300, 328
Attempt 2, 28, 264
Attention deficit hyperactivity disorder (ADHD) 241-242
Attrition 21-22, 27, 37, 55, 61, 127, 187, 193, 211, 226, 229, 250-251, 284, 288
Attrition rate 22-23, 27, 62, 64-65, 129, 140, 193, 201, 222, 227, 240, 251, 261, 276, 290
Benchmarks 98-99, 321
Biology grade 52, 73, 101
Bonus points 273-274
Caputi Model for NCLEX Success 297-298, 328
Caring 11, 39, 41, 116, 139, 197, 206-207, 222, 243, 267, 316
Caring curriculum 12, 15, 206-207, 215, 222
Case study 8-9, 89, 173, 183, 185-186, 204, 213, 217, 226-264, 309, 318
Categories on NCLEX-RN test plan 311, 316-317, 331

Certification as nursing assistant 53
Certified nursing assistant (CNA) 53, 69, 94, 231-232, 260, 281
Characteristics of nursing students 17, 21
Chemistry grade 52, 73, 101
Child care 39-40, 44, 84, 87, 105, 123, 191, 114
Choke points 78-79, 94-95, 99, 109-110, 115-116, 119, 128, 142-143, 198, 208, 216, 218, 220
CITE Learning Styles Instrument 88, 90
Classroom aspects 275
Clinical aspects 275
Clinical contract 200
Clinical evaluation 31, 44, 94, 177, 187, 259, 331
Clinical experience assessment 187-188
Clinical ratio 231
Clock hours 140, 232
Cognitive leaps 175-176
Cognitive restructuring 344
Collaboration skills 165, 168
Collaborative testing 12, 164-168
College resources 122
Commercials 244, 246
Communication skills 166-167, 190, 243, 249, 307
COMPASS® 237-240
Completion rates 251, 256-258, 260
Computer programs 200, 212, 235, 237, 269, 314
Computer-assisted instruction 169, 181, 194, 237, 301-302, 307, 340
Concentration 82-83, 106, 123, 161
Concept mapping 120, 186, 244, 247, 254, 304, 309, 331
Concept maps 6, 12, 120-122, 125, 170, 186, 247-249, 304, 307, 310-311, 330-331, 342, 360
Conditional acceptance 53
Confidence 23-24, 39, 159-160, 163, 166-167, 172, 174, 211, 238, 272, 320, 339, 344, 346, 354, 360
Connecting with faculty 118, 125
Conversation circles 9, 194, 196-197
Counseling 24, 40, 44, 72, 84, 86, 96-97, 99, 104, 106, 108, 110, 112, 130, 135, 139, 155, 159, 191-192, 202, 209, 214-216, 218, 267, 278, 281, 302, 360
Counselor 97, 130, 192, 210, 216, 344
Course content 41, 118, 169-170, 173, 182, 186, 213, 274, 310, 323, 351, 357
Course evaluation tool 203-204, 206-207, 219
Courses 4, 26-27, 29-34, 38-39, 41-43, 51, 55-57, 61, 63-65, 67-68, 73-75, 82-83, 94, 96, 98-102, 106, 118-120, 127-128, 141-142, 145-146, 178-182, 184-186, 201, 207-209, 212, 214-215, 217, 222, 232-233, 237, 239-240, 243, 248-249, 251, 257, 259, 275-278, 281, 290, 291-293, 299-301, 304, 309, 324, 326, 333, 348, 351, 353-356, 358-359, 361
Coursework grades 54, 58
Creative calendar planning 249-250
Creative class scheduling 146, 210

Index

Credit hours 19, 40, 44, 84, 117, 133, 140, 231-232, 235, 338, 361
Critical thinking skills 32, 121, 145, 167, 173-174, 179-180, 213, 306-308, 333, 342, 355-356
Critical thinking test items 235, 310, 320, 359
Critical thinking tools 187, 190, 200, 309-311, 330
Cultural considerations 145-146, 193, 209, 215
Cultural differences 195, 198, 215
Cultural diversity 195
Culturally diverse nursing program 195
Culturally sensitive teaching and learning 197
Curriculum 4, 6, 12, 14-15, 29, 32, 79, 90, 91, 96, 98, 110, 116, 119-121, 128, 176-179, 181, 185, 206-207, 215, 221-222, 231-232, 240, 248, 250, 259, 262, 306, 310, 315, 317, 320-321, 323-324, 328, 330-331, 341, 346, 349, 351, 359
Curriculum choke point 78, 94, 109-110, 115-116, 119, 128, 142-143, 201, 208, 216, 218, 220, 301
Data 2-3, 5-6, 9, 11, 13, 17, 27, 43, 45-46, 57, 63-65, 68-69, 72, 74, 78-81, 83-86, 90, 94, 99-100, 102-103, 105-109, 111-112, 115-116, 118, 127, 132, 135-136, 139, 142, 145-148, 152, 164, 166, 175-176, 185-186, 193, 198, 201-202, 207-209, 213, 216, 219, 226, 228-232, 236, 240, 244, 250-251, 255-256, 258, 260, 271, 276-277, 284-288, 290, 292-293, 300, 306, 308-309, 311, 313-315, 319, 324-325, 327-328, 341-342, 347
Data analysis 136, 193, 219, 229
Data interpretation 229-230
Definition of at-risk student 28-32
Delaying NCLEX 296
Demographics 1, 3, 82-83, 106, 123, 347
Description of nursing program 231
Descriptive study 227
Developing a readmission policy 264, 285, 289
Development of the success program 230, 235, 252
Difficult content 94-95, 109, 301
Disclosure 130, 230
Discussion board 243
Diversity 19, 25, 29, 37, 67, 71, 75, 173, 193, 195, 197
[in] learning environment 195
[in] populations 71
Drop-out 264
Due process 267
Electronic whiteboards 243
Employer satisfaction 257
English skills 9, 18, 24, 26-27, 34, 58, 62, 72, 96, 152, 158, 164, 169, 193-194, 196, 251, 292, 299, 302, 355-356
English-as-a-Second-Language (ESL) 30, 125, 187, 193, 299, 302, 354, 356
Entrance examinations 56
Entry 4, 38, 40, 44, 55, 63, 84, 105, 116, 178-179, 230, 233, 239, 281, 288, 295-296, 307

Environmental factors 23-25, 39, 102, 107, 110
Error in measurement 273
Essay 54, 57-58, 161, 178, 185
Evaluate readmission policy 288-289
Evaluating critical thinking 179
Evaluation 23, 31, 44-46, 57, 69, 75, 79, 83, 86, 94, 127-128, 130, 132, 145, 155, 172, 177, 179, 182, 184-185, 187, 200-204, 206-210, 214, 216-220, 222, 232, 241, 246-247, 253, 259, 262, 288, 290, 293-295, 297, 301-302, 310-312, 318, 324, 329-332, 339, 343, 346, 358, 360
Evidenced-based practice 10-11, 306
Exam analysis 151-153, 157, 159, 164, 200, 212
Exam analysis procedure 152, 155
Exam analysis worksheet 152, 155-156
Exam anxiety 152, 159, 163
Exam performance 152, 155, 162, 164, 217, 353, 355
Exam reviews 151
Exam skills 153, 155, 160-161, 163
Exam techniques 152-153, 155, 159
Exit exams 235-236
Exit interview 187, 213, 216, 218, 233, 284-285, 358
Factors affecting student success 5
Factors needing improvement 81, 85, 106-107
Faculty advising 150, 203
Faculty assignments 249
Faculty development 108, 187, 195, 221-222, 235, 243-244, 248, 252, 259, 262
Faculty learning styles assessment 92

Faculty office hours 108, 149, 212
Faculty retention 130, 132, 134
Failing 9, 17, 21, 27-28, 43, 46, 55, 59, 128, 139, 141, 150-151, 200, 233, 264-294, 321
Financial aid 67, 112, 123, 136-137, 190, 214, 276, 192
First time pass rate 67, 296-297, 325
Flexible scheduling 120
Follow up contract 150
Full-time faculty 97, 231
General program overview 109
Grade point average (GPA) 26-27, 30, 31, 33-34, 40, 43-44, 50, 52, 54-58, 61-62, 68, 71-74, 78-81, 84, 100, 101-103, 106, 116, 141, 233, 239-240, 260, 281, 287, 299, 320, 353-355
Grades 26, 30, 32, 45, 54-55, 57-58, 61, 63, 73-75, 94, 97, 101-103, 110, 130, 136, 141-142, 149, 165, 168, 201, 216, 218, 220, 233, 236, 239-240, 271, 274, 283-285, 299-300, 319, 331, 333, 353-356
Grading 6, 31, 119, 122, 130, 136, 168, 179, 182, 185, 209, 272, 274, 276, 300, 311, 320
Grading options 149, 211
Grading policies 271
Graduation 4, 41-42, 50, 63, 71, 99, 120, 129, 131-132, 140, 178-179, 185, 187, 216, 218, 232, 243, 257, 264, 281, 284, 293, 296-297, 321-322, 325, 333, 339, 344-347, 349, 351, 353-354, 358, 360
Graduation rate 38, 63-64, 99, 129, 198, 201, 208, 258

Group remediation 136-137, 341
Hard criteria 57
Health Education Systems, Incorporated (HESI) 30, 54, 56, 58, 74, 95-98, 178, 221, 235-236, 222-224, 339, 350, 357-360
Health habits 82-83
Illinois Eastern Community Colleges (IECC) 227-231, 234-237, 249-251, 253, 256-257, 259, 261
Inactive status 264-265
Indicators of success 38, 42, 63, 66, 78, 99-100, 110, 128, 201-202, 207, 216, 218, 221
Individual remediation 137, 340
Inform early when failing 150
Instructional strategies 11, 88, 108, 110, 112, 147, 215, 236, 244, 248-249, 261
Integrative review 6, 8-13, 15, 61, 121-122, 164-165, 167-168, 170-173, 186
Interaction recordings 247
Interventions (that helped students) 5-6, 9, 45, 62, 66, 79, 85, 89, 95, 99, 111, 125, 127, 145-146, 150-151, 153, 155, 157-161, 187, 195, 198-204, 207, 209, 211, 216, 219-220, 221-222, 226, 234-235, 241-242, 253, 261, 267-268, 279, 294, 320, 328, 333, 349, 360
Key element 343
Key words 125, 137, 152-153, 159-160, 162, 164, 343
Ladder curriculum 231
Language development 193
Language proficiency 193, 302

Language skills 26-27, 158, 196, 353, 355
Learning contract 267, 270, 275
Learning environments 120, 128, 197
Learning needs 95, 108, 133, 169, 171, 174, 187, 194, 196, 199, 211, 236, 238, 241, 249-250, 262, 308, 340
Learning Skills Center 168-169, 209, 228, 230, 232, 238, 240-241, 252-254, 262
Learning style 88-94, 111-112, 115, 123, 138, 210, 254-255, 301, 348
Learning style inventory 78, 90-91, 108-109, 112, 234, 252, 254
Leave of absence 264-265, 278, 280, 282
Liaison for nursing students 192
Licensed practical nurse program 295, 309
Literature review 6-7, 193
LLUSN-LAP Exam Analysis Program 212, 216, 332
Math 29, 31, 33, 40, 44, 56, 58, 68, 72, 74, 79, 96-97, 106, 110-111, 118, 124, 145-146, 169, 209, 212, 234, 238-239, 244-245, 254-255
Math computational ability 54, 58, 72, 74, 100, 102, 106, 108, 118, 141
Math review 234, 244
Math skills course 234
Math test score 40, 44, 68, 71, 73-74, 81, 84, 100-103, 106
Measurement 60, 182, 203, 260, 273-274
Model for NCLEX success 67, 297-298, 328

Multiple choice questions 152-153, 177-178, 348, 350
Multitasking skills 253
National Education Consultants (NEC) 235, 259
National League for Nursing Accrediting Commission (NLNAC) 22, 260
National organizations 315, 317
NCLEX 1-6, 9, 15, 34-35, 64, 67-68, 72, 83, 94, 96, 98, 119, 142, 151, 177, 208, 217-218, 226, 232-233, 235-236, 240, 242, 257-259, 261-262, 271, 288, 295-333
NCLEX failure 258, 296-297, 300-301, 328, 375
NCLEX-style questions 314, 343, 360
NCLEX-style test item 273, 349, 359
NCLEX pass rate 64-65, 99, 111, 138, 198, 217, 219-220, 226, 232, 237, 256-258, 261, 296-297, 332, 338, 346, 359-360
NCLEX review books 314, 326, 340, 345, 359
NCLEX review course 218, 235, 341, 249-250, 352, 359
NCLEX success 2, 4, 6, 9, 63-64, 67, 258, 295-300, 302, 304, 321-322, 324, 328-329, 331-333, 338
NCLEX success course 328, 338-361
NCLEX test plan 186, 273, 311, 315-316, 318, 329, 331
NCLEX-PN 295
NCLEX-RN 162-163, 232, 234, 295-296, 315, 320-321, 323, 357
NCLEX-RN pass rate 227-228, 321

Negative factors 40, 44, 84-86, 106, 123-124, 146, 216, 328
Negative influences 19, 38
Non-academic variables 297, 355
Non-academic factors 302
Non-academic support 145-146, 190, 209, 214
Non-English language background 9, 24, 103
Nontraditional student 18, 20-21, 35
Note-taking 24, 82-83, 106, 123, 125, 134, 210
Number of readmissions 276-277, 281, 286-287
Number one reason students are at-risk 32
Nursing curriculum 90, 119, 331, 346
Nursing faculty behaviors 39
Nursing knowledge 34, 295, 297, 315, 318, 328, 331-332
Nursing shortage 17, 23, 62, 75, 129
Nursing skills laboratory aspects 275
Objective exam analysis worksheet 152, 156
Ongoing communication 249, 201
Online grade books 243
On-time completion 131
On-time completion rate 71
On-time graduation 42, 50, 140, 198, 264
Open door policy 27, 62, 65-66, 137
Oral expressiveness 254-255
Orientation 95-98, 134, 136-137, 148, 174, 204-205, 210, 214-215, 248, 271
Outcome criteria 78, 94, 99
Part-time employment 191, 214

Part-time faculty 231
Pass rate 2, 4, 64-65, 67-68, 97, 99, 111, 138, 198, 217, 219-220, 226-229, 231-232, 237, 256-258, 261, 296-297, 300, 321, 325, 327, 332, 338, 346, 358, 359-360
Peer tutoring 12, 110-111, 134, 170-173, 199
Peer tutors 106-107, 170-173, 213, 240
Persistence rate 99, 131, 135, 138
Personal concerns 191, 202, 253
Personal contact 243
Personal factors 24-25, 39-40, 44, 84, 102, 104, 124
Personal interest inventory 54
Personal interview 54, 57-58
Phenomena 13
Phenomenological study 8-9
Positive factors 25, 41, 81, 83, 85, 102, 107, 124, 118
Positive influences 19
Positive predictors for success 25-26, 61
PowerPoint® 243
Practice analysis 215-216, 231
Practice tests 343, 358
Preceptors 231, 351
Predict NCLEX success 9, 63, 297, 321-322
Predictor exam 322, 325, 332, 339-342, 344, 346, 360-361
Predictors of student success 37
Preferred learning styles 88
Pre-nursing student support 133
Pre-nursing success course 75, 117-118, 121, 134, 140-143
Preparing for class 118, 125

Prerequisite 4, 6, 26, 31, 58, 133, 141, 240, 286
Prerequisite courses 51, 53, 55-57, 61, 65, 68, 73, 100, 102, 106, 119, 141, 299
Previous college degree 52, 71, 103, 108
Previous college experience 73, 101
Previous coursework grades 54, 58
Proactive efforts 134
Professional references 54, 57-58
Program outcomes 6, 45, 100, 110, 120, 207, 251, 256-257, 259
Program plan for student success 1-2, 5-6, 13-14
Program policies 4, 15, 266, 275
Program success 4, 6
Progression 4, 95, 120, 231-232, 321-322, 324
Progression policies 119, 321, 332, 340
Purpose 4, 10, 11, 38, 45, 61, 63, 66-67, 71, 76, 81, 89, 98, 105-106, 117-119, 124, 150, 152, 164, 171, 199, 203, 210, 216, 226-228, 232, 243, 246, 251, 276, 285, 288, 290, 291-292, 294, 311, 315, 322, 338-340
Purposeful selection 229
Quality assurance 5-6
Ranking 58, 238-239, 282, 316
Ranking system for admission 238
Rationale 66, 76, 83, 92, 148, 166-168, 178, 184, 206, 217, 240, 281-282, 286, 288, 304-305, 310, 314, 319, 345, 359-360
Reactive efforts 134

Reading 29, 31, 34, 40, 44, 56-58, 65, 68, 71-72, 81-84, 92, 96-97, 100, 103, 106, 110-111, 118, 123-126, 134, 138, 142, 158, 162-164, 168-170, 181, 193, 196, 209, 212, 229, 233-234, 242, 253, 255, 269, 302, 343, 354

Reading comprehension 24, 29, 33, 56, 158, 302, 353-356

Reading score 45, 52, 54, 58, 74, 100, 141

Reading speed 158

Reading strategies 193

Readmission 57, 124, 264-265, 276-279, 281-283, 286-288, 290-294

Readmission policy 119, 264, 266, 276-278, 281, 283, 285-289, 291-294, 301

Readmission request 279, 285

Readmission requirements 287

Referrals 155, 192, 199, 253, 268, 302

Reinstatement 265

Relaxation strategies 138, 343

Reliable test 273

Remediating content 339

Remediation 4, 6, 19, 31, 55, 57, 81-82, 96, 98-99, 124, 136-137, 153, 169, 208, 211, 238, 274, 278, 287, 300-301, 303-304, 320-326, 338-342, 346, 351-352, 356-359, 361

Repeat a course 22, 276

Repeating a nursing course 301

Research 1, 3, 7-8, 10, 11, 15, 18, 27-28, 37, 45, 55, 61, 69, 75, 89, 93-95, 99, 121, 130, 136, 153, 165-167, 171-172, 182, 185-186, 214, 226-230, 232, 237, 251, 254, 256, 261, 299, 306, 316, 318, 339

Research method 227-228

Research questions 121, 165, 171, 227-229

Research studies 6, 8-11, 15, 61, 165, 338, 361

Research study 9, 57, 61, 89, 95, 176, 228, 321, 338, 349

Researcher actions 230

Retention 2, 17, 22, 25, 28, 37-38, 41, 46, 79, 95, 111, 117-118, 129-132, 134-140, 152, 157, 187, 198, 203, 207-208, 211, 227, 251-252, 262, 284, 286

Retention of information 157

Retention rate 22, 38, 42, 46, 61, 65, 67, 99, 110, 131-132, 140, 172, 201-202, 208, 216, 218, 220, 240, 260, 261, 264

Retention specialist 122, 128-141, 143, 149, 198-199, 208, 210, 211-213, 216, 219, 221, 328-329, 332

Retention strategies 111, 193, 198

Review 6-13, 15, 23, 43, 50, 54, 56, 60-61, 82, 92, 94, 96-98, 108-111, 116, 121-122, 124, 128, 134, 136-137, 142, 145, 151-152, 157, 159, 162-165, 167-173, 176, 180, 185-187, 192-193, 196, 199, 201, 203, 205, 207-208, 210-213, 215-220, 230-236, 238, 244-247, 254, 258-259, 266, 268-269, 271, 279-280, 293, 299-300, 303-305, 314, 316, 320, 322-326, 328, 331-333, 338-345, 347, 349-355, 357-360

Review course 213, 218, 232-233, 235-236, 323-324, 326, 341-342, 347, 349-353, 355, 357-360
Revision 37, 69, 78, 100, 116, 145, 151, 204, 207-208, 219-220, 246, 250, 286, 288, 293, 305, 324, 341
Role-play 182, 186, 247, 307
Rubric for ranking applicants 239
Science 8, 10, 11-12, 26, 29, 31, 33-34, 40, 44-45, 54-55, 61, 84, 98, 103, 134, 141, 222, 238-240, 274, 354-355
Science courses 31-32, 55, 68, 102, 106, 141, 239-240, 299, 354
Scientific test analysis 319
Selective admission 51, 58, 62-63, 65-66, 68, 72, 79, 108
Selective criteria 36, 38-39, 45, 50, 52-54, 57, 60-62, 64, 68-69, 71, 73-75, 78, 80-81, 86, 99-103, 106, 108-110, 115-116
Selective criteria score 52-53, 60, 73, 101-103, 108
Self efficacy 26, 39-40, 44, 84, 105, 124
Self-assessment 26, 72, 75, 78, 81-83, 85-86, 100, 103, 106-107, 112, 118, 123, 146, 169, 214, 301, 328
Skill performance deficiency 269
Skits 181, 185-186, 244, 246
Small group work 244-245
Soft criteria 57, 60
Standard for passing 276
Standardized examinations 320, 322
Standardized testing 4, 96, 178, 320
Standardized tests 54, 178-179, 183, 353, 359

Start Right in Nursing School: A Self-Assessment Tool ™ 46, 72, 82-83, 106-107, 123, 146, 214, 301, 328
Stop-out 63, 71, 99, 192, 201, 208, 265, 277, 279, 281
Strategies for Success course 234
Stress 19-20, 23, 27, 29, 40, 44, 84-85, 88, 104, 106, 108, 110-111, 124, 126-127, 130, 133, 150, 159, 163, 178, 190, 192, 198, 216, 241, 253, 258, 267, 303-304, 314, 328-329, 344-345, 350, 353-354, 356
Stress management 24, 97, 118, 126, 134, 137, 234
Stress reduction 106, 127, 253, 344, 350
Student at-risk 9, 21, 28, 36, 43, 46, 55, 328
Student characteristics 5, 37, 45, 73, 99, 135, 250, 259-260, 295, 297-298, 301-302, 328-329
Student enrollment 257-258
Student handbook 119, 266
Student learning need 169, 200, 211, 236, 238, 250, 262
Student learning styles 89-91, 228-229, 254, 256, 261
Student Learning Styles Assessment Survey 91
Student perspective on success 164, 203
Student preparedness 233, 321
Student progress 94, 150, 185, 187, 202, 211, 216, 259, 300, 328
Student satisfaction 111, 132, 136, 217, 219-220, 257
Student self-assessment 4, 78, 86, 106

Student Self-Checklist for NCLEX Success 302, 304, 328-329, 332
Student success 1-15, 17, 25, 37, 41, 59, 63, 68-69, 71, 76, 78-112, 115-143, 145-222, 235, 237, 243, 250, 252, 259, 261-262, 277, 284, 291, 295, 297, 315
Student Success Program 9, 17, 69, 78-112, 115-143, 145-222, 252, 262, 268, 284, 291, 293, 295, 298, 328, 333, 338, 360
Student support courses 186
Student support in clinical practice 187
Student surveys 259
Study 2, 8, 9, 18-19, 22, 26-30, 32-36, 46, 56-57, 59, 61-63, 75, 78-79, 82-83, 85-86, 88-89, 95-97, 99, 103, 107-109, 116, 118, 120, 124-126, 134-136, 138-139, 142, 148, 153, 157-158, 162, 164, 166, 169-170, 172-174, 176, 180-183, 185-186, 191-193, 195, 198, 202, 204, 210, 211, 213, 218, 226-262, 268, 270, 274, 286, 292, 299-301, 303-304, 308-309, 317-318, 321-323, 326, 328-329, 339, 342-345, 347-349, 351-352, 354-357, 359-361
Study groups 25, 87, 122, 163, 194, 203, 302, 340-341
Study skills 23-24, 33, 81-83, 86, 96-97, 107, 110-112, 118, 123, 130, 137, 172, 198, 212, 217, 219-220, 234, 253, 260, 278, 292, 357, 359
Studying 19, 27, 34, 36, 83, 85, 88-89, 125-126, 135, 138, 178, 202, 255, 292, 303-304, 317, 344-345, 355, 357

Success 1-15, 17-18, 21-22, 25-28, 36-39, 41-42, 45, 51, 55, 57, 59, 61-64, 66-69, 71-72, 75-76, 78-112, 115-143, 145-222, 226-262, 265, 267, 277-279, 284, 286, 288, 290-333, 338-361
Success program 17, 69, 78-112, 115-143, 145-222, 226-262, 268, 284, 291, 293, 298, 328, 333, 338, 360
Success program components 96
Support services 4, 21, 36-37, 62, 136, 212
Survey at-risk nursing students 28
Syllabus 119, 204, 247
Tactile concrete 254
Teaching critical thinking 174, 180
Teaching strategies 89, 92-93, 111, 120, 208, 221, 243-244, 262, 295, 297, 301-302, 307-308, 318, 329-331
Teaching-learning strategies 228-229, 255-256
Technology 91, 179, 236, 243, 251-252
Test anxiety 23-24, 40, 44, 64, 84, 127, 134, 138, 166, 192, 258, 302, 304, 329, 343, 353-354, 356, 360
Test bank 244
Test blueprint 208, 244, 273, 310-312, 319
Test construction and scoring 272
Test items 83, 109, 134, 137, 166-168, 174, 201, 208, 217-218, 221, 235, 244, 259, 272-273, 302, 304, 310-311, 314, 316, 319-320, 330-333, 349, 357, 359
Test preparation 83, 106, 304

Testing 4, 6, 12, 29, 33, 83, 96, 98-99, 104, 107, 118, 136-137, 148, 150-152, 164-168, 177-178, 184-186, 188, 192, 196, 199, 205, 232, 237-238, 241-242, 253, 255, 258-259, 272-273, 278, 286, 295-297, 302, 304-306, 310, 318-320, 324, 329-330, 332, 339-340, 342-347, 354, 357, 359-360
Testing policy 95, 273
Testing time 196, 253
Testing/evaluation 297, 302, 310, 318, 329-330, 332
Test-taking analysis and strategies 151, 212
Test-taking anxiety 167
Test-talking skills 99, 104, 107, 110-111, 118, 130, 167, 172, 202, 234, 262, 342, 353-355
Textbook resources 169
NCLEX Experience: Interview Protocol, The 346-348
Theory examination advisement 268
Think, pair, share 243
Thinking skills 32, 120-121, 145, 167, 173-174, 179-180, 183, 213, 295, 297, 306-308, 310-311, 316, 318, 328-330, 333, 342, 355-356
Time management 24, 40, 54-55, 72, 82-84, 104, 106-107, 110-111, 118, 122-123, 126, 134, 137, 141-142, 148, 173, 198, 218, 234, 253, 278, 328
Title III grant 228, 236, 238, 251-252, 262
Traditional student 17
Transcripts 74, 229-230
Transfer students 31, 37, 282-283, 293
Transparent overlay 241
Tutoree 172-173
Tutorial 35, 238, 295, 301, 309, 330, 344
Tutorial for COMPASS 238
Tutoring 12, 59, 96-99, 110-111, 123, 130, 134, 145, 155, 157, 169-173, 199, 202-203, 209, 213, 217, 219-221, 240-241, 253, 326
Tutors 96, 106-107, 170-173, 203, 213, 235, 240-241
Unsafe performance 290
Valid test 6, 208, 272-274
Videotaping 244, 246-247
Visual aids 244-246
Visual numeric 254
Vocabulary 56, 158, 163, 193-194, 302
Withdrawal-failing (WF) 265-266
Withdrawal-passing (WP) 265-266
Withdrawing 265-266, 284, 292
Work experience 54, 57-58, 232